AF412716

Itch – Management in Clinical Practice

Current Problems in Dermatology

Vol. 50

Series Editors

Peter Itin Basel
Gregor B.E. Jemec Roskilde

Itch – Management in Clinical Practice

Volume Editors

Jacek C. Szepietowski Wrocław
Elke Weisshaar Heidelberg

28 figures, 26 in color, and 36 tables, 2016

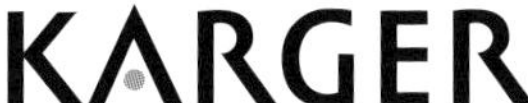

Basel · Freiburg · Paris · London · New York · Chennai · New Delhi ·
Bangkok · Beijing · Shanghai · Tokyo · Kuala Lumpur · Singapore · Sydney

Current Problems in Dermatology

Jacek C. Szepietowski
Department of Dermatology,
Venereology and Allergology
Wrocław Medical University
Wrocław (Poland)

Elke Weisshaar
Department of Clinical Social Medicine,
Occupational and Environmental Dermatology
Heidelberg University Hospital, Ruprecht Karls University
Heidelberg (Germany)

Library of Congress Cataloging-in-Publication Data

Names: Szepietowski, Jacek, editor. | Weisshaar, Elke, editor.
Title: Itch - management in clinical practice / volume editors, Jacek C.
  Szepietowski, Elke Weisshaar.
Other titles: Current problems in dermatology ; v. 50. 1421-5721
Description: Basel : Karger, [2016] | Series: Current problems in
  dermatology, ISSN 1421-5721 ; vol. 50 | Includes bibliographical
  references and indexes.
Identifiers: LCCN 2016027847| ISBN 9783318058888 (hard cover : alk. paper) |
  ISBN 9783318058895 (electronic version)
Subjects: | MESH: Pruritus--therapy
Classification: LCC RL721 | NLM WR 282 | DDC 616.5--dc23
LC record available at https://lccn.loc.gov/2016027847

Bibliographic Indices. This publication is listed in bibliographic services, including Current Contents® and Index Medicus.

Contents

Preface

Itching is a very common symptom in dermatology as well as in other fields of medicine such as internal medicine, psychosomatics, neurology, and even oncology. Whereas itching has been underresearched for hundreds of years, the community of itch researchers can be proud to state that a lot of knowledge has been acquired in clinical aspects of acute and chronic itch within the last 15 years. This has resulted in many publications including several itch books in recent years. All of them are a great pleasure to read and a real enrichment for the itch community.

With this volume, we aim to address the management of chronic itch, which is an important issue for daily clinical practice, especially in dermatology. Whereas all the other books have focused on experimental aspects and diagnostics such as new research on receptors, neuroimaging of itch, cytokines, and chemokines (all of which are very important aspects of itch), this volume focuses on itch management in consideration of general aspects as well as in relation to special age groups, special body regions, and specific diseases. With this book, we hope to summarize the knowledge of recent research in itch management. We also set out to address dermatologists in training who wish to get a good overview of the great variety of treatments available, topically as well as systemically. We do not want to forget to mention that in most of the cases, the combination of, for instance, topical, systemic, and UV phototherapy may be necessary to fight this intractable symptom. Furthermore, psychological aspects should be considered. We aim to direct the readers' attention to the fact that fighting the symptom of chronic itch means a variable, broad, and all-embracing therapy that includes dermatological expertise and treatment as well as interdisciplinary cooperation.

We want to thank all the experts who contributed to this volume. None of these chapters could have been written without the help of experts and friends worldwide. We also thank Frau Hausmann and Frau Braun, Karger Verlag, for their continuous and quick support. Furthermore, we particularly thank all our itch patients who shared their history, disease, and suffering with us, and thus made it possible to accumulate such an amount of rich experience and knowledge. May this book be a great inspiration and help for the reader to find the best possible treatment of itch.

Jacek C. Szepietowski, Wrocław
Elke Weisshaar, Heidelberg

Szepietowski JC, Weisshaar E (eds): Itch – Management in Clinical Practice.
Curr Probl Dermatol. Basel, Karger, 2016, vol 50, pp 1–4 (DOI: 10.1159/000446009)

Classification of Itch

Sonja Ständer

Department of Dermatology and Center for Chronic Pruritus, University Hospital Münster, Münster, Germany

Abstract

Chronic pruritus has diverse forms of presentation and can appear not only on normal skin [International Forum for the Study of Itch (IFSI) classification group II], but also in the company of dermatoses (IFSI classification group I). Scratching, a natural reflex, begins in response to itch. Enough damage can be done to the skin by scratching to cause changes in the primary clinical picture, often leading to a clinical picture predominated by the development of chronic scratch lesions (IFSI classification group III). An internationally recognized, standardized classification system was created by the IFSI to not only aid in clarifying terms and definitions, but also to harmonize the global nomenclature for itch.

© 2016 S. Karger AG, Basel

Chronic pruritus (CP) is described as an unpleasant sensation that persists for 6 weeks or more. A common problem presented by many patients in daily medical practice, CP is now considered to be an interdisciplinary symptom requiring a proper diagnosis and treatment. The treating physician must be conscious of the individual presentation of CP in the patient before delving into diagnostics. Various diseases are capable of inducing CP, but without additional clarification of the clinical groups with CP, further diagnostics remain too comprehensive and time-consuming. These same clinical groups are defined by means of dermatological examinations. Although pruritic dermatoses can be diagnosed without difficulty, pruritus on normal, unaltered skin and pruritus accompanied by chronic, secondary scratch lesions often do not signify the underlying disease, in which case a specific laboratorial and radiological examination is required. A clinical classification system was developed by the International Forum for the Study of Itch (IFSI) in 2007 in order to better assist in the diagnostics of CP patients and improve communication with colleagues [1]. Furthermore, definitions of medical terms have been updated and refined by the IFSI in order to prevent confusion with older, more general terms.

Clinical Classification of Pruritus: Clinical Group

Distinguishing between disorders with and without primary or secondary skin lesions, this classification system addresses primarily the patient's clinical presentation. The skin and background of patients with pruritus are used to classify three groups of conditions found in the first part of this classification system.

First Group (IFSI Group I): Pruritus on Diseased Skin

This group is characterized by pruritic skin diseases and comprised of inflammatory, infectious, and autoimmune cutaneous diseases; genodermatoses; adverse drug reactions (with rash); dermatoses of pregnancy, and skin lymphomas. Each of these causes specific changes to the skin.

Second Group (IFSI Group II): Pruritus on Nondiseased Skin

This group consists of conditions caused by systemic diseases. These include endocrine and metabolic disorders, hematological and lymphoproliferative diseases, infections, solid neoplasms, psychiatric diseases, drug-induced pruritus, and neurological diseases. The term 'pruritus sine materia' was once used to describe this condition, but is no longer suitable for use due to multiple interpretations by different authors.

Third Group (IFSI Group III): Chronic Scratch Lesions

This group includes for example prurigo nodularis and lichen simplex chronicus. Pinching, rubbing, and scratching are mechanical reactions frequently induced by CP. This group is characterized by scratching and its resulting damage to the skin. Said damage can include excoriations, papules and nodules, lichenification, and crusts. Atrophic scars and hyper- and hypopigmentation often remain on the skin even after lesions have healed. In CP, multiple lesions may coexist in different stages. An underlying origin may be found in a systemic or dermatological disease. Many patients from group III usually suffer from long-term CP and are unable to recall initial skin changes.

Clinical Classification of Pruritus: Underlying Category

Following the initial clinical examination, further laboratorial and radiological examinations are carried out with the aim to pinpoint any underlying pruritogenic disease. In order to provide a differential diagnostic tool in this process, we recommend the following categories of underlying diseases (table 1): category I = dermatological diseases, category II = systemic diseases, including diseases of pregnancy and drug-induced pruritus (without rash), category III = neurological diseases, and category IV = psychiatric diseases. Multiple underlying diseases can also contribute to itch in some patients and are thus categorized as 'mixed' (category V; e.g. CP in xerosis, renal failure). Because an underlying disease can remain unidentifiable in some patients, the category 'others' (category VI) was created. Epidemiological data on diseases causing CP, excluding single diseases, is greatly lacking, and empirical data serves only to highlight the high estimated percentage of patients suffering from this symptom. Therefore, there is currently no precise data on the prevalence and incidence of pruritogenic diseases.

General Definitions

The definitions of pruritogenic entities are regularly discussed and refined by the IFSI [1, 2]. The following points include more recent definitions and terms.

- Pruritus is described as either 'acute' (lasting up to 6 weeks) or 'chronic' (lasting 6 weeks or more).

Table 1. Categories of underlying diseases [1]

Category	Diseases
I. Dermatological	Dermatoses such as psoriasis, xerosis, atopic dermatitis, scabies, and urticaria
II. Systemic	Systemic diseases involving the liver (e.g. primary biliary cirrhosis), kidneys (e.g. chronic renal failure), blood (e.g. Hodgkin's lymphoma), and certain drugs
III. Neurological	Diseases or disorders of the central of peripheral nervous system, e.g. nerve damage, compression, or irritation
IV. Psychological/psychosomatic	Includes somatoform pruritus with comorbidities associated with psychiatric and psychosomatic diseases
V. Mixed	The overlapping and coexistence of multiple diseases causing pruritus
VI. Other	Of undetermined origin

- It is generally agreed upon that 'pruritus' and 'itch' may be utilized synonymously.

Terms Related to the Origin of the Pruritus [1]

- 'Atopic pruritus' is pruritus along with atopic dermatitis.
- 'Diabetogenic pruritus' is pruritus in diabetes mellitus type I or II.
- 'Hepatic pruritus' and 'cholestatic pruritus' are terms representing itch in liver disease.
- 'Neuropathic pruritus' describes damage to nerve fibers found, e.g. in brachioradial pruritus and notalgia paresthetica.
- 'Paraneoplastic pruritus' is pruritus in the context of a malignant underlying disease.
- 'Premonitory pruritus' can appear months or years before a diagnosis of the underlying disease.
- 'Pruritus of unknown origin' and 'pruritus of undetermined origin' are two terms used to describe patients with CP of an unknown origin. Both may be used interchangeably together with 'itch of undetermined origin', or (1) also for patients for whom diagnostics have yet to be performed and whose history suggests no origin of the pruritus, and (2) in patients with pruritus of unknown origin after diagnostics. 'Pruritus sine materia' is a term that has caused much confusion since it was previously associated with diverse conditions (e.g. pruritus in systemic diseases, pruritus on non-diseased skin). Therefore, the use of this term should be avoided.
- 'Senile pruritus' may be substituted with 'pruritus of advanced aging' or 'pruritus in the elderly'.
- 'Somatoform pruritus' is a term utilized for identifying pruritus of psychosomatic or psychiatric origin.
- 'Uremic pruritus', 'chronic pruritus associated with CKD', and 'nephrogenic itch' may be used to identify pruritus in chronic kidney failure.

Terms Related to Trigger Factors

- Alloknesis: a normally nonpruritogenic stimulus (e.g. light stroke with a cotton swab) induces itching.

- Hyperknesis: a normally nonpruritogenic stimulus (e.g. by pin-prick inducing normally a pricking sensation) induces a strong itching.
- Aquagenic pruritus: pruritus after contact with water.
- Aquadynia: pruritus and pain after contact with water.

Neurophysiological Classification of Pruritus

In 2003, a neurophysiologically based classification system was proposed Twycross et al. [3]. Itch was classified by in accordance with its origin.

- 'Neurogenic itch' is itch induced by mediators acting centrally in the absence of neural damage.
- 'Neuropathic itch' is comprised of diseased or lesioned pruritic neurons generating itch.
- 'Pruritoceptive itch' consists of pruritic nerves activated by pruritogens at their sensory endings.
- 'Psychogenic itch' is defined as pruritus of psychosomatic or psychiatric origin.

This classification system is important not only for the significance it carries for neurobiological research, but also for its use in describing the neuroanatomical mechanisms that underlie pruritus. Despite this, this system should not be implemented for clinical application because many diseases fall under multiple categories, for example, atopic dermatitis and cholestatic pruritus.

References

1 Ständer S, Weisshaar E, Mettang T, Szepietowski JC, Carstens E, Ikoma A, et al: Clinical classification of itch: a position paper of the International Forum for the Study of Itch. Acta Derm Venereol 2007;87:291–294.

2 Weisshaar E, Szepietowski JC, Darsow U, Misery L, Wallengren J, Mettang T, et al: European guideline on chronic pruritus. Acta Derm Venereol 2012;92:563–581.

3 Twycross R, Greaves MW, Handwerker H, Jones EA, Libretto SE, Szepietowski JC, et al: Itch: scratching more than the surface. QJM 2003;96:7–26.

Prof. Dr. Dr. Sonja Ständer
Department of Dermatology and Center for Chronic Pruritus, University Hospital Münster
Von-Esmarch-Strasse 58
DE–48149 Münster (Germany)
E-Mail sonja.staender@uni-muenster.de

Szepietowski JC, Weisshaar E (eds): Itch – Management in Clinical Practice.
Curr Probl Dermatol. Basel, Karger, 2016, vol 50, pp 5–10 (DOI: 10.1159/000446010)

Epidemiology of Itch

Elke Weisshaar

Department of Clinical Social Medicine, Occupational and Environmental Dermatology, Heidelberg University Hospital, Ruprecht
Karls University, Heidelberg, Germany

Abstract

Epidemiology is the study of disease frequency and the
associations between risk factors and outcome in a population. Clinical populations are highly selective and de-
pend for instance on perceived severity of symptoms and
access to health services. Assessment of a disease in the
community and in specific populations is an important
measure for the purpose of health planning as well as for
the understanding of associations between disease and
factors in the environment. Itch is definitely the most frequent symptom of the skin and can occur in acute and
chronic skin diseases and other diseases like end-stage
renal disease, cholestasis, and hematological, neurological, and psychiatric diseases. This diversity may explain
why research on the epidemiology of itch was disregarded for a long time. A recent European study demonstrated that the prevalence of itch among dermatological patients is 54.4%. The prevalence of acute itch in the
general population is 8.4% and for chronic itch it is 13.5%;
however, with a recurrent symptom it is important to
consider different prevalence estimates (point, 12-month,
and lifetime prevalence). The lifetime prevalence of
chronic itch in the general populations is 22%, demonstrating that more than 1 in 5 people experience chronic
itch once in their life. This shows that research in this field
should not only focus on patients. This chapter briefly
summarizes major facts on the epidemiology of itch in
the general population and in some patient populations.

Dermatoepidemiology is a new and important
emerging field in dermatology. Though itch is a
very frequent symptom of the skin, the epidemiology of itch has been disregarded in the past and
the number of true epidemiological studies on
itch is limited. The frequency and the causes of
itch vary greatly depending on age, ethnicity,
characteristics, underlying diseases, and access to
the regional health care system [1]. In addition,
chronic itch (CI; >6 weeks) can be of multifactorial origin or may be of an undetermined origin
despite intensive diagnostic measures [1]. Due to
differing methodologies and the lack of standardized measures, it is still difficult to compare exist-
ing studies; however, a questionnaire measuring
the prevalence of CI was developed and validated,
and has meanwhile been utilized in a number of
population-based studies [2–7]. With a recurrent
symptom it is important to consider different

prevalence estimates like point (current itch), 12-month, and lifetime prevalence (itch ever experienced in life). During the last years the number of studies has increased, demonstrating that itch is highly prevalent [6–22].

Itch in the General Population

A population survey from 2004 assessing the prevalence of skin complaints among 40,888 adults (females and males) in Oslo showed a prevalence of acute itch (<6 weeks) of 8.4% [9]. Individuals reporting itch were younger and had a lower household income [9]. In this study itch was the most prevalent symptom of all reported symptoms from the skin. The prevalence of itch was 8.8% among adolescents, with mental distress and eczema contributing the most to the distribution of itch in adolescents [10].

The point prevalence of CI (>6 weeks) among employees (n = 11,730) voluntarily participating in a skin cancer detection program was 16.7% [16]. The Heidelberg Pruritus Prevalence Study (n = 2,540), using a previously validated questionnaire [3], showed a point prevalence of 13.5%, a 12-month prevalence of 16.4%, and a lifetime prevalence of 22% of CI in the general populations [4]. In the follow-up of this German study, the 12-month cumulative incidence of CI was 7% and the lifetime prevalence was 25.5% [5]. In this study, women were more affected than men, but a significant sex difference was only found for the lifetime prevalence [4]. Female sex was associated with an increased but nonsignificant risk for incident CI during the past 12 months [5].

Itch in Dermatology

A large survey in dermatological outpatient clinics was conducted in 13 European countries assessing the distribution of skin conditions among dermatological patients. In this sample of 4,994 adult participants, the prevalence of itch among dermatological patients was 54.4%, and among controls it was 8%. The intensity was highest among patients with prurigo (7.4 ± 2.3) [11]. The point prevalence of itch in a dermatological practice in Germany in a 1-week period was 36.2% (87.6% of whom had CI) [15].

There are no epidemiological studies investigating the prevalence of itch in children, but in this group itch is mainly caused by atopic dermatitis, especially in Western countries. As atopic dermatitis is the most frequent skin disease in childhood, its prevalence can be used as a point of reference. The prevalence rates of atopic dermatitis vary from 17 to 22% in highly affected countries like Japan, USA, and Denmark, to 7% in Tanzania. This most likely explains the differing prevalence rates of itch in children throughout the world [1].

Itch is described to be the main dermatological symptom in pregnancy and is reported to occur in approximately 18% of pregnancies [1]. There are no epidemiological studies clearly focusing on the prevalence of itch during pregnancy related and unrelated to skin diseases. It is most likely that itch in pregnancy is mainly related to dermatoses, with atopic eruption of pregnancy being the most common dermatosis of pregnancy [23]. In a French prospective study of 3,192 pregnant women, 1.6% suffered from itch, and most of these women had pregnancy-specific dermatoses [24]. The prevalence of itch in pregnancy was 4.6% in an Indian study of 500 pregnant women, and with the exception of 4 cases, all suffered from specific dermatosis of pregnancy [25]. Intrahepatic cholestasis is higher in Chile, depending on ethnic predisposition and dietary factors. A prevalence rate of 13.2% was found for pruritus gravidarum and 2.4% for cholestatic jaundice of pregnancy [26].

According to a survey by questionnaire among 17,000 members of the American Psoriasis Foundation, itch was the second most frequent symptom, experienced by 79% of the interviewed psoriasis patients [27]. In a study in Singapore with 101 psoriasis patients, 84% reported generalized itch, 77% of them with daily occurrence [21]. Itch in psoriasis was underestimated in the past, which may be due to the fact that it is frequently not so severe compared to other dermatoses. Furthermore, psoriasis patients tend to be more restrained, but fortunately this topic has meanwhile become a topic of research [28].

In teenagers with acne, 13.8–70% (depending on ethnic origin) suffered from episodes of acute itch. A direct association of acne severity and itch in adolescents was demonstrated and the prevalence of itch increased with greater acne severity [29–31].

According to a Turkish study that investigated 4,099 elderly patients, itch ranked first among skin diseases, with 11.5% complaining about itch. Females were more affected (12.0%) than men (11.2%) [20]. Concerning age, patients older than 85 years were the most affected (19.5%). In consideration of season variations, itch was among the five most frequent diagnoses in all seasons, being most frequent in winter (12.8%) and autumn (12.7%) [18, 20]. Pruritic diseases were the most common in a study from Thailand (41%), which identified xerosis (which was for the authors identical with senescent itch) as the most frequent disease (38.9%) in a total of 149 elderly patients [32]. A very recent study investigated CI in a Hispanic geriatric population (n = 301) and showed 25% to be affected [18]. Of those with CI, 69% showed xerosis and 28% itch-related dermatoses. The prevalence of CI in this population was significantly correlated with xerosis, diabetes, and venous insufficiency [18]. However, there is still a need for epidemiological research in order to establish an evidence base for the claim that itch is more frequent in the elderly [33].

The prevalence of itch was reported to be higher in darker skin types [34], and differences in prevalence, clinical characteristics, and itch pathways across ethnicity were also reported. Although the current knowledge about itch is too limited to explain these differences, especially in perception, cultural and lifestyle differences are thought to contribute [34, 35]. There are no epidemiological data on itch in African countries like Uganda, but according to the high frequency of skin diseases among HIV individuals the prevalence is supposedly high. One study showed that 81% of a total of 84 patients suffered from itch caused by dermatoses, and there was no patient diagnosed to have an underlying systemic disease [19].

Itch in Specific Diseases

There is a worldwide variation in the epidemiology of itch in systemic diseases, which is mainly explained by differing life expectancies and as a result different populations of the elderly [1]. Some studies in patients attending a dermatologic clinic may find systemic diseases to be less frequent as a cause of itch compared to dermatological diseases, and results may therefore be different in comparison, for example, to an internal medicine department [19]. There are not many studies in this field because research regarding systemic causes of CI is rather limited.

In 10–50% of itch patients, a systemic disease can be found resembling the underlying etiology [19, 1]. In about 8–35% of the patients, the cause of itch remains unclear in spite of intensive diagnostic investigations [1]. American studies have shown that 22–30% of patients with generalized pruritus had an underlying systemic disease [1]. In a German study population, 36% had an underlying systemic disease, while no pruritus patients in Uganda had one [19]. The lack of systemic pruritus in Uganda can be explained by the Ugandan health care situation and reduced life expectancy [19]. Two recent studies significantly added to the understanding of itch in systemic disease [36, 37]. A recent population-based cohort study in 8,744 patients with CI showed that CI without concomitant skin changes is a risk factor for having undiagnosed hematological and bile duct malignancies. The authors concluded that screening for malignancy should be limited to the evaluation of bile duct and hematological malignancies [36]. A nationwide Danish cohort study based on registry data investigated the association between hospital inpatient and outpatient diagnosis of itch and cancer incidence [37]. The 1-year absolute cancer risk was 1.63%. Among patients with itch, a 13% higher than expected number of cases with hematological and various solid cancers were found. This refers especially to hematological cancers, above all Hodgkin's lymphoma [37]. However, the study was unable to differentiate between acute and chronic itch.

Itching in cholestasis is described by up to 100% of patients. In 25–70% it is a presenting symptom of primary biliary cirrhosis, and in around 15% it is a symptom of hepatitis C virus infection [1]. Distinct epidemiological studies about the prevalence of acute and CI in liver diseases are missing.

CI in patients with end-stage renal disease is a considerable problem, and itch in hemodialysis (HD) used to be reported by up to 85% of these patients in the 1970s and 1980s; however, in the last years it has been reported to have decreased, mainly because of improved dialysis techniques [1]. According to recent studies, regional differences need to be taken into account [1, 14, 17, 22]. However, comparison of studies is difficult because of the undulating pattern of itch, a lack of defining prevalence periods, and definitions of itch. In addition, dialysis quality standards vary among countries, which can explain the large variations in reported prevalence of itch in HD [1]. To close this gap, a representative cross-sectional prospective prevalence study on CI in 860 HD patients (GEHIS: German Epidemiological Hemodialysis Itch Study) was initiated [6]. CI affected 25.2% (point prevalence) of HD patients. 27.2% reported CI within the past 12 months, and 35.2% reported CI at least once in their life (lifetime prevalence). No significant differences in prevalence estimates were shown in relation to ethnic origin, schooling, or patients' marital status [6]. There was a significant association between the prevalence of CI (point prevalence) and age: those aged <70 years were significantly more affected by CI than those ≥70 years. The 12-month, lifetime, and point prevalence of CI were significantly higher in HD patients with self-reported eczema and dry skin. There was a significant association of the time since HD treatment started and the occurrence of CI [6]. Dialysis quality measured as Kt/V was not associated with the presence of CI [7]. 43.5% of HD patients suffering from CI had normal looking skin, 37.9% had secondary scratch lesions, and 18.6% had a skin disease [2]. GEHIS also demonstrated that the provision of care in HD patients suffering from CI is rather poor because only 32.4% had ever received any treatment for itch [2].

Itch in diabetes mellitus was reported as localized itch, especially in the genital and perianal areas, was significantly more common in diabetic women, and significantly associated with poor diabetes control [38]. Most of the studies miss control groups and it is not clear if itch is significantly more frequent in diabetic patients. Pruritus vulvae was significantly more common in diabetic women (18.4%) than in controls (5.6%). In Israel, 2% of diabetes patients were affected by itch [39]. Quite interestingly, diabetes was the only comorbidity that was associated with the occurrence of CI in HD patients, but interestingly with less CI [7]. This result needs further investigation but may suggest that CI in HD patients is of possible multifactorial origin and plays a different role compared to a population without any renal disease. CI was significantly associated with diabetes mellitus in Hispanic geriatric patients [18].

CI is reported to be frequent in HIV patients. In African patients it is most frequently associated with prurigo nodularis [1, 19]. In a study on HIV-positive patients who were surveyed in a large clinic in the Southeastern USA, 45% reported itch, making it the most common skin complaint in this group of patients [12].

CI was reported in patients suffering from neurotic excoriations, obsessive-compulsive disorders, delusion of parasitosis, anxiety disorder, and depression [1]. A study of 109 inpatients with CI showed that more than 70% had a psychiatric comorbidity [40]. 32% of 111 patients in a mental health center reported itching [13]. 17.5% of patients with depression experienced itching during depressive episodes [41].

Itch and Drugs

Acute drug-induced itch is usually accompanied by specific skin lesions (e.g. urticarial eruptions). Chronic drug-induced itch usually presents without any skin lesions and should be considered in patients presenting with itch of so far undetermined origin [42]. In an American prospective study with hospitalized patients, itch without any skin lesions occurred in 5% of patients with drug-induced cutaneous side effects [43]. Hydroxyethyl-starch-induced itch, which may occur in up to 50% of the patients treated with hydroxyethyl starch, and new chemotherapies, such as multityrosine inhibitors, need to be considered in CI [1, 42]. With regard to the demographical situation and the increasing number of patients with multiple drug intakes, drug-induced itch may play an increasing role, especially in the elderly population [42].

References

1 Weisshaar E, Dalgard F: The epidemiology of itch: adding to the burden of skin morbidity. Acta Derm Venereol 2009; 89:339–350.
2 Hayani K, Weiss M, Weisshaar E: Clinical findings and provision of care in haemodialysis patients with chronic itch: new results from the German Epidemiological Haemodialysis Itch Study. Acta Derm Venereol 2016;96:361–366.
3 Matterne U, Strassner T, Apfelbacher CJ, Diepgen TL, Weisshaar E: Measuring the prevalence of chronic itch in the general population: development and validation of a questionnaire for use in large-scale studies. Acta Derm Venereol 2009;89:250–256.
4 Matterne U, Apfelbacher CJ, Loerbroks A, Schwarzer T, Büttner M, Ofenloch R, Diepgen TL, Weisshaar E: Prevalence, correlates and characteristics of chronic pruritus: a population-based cross-sectional study. Acta Derm Venereol 2011; 91:674–679.
5 Matterne U, Apfelbacher CJ, Vogelgsang L, Loerbroks A, Weisshaar E: Incidence and determinants of chronic pruritus: a population-based cohort study. Acta Derm Venereol 2013;93:532–537.
6 Weiss M, Mettang T, Tschulena U, Passlick-Deetjen J, Weisshaar E: Prevalence of chronic itch and associated factors in hemodialysis patients: a representative cross-sectional study. Acta Derm Venereol 2015;98:816–821.
7 Weisshaar E, Weiss M, Passlick-Deetjen J, Tschulena U, Maleki K, Mettang T: Laboratory and dialysis characteristics in hemodialysis patients suffering from chronic itch – results from a representative cross-sectional study. BMC Nephrol 2015;16:184.
8 Dalgard F, Svensson A, Holm JØ, Sundby J: Self-reported skin complaints: validation of a questionnaire for population surveys. Br J Dermatol 2003;149:794–800.
9 Dalgard F, Svensson Å, Holm JØ, Sundby J: Self-reported skin morbidity in Oslo: associations itch socio-demographic factors among adults in a cross sectional study. Br J Dermatol 2004;151:452–457.
10 Halvorsen JA, Dalgard F, Thoresen M, Thoresen M, Bjertness E, Lien L: Itch and mental distress: a cross-sectional study among late adolescents. Acta Derm Venereol 2009;89:39–44.
11 Halvorsen JA, Kupfer J, Dalgard F: The prevalence and intensity of itch among dermatological patients in 13 European countries (abstract). Acta Derm Venereol 2013;91:620–621.
12 Kaushik SB, Cerci FB, Miracle J, Pokharel A, Chen SC, Chan YH, Wilkin A, Yosipovitch G: Chronic pruritus in HIV-positive patients in the southeastern United States: its prevalence and effect on quality of life. J Am Acad Dermatol 2014;70:659–664.
13 Mazeh D, Melamed Y, Cholostoy A, Aharonovitzch V, Weizman A, Yosipovitch G: Itching in the psychiatric ward. Acta Derm Venereol 2008;88:128–131.
14 Mistik S, Utas S, Ferahbas A, Tokgoz B, Unsal G, Sahan H, Ozturk A, Utas C: An epidemiology study of patients with uremic pruritus. J Eur Acad Dermatol Venereol 2006;20:672–678.
15 Kopyciok ME, Ständer HF, Osada N, Steinke S, Ständer S: Prevalence and characteristics of pruritus: a one-week cross-sectional study in a German dermatology practice. Acta Derm Venereol 2016;96:50–55.
16 Ständer S, Schäfer I, Phan NQ, Blome C, Herberger K, Heigel H, Augustin M: Prevalence of chronic pruritus in Germany: results of a cross-sectional study in a sample working population of 11,730. Dermatology 2010;221:229–235.

17 Suseł J, Batycka-Baran A, Reich A, Szepietowski JC: Uraemic pruritus markedly affects the quality of life and depressive symptoms in haemodialysis patients with end-stage renal disease. Acta Derm Venereol 2014;94:276–281.

18 Valdes-Rodriguez R, Mollanazar NK, González-Muro J, Nattkemper L, Torres-Alvarez B, López-Esqueda FJ, Chan YH, Yosipovitch G: Itch prevalence and characteristics in a Hispanic geriatric population: a comprehensive study using a standardized itch questionnaire. Acta Derm Venereol 2015;95:417–421.

19 Weisshaar E, Apfelbacher CJ, Jäger G, Zimmermann E, Bruckner T, Diepgen TL, Gollnick H: Pruritus as a leading symptom – clinical characteristics and quality of life in German and Ugandan patients. Br J Dermatol 2006;155:957–964.

20 Yalçin B, Tamer E, Toy GG, Oztaş P, Hayran M, Alli N: The prevalence of skin diseases in the elderly: analysis of 4,099 geriatric patients. Int J Dermatol 2006;45:672–676.

21 Yosipovitch G, Goon A, Wee J, Chan YH, Goh CL: The prevalence and clinical characteristics of pruritus among patients with extensive psoriasis. Br J Dermatol 2000;143:969–973.

22 Zucker I, Yosipovitch G, David M, Gafter U, Boner G: Prevalence and characterization of uremic pruritus in patients undergoing hemodialysis: uremic pruritus is still a major problem for patients with end-stage renal disease. J Am Acad Dermatol 2003;49:842–846.

23 Vaughan Jones S, Ambros-Rudolph C, Nelson-Piercy C: Skin disease in pregnancy. BMJ 2014;348:g3489.

24 Roger D, Vaillant L, Fignon A, Pierre F, Bacq Y, Brechot JF, Grangeponte MC, Lorette G: Specific pruritic dermatoses of pregnancy. A prospective study of 3,192 pregnant women. Arch Dermatol 1994;130:734–739.

25 Shanmugam S, Thappa DM, Habeebullah S: Pruritus gravidarum: a clinical and laboratory study. J Dermatol 1998; 25:582–586.

26 Reyes H, Gonzalez MC, Ribalta J, Aburto H, Matus C, Schramm G, Katz R, Medina E: Prevalence or intrahepatic cholestasis of pregnancy in Chile. Ann Int Med 1978;88:487–493.

27 Krueger G, Koo J, Lebwohl M, Menter A, Stern RS, Rolstad T: The impact of psoriasis on quality of life. Results of a 1998 National Psoriasis Foundation patient membership survey. Arch Dermatol 2001;137:280–284.

28 Szepietowski JC, Reich A: Pruritus in psoriasis: an update. Eur J Pain 2016;20: 41–46.

29 Lim YL, Chan YH, Yosipovitch G, Greaves MW: Pruritus is a common and significant symptom of acne. J Eur Acad Dermatol Venereol 2008;22:1332–1336.

30 Reich A, Trybucka K, Tracinska A, Samotij D, Jasiuk B, Srama M, Szepietowski JC Acne itch: do acne patients suffer from itching? Acta Derm Venereol 2008; 88:38–42.

31 Dalgard F, Halvorsen JA, Kwatra SG, Yosipovitch G: Acne severity and itch are associated: results from a Norwegian survey of 3775 adolescents. Br J Dermatol 2013;169:215–216.

32 Thaipisuttikul Y: Pruritic skin diseases in the elderly. J Dermatol 1998;25:153–157.

33 Weisshaar E, Matterne U: Epidemiology of itch; in Carstens E, Akiyama T (eds): Itch: Mechanisms and Treatment. Boca Raton, CRC Press, 2014.

34 Hajdarbegovic E, Thio HB: Itch pathophysiology may differ among ethnic groups. Int J Dermatol 2012;51:771–776.

35 Tey HL, Yosipovitch G: Itch in ethnic populations. Acta Derm Venereol 2010; 90:227–234.

36 Fett N, Haynes K, Propert KJ, Margolis DJ: Five-year malignancy incidence in patients with chronic pruritus: a population-based cohort study aimed at limiting unnecessary screening practices. J Am Acad Dermatol 2014;70:651–658.

37 Johannesdottir SA, Farkas DK, Vinding GR, Pedersen L, Lamberg A, Lamberg A, Sørensen HT, Olesen AB: Cancer incidence among patients with a hospital diagnosis of pruritus: a nationwide Danish cohort study. Br J Dermatol 2014; 171:839–846.

38 Neilly JB, Martin A, Simpson N, MacCuish AC: Pruritus in diabetes mellitus: investigation of prevalence and correlation with diabetes control. Diabetes Care 1986;9:273–275.

39 Yosipovitch G, Hodak E, Vardi P, Shraga I, Karp M, Sprecher E, David M: The prevalence of cutaneous manifestations in IDDM patients and their association with diabetes risk factors and microvasculature complications. Diabetes Care 1998;21:506–509.

40 Schneider G, Driesch G, Heuft G, Evers S, Luger TA, Ständer S: Psychosomatic cofactors and psychiatric comorbidity in patients with chronic itch. Clin Exp Dermatol 2006;31:762–767.

41 Pacan P, Grzesiak M, Reich A, Szepietowski JC: Is pruritus in depression a rare phenomenon? Acta Derm Venereol 2009;89:109–110.

42 Maleki K, Weisshaar E. Drug-induced pruritus. Hautarzt 2014;65:436–442.

43 Bigby M, Jick S, Jick H, Arndt K: Drug-induced reactions. A report from the Boston Collaborative Drug Surveillance Program on 15,438 consecutive inpatients, 1975 to 1982. JAMA 1986;256: 3358–3363.

Prof. Elke Weisshaar, MD, PhD
Department of Clinical Social Medicine, Occupational and Environmental Dermatology
Heidelberg University Hospital, Ruprecht Karls University
Thibautstrasse 3, DE–69115 Heidelberg (Germany)
E-Mail elke.weisshaar@med.uni-heidelberg.de

Szepietowski JC, Weisshaar E (eds): Itch – Management in Clinical Practice.
Curr Probl Dermatol. Basel, Karger, 2016, vol 50, pp 11–17 (DOI: 10.1159/000446011)

Central Mechanisms of Itch

Earl Carstens[a] · Tasuku Akiyama[b]

[a]Department of Neurobiology, Physiology and Behavior, University of California, Davis, Davis, Calif., and [b]Temple Itch Center,
Departments of Dermatology and Anatomy and Cell Biology, Temple University, Philadelphia, Pa., USA

Abstract

This chapter summarizes recent findings regarding the central transmission of acute and chronic itch. Itch is transduced by cutaneous pruriceptors that transmit signals to neurons in the superficial spinal cord. Spinal itch-signaling circuits utilize several neuropeptides whose receptors represent novel targets to block itch transmission. Itch is relieved by scratching, which activates spinal interneurons to inhibit itch-transmitting neurons. Spinal itch transmission is also thought to be modulated by descending pathways. Itch is transmitted rostrally via ascending pathways to activate a variety of brain regions involved in sensory discrimination of affective and motor responses to itch. The pathophysiological mechanisms of chronic itch are poorly understood but likely involve sensitization of itch-signaling pathways and/or dysfunction of itch-inhibitory circuits. Improved understanding of central itch mechanisms has identified a number of novel targets for the development of antipruritic treatment strategies.   © 2016 S. Karger AG, Basel

Itch is defined as an unpleasant sensation associated with the desire to scratch. Chronic itch decreases the quality of life [1] and imposes a high economic burden [2, 3]. This chapter reviews recent breakthroughs in our understanding of the central processing of itch and novel therapeutic approaches to block itch transmission or enhance the inhibition of itch at peripheral, spinal, and supraspinal sites. We also address the poorly understood pathophysiology of chronic itch and potential interventions.

Peripheral Encoding of Itch

Pruritic stimuli activate at least two distinct classes of itch-signaling nerve fibers (fig. 1). Histamine activates mechanically insensitive C-fibers [4, 5] via H_1/H_4 receptors and transient receptor potential cation channel V1 (TRPV1) [6], while non-histaminergic pruritogens activate polymodal nociceptors [7, 8] via TRPA1 [9]. Figure 1 provides a list of many pruritogens and their receptors. The participation of TRP channels in itch

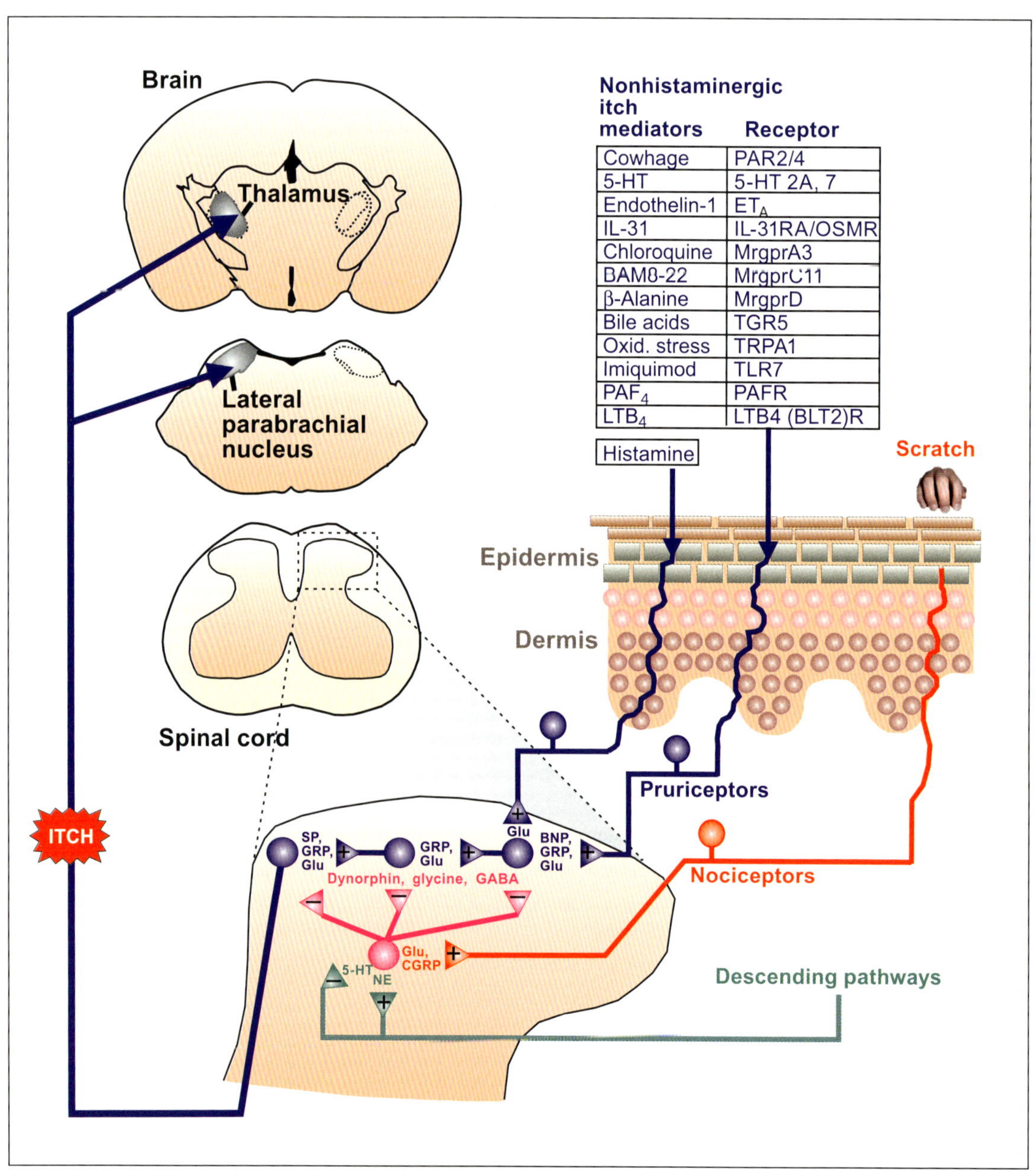

Fig. 1. Schematic drawing of the neural pathway for itch. 5-HT = 5-Hydroxytryptamine (serotonin); CGRP = calcitonin gene-related peptide; ET_A = endothelin-A receptor; Glu = glutamate; IL = interleukin; LTB_4 = leukotriene B_4; Mrgpr = Mas-related G protein-coupled receptor; NE = norepinephrine; OSMR = oncostatin M receptor; Oxid. stress = oxidative stress; PAF = platelet-activating factor; PAR = protease-activated receptor; PAFR = platelet-activating factor receptor; SP = substance P; TGR5 = G protein-coupled bile acid receptor; TLR = Toll-like receptor.

provides an avenue to allow the small local anesthetic QX-314 to enter into pruriceptive afferent fibers and block conduction, thereby silencing itch transmission [10]. Additional details concerning peripheral mechanisms of itch may be found in the chapter by Azimi et al. [this vol., pp. 18–23].

Spinal/Trigeminal Encoding of Itch

The central branches of pruriceptors terminate in superficial layers of the spinal or medullary dorsal horn to activate second-order neurons. Candidate neurotransmitters released from the central terminals of pruriceptors include glutamate [11] and the neuropeptides gastrin-releasing peptide (GRP), substance P, and brain natriuretic peptide (BNP) [12–15] (fig. 1). BNP is released from pruriceptors and is necessary for both histaminergic and nonhistaminergic itch [15]. MrgprA3-expressing pruriceptor terminals directly contact spinal neurons expressing the GRP receptor, implicating GRP as a neuropeptide released from pruriceptors [16]. GRP is also released from excitatory spinal interneurons. Neurotoxic ablation of neurons expressing neurokinin 1 (NK1), the receptor for substance P, also reduced itch behavior [14]. Nearly all spinal neurons with ascending axonal projections to the thalamus and parabrachial nucleus (see below) express NK1 [17]. These data suggest a spinal itch-signaling pathway in which BNP is released from pruriceptors to serially activate interneurons that release GRP, and then substance P, to activate NK1 receptor-expressing neurons that transmit itch signals to the brain (fig. 1). A cocktail of antagonists for NK1, GRP, and glutamate (AMPA; α-amino-3-hydroxy-5-methyl-4-isoxazolepropionic acid) receptors completely inhibited scratching behavior and activation of dorsal horn neurons elicited by chloroquine (MrgprA3 agonist), whereas individual or pairs of antagonists were less effective [11]. In contrast, the AMPA antagonist alone was sufficient to block histamine-evoked itch and excitation of dorsal horn neurons. These data implicate multiple spinal neuropeptides in mediating nonhistaminergic itch, and glutamate as the primary neurotransmitter for histamine-mediated itch. The use of combinations of antagonists for NK1, GRP, BNP, and glutamate (AMPA) receptors may prove useful to relieve itch.

Scratch Inhibition of Itch

It is well known that scratching relieves itch. Scratching within or adjacent to the receptive field area of spinal neurons inhibits their pruritogen-evoked activity [18, 19]. This effect is state dependent in that only pruritogen- but not algogen-evoked firing is suppressed by scratching. The inhibitory neurotransmitters GABA (γ-aminobutyric acid) and glycine mediate scratch inhibition [20], and mice lacking spinal glycine exhibited excessive scratching [21]. A specific class of inhibitory interneurons expressing the transcription factor Bhlhb5 (and co-expressing the somatostatin 2A receptor and galanin or neuronal nitric oxide synthase) is crucial for inhibition of itch. Genetic ablation of these inhibitory interneurons resulted in abnormally increased itch behavior [22]. The inhibitory interneurons are thought to release dynorphin, which acts at κ-opioid receptors presumably expressed by itch-signaling neurons [23]. Indeed, κ-opioid agonists such as nalfurafine suppressed itch behavior in mice [23, 24] and relieved itch from chronic kidney disease in human patients [25]. In mice lacking Bhlhb5, excessive scratching was significantly attenuated and skin lesions improved following spinal transplantation of GABAergic neurons [26]. These data thus indicate that GABA, glycine, and dynorphin modulate the spinal transmission of itch signals and that agonists of these inhibitory neurotransmitters may prove useful in treating itch.

Ascending Transmission of Itch

Itch-signaling neurons send ascending axons to the contralateral ventrobasal thalamus (spinothalamic tract) and to the lateral parabrachial nucleus bilaterally (spinoparabrachial tract) (fig. 1). In primates, separate subpopulations of spinothalamic tract neurons responded to histamine versus cowhage [27], a bean plant whose seed pods have spicules containing proteases that elicit nonhistaminergic itch [28]. This distinction is less evident in rodents, whereby most spinal neurons respond to histamine as well as nonhistaminergic pruritogens (fig. 1). In rodents, many spinothalamic and spinoparabrachial neurons respond to multiple pruritogens [29–31]. Interestingly, most or all pruritogen-responsive neurons are also excited by the algogens capsaicin and mustard oil, as well as other pain-producing stimuli. This presents a problem in terms of understanding how the nervous system discriminates between itch and pain. One possibility is that pruritogen-responsive neurons signal itch (even though they can be activated by noxious stimuli), while pain is signaled by a larger population of nociceptive neurons that is insensitive to pruritogens. This is consistent with a report that capsaicin, which normally elicits pain behavior, instead elicits itch behavior in mice lacking the capsaicin-sensitive receptor TRPV1, in whom TRPV1 was genetically inserted selectively back into sensory neurons expressing MrgprA3 [16].

Descending Modulation of Itch

Spinal itch transmission is thought to be under descending modulation from the brain, although to date there is limited data. Depletion of spinal cord levels of norepinephrine increased itch behavior, indicating a role for noradrenergic pathways descending from locus coeruleus and adjacent regions to inhibit itch transmission, possibly by activating inhibitory interneurons [32] (fig. 1).

Depletion of supraspinal serotonin reduced itch behavior, indicating that serotonergic pathways descending from the rostral ventromedial medulla may tonically facilitate itch [33] (fig. 1).

Supraspinal Processing of Itch

To date, little is known regarding the functional properties of neurons in the ventrobasal thalamus or parabrachial nuclei that receive direct ascending pruriceptive input. However, numerous functional imaging studies in humans have revealed a variety of brain regions that are activated during itch [34]. These include (1) the thalamus, primary and secondary somatosensory cortex, areas involved in recognition of and attention to itch, and localization and intensity rating of itch, (2) the cingulate and insular cortex, areas associated with cognition, motivation to act (scratch), and awareness of emotional state and body feeling, (3) the medial parietal cortex, posterior cingulate cortex, and precuneus, areas possibly associated with the subjective sensation of itch, and (4) motor-related areas, including the supplementary, premotor, and primary motor cortices, striatum and cerebellum, areas potentially involved in planning motor responses (e.g. scratching) to itch and affective aspects such as the desire to scratch.

Itch relief by scratching and the act of scratching itself have been suggested to be pleasurable. It is interesting that scratching during itch activates brain areas associated with reward including the midbrain striatum, medial prefrontal cortex, anterior cingulate cortex, and orbitofrontal cortex [34].

Humans often perceive itch and scratch themselves when observing other people scratching, a phenomenon called contagious itch [35]. Contagious scratching has also been observed in monkeys [36]. Interestingly, contagious itch is associated with activation of the same brain areas that are active during histamine-evoked itch [37].

Chronic Itch

Chronic itch arises from a variety of skin conditions, such as atopic dermatitis or psoriasis, from systemic kidney or liver disease, nerve damage, and many other sources, and is usually resistant to antihistamine treatment, implying dysfunction of the nonhistaminergic itch pathways. Chronic itch could be due to altered skin physiology or damage causing sensitization of pruriceptors, central sensitization of spinal/trigeminal transmission, disruption of spinal itch-inhibition, disruption of descending itch modulation, altered supraspinal processing of itch signals, or combinations thereof. Symptoms of chronic itch include ongoing (spontaneous) itch, increased itch to a normally pruritic stimulus (hyperknesis), and itch elicited by low-threshold tactile stimulation (alloknesis). In rodent models of atopic dermatitis, dry skin itch, and contact hypersensitivity, animals exhibited spontaneous scratching behavior, alloknesis, and enhanced scratching elicited by nonhistaminergic pruritogens (chloroquine, serotonin, proteases), but not histamine [38–40]. Primary and second-order sensory neurons with input from dry skin exhibited significantly enhanced responses to nonhistaminergic itch mediators, but not to histamine [38, 41], suggesting peripheral and possibly central sensitization of nonhistaminergic itch-signaling neurons in this dry skin model.

Mice lacking a subset of spinal inhibitory interneurons (see above) exhibited enhanced spontaneous scratching and hyperknesis [22], suggesting that dysfunction of spinal inhibition contributes to this genetic model of neuropathic itch.

Human patients suffering from itch of end-stage renal disease exhibited greater baseline activation in the anterior cingulate cortex, insula, claustrum, hippocampus, and nucleus accumbens, as well as reduced cowhage-evoked activation of primary somatosensory cortex and other areas, compared to healthy control subjects [42]. This suggests that chronic itch results in altered supraspinal processing of itch signaling.

Conclusions

Our understanding of the central transmission of itch has increased dramatically in recent years, revealing a number of attractive targets for future development of novel therapeutics to block itch transmission or enhance itch inhibition at peripheral, spinal, and supraspinal sites. Less is known regarding pathophysiological mechanisms underlying chronic itch. However, with the availability of animal models for many types of chronic itch, we can expect dramatic advances to be made in our knowledge of the pathophysiology of chronic itch with the advent of new evidence-based treatment strategies.

Acknowledgements

The authors' cited work was supported by grants from the National Institutes of Health (AR063228, DE021183, AR057194).

References

1 Halvorsen JA, Dalgard F, Thoresen M, Bjertness E, Lien L: Itch and pain in adolescents are associated with suicidal ideation: a population-based cross-sectional study. Acta Derm Venereol 2012; 92:543–546.

2 Thorpe KE, Florence CS, Joski P: Which medical conditions account for the rise in health spending? Health Aff (Millwood) 2004;Suppl Web Exclusives:W4-437-445.

3 Bickers DR, Lim HW, Margolis D, Weinstock MA, Goodman C, Faulkner E, Gould C, Gemmen E, Dall T: The burden of skin diseases: 2004. A joint project of the American Academy of Dermatology Association and the Society for Investigative Dermatology. J Am Acad Dermatol 2006;55:490–500.

4   Schmelz M, Schmidt R, Bickel A, Handwerker HO, Torebjörk HE: Specific C-receptors for itch in human skin. J Neurosci 1997;17:8003–8008.
5   Namer B, Carr R, Johanek LM, Schmelz M, Handwerker HO, Ringkamp M: Separate peripheral pathways for pruritus in man. J Neurophysiol 2008;100:2062–2069.
6   Shim WS, Tak MH, Lee MH, Kim M, Koo JY, Lee CH, Kim M, Oh U: TRPV1 mediates histamine-induced itching via the activation of phospholipase A2 and 12-lipoxygenase. J Neurosci 2007;27:2331–2337.
7   Johanek LM, Meyer RA, Friedman RM, Greenquist KW, Shim B, Borzan J, Hartke T, LaMotte RH, Ringkamp M: A role for polymodal C-fiber afferents in nonhistaminergic itch. J Neurosci 2008;28:7659–7669.
8   Ringkamp M, Schepers RJ, Shimada SG, Johanek LM, Hartke TV, Borzan J, Shim B, LaMotte RH, Meyer RA: A role for nociceptive, myelinated nerve fibers in itch sensation. J Neurosci 2011;31:14841–14849.
9   Wilson SR, Gerhold KA, Bifolck-Fisher A, Liu Q, Patel KN, Dong X, Bautista DM: TRPA1 is required for histamine-independent, Mas-related G protein-coupled receptor-mediated itch. Nat Neurosci 2011;14:595–602.
10 Roberson DP, Gudes S, Sprague JM, Patoski HA, Robson VK, Blasl F, Duan B, Oh SB, Bean BP, Ma Q, Binshtok AM, Woolf CJ: Activity-dependent silencing reveals functionally distinct itch-generating sensory neurons. Nat Neurosci 2013;16:910–918.
11 Akiyama T, Tominaga M, Takamori K, Carstens MI, Carstens E: Roles of glutamate, substance P, and gastrin-releasing peptide as spinal neurotransmitters of histaminergic and nonhistaminergic itch. Pain 2014;155:80–92.
12 Sun YG, Chen ZF: A gastrin-releasing peptide receptor mediates the itch sensation in the spinal cord. Nature 2007;448:700–703.
13 Sun YG, Zhao ZQ, Meng XL, Yin J, Liu XY, Chen ZF: Cellular basis of itch sensation. Science 2009;325:1531–1534.
14 Carstens EE, Carstens MI, Simons CT, Jinks SL: Dorsal horn neurons expressing NK-1 receptors mediate scratching in rats. Neuroreport 2010;21:303–308.
15 Mishra SK, Hoon MA: The cells and circuitry for itch responses in mice. Science 2013;340:968–971.

16 Han L, Ma C, Liu Q, Weng HJ, Cui Y, Tang Z, Kim Y, Nie H, Qu L, Patel KN, Li Z, McNeil B, He S, Guan Y, Xiao B, Lamotte RH, Dong X: A subpopulation of nociceptors specifically linked to itch. Nat Neurosci 2013;16:174–182.
17 Al-Khater KM, Todd AJ: Collateral projections of neurons in laminae I, III, and IV of rat spinal cord to thalamus, periaqueductal gray matter, and lateral parabrachial area. J Comp Neurol 2009;515:629–646.
18 Akiyama T, Tominaga M, Carstens MI, Carstens EE: Site-dependent and state-dependent inhibition of pruritogen-responsive spinal neurons by scratching. Eur J Neurosci 2012;36:2311–2316.
19 Davidson S, Zhang X, Khasabov SG, Simone DA, Giesler GJ Jr: Relief of itch by scratching: state-dependent inhibition of primate spinothalamic tract neurons. Nat Neurosci 2009;12:544–546.
20 Akiyama T, Iodi Carstens M, Carstens E: Transmitters and pathways mediating inhibition of spinal itch-signaling neurons by scratching and other counterstimuli. PLoS One 2011;6:e22665.
21 Foster E, Wildner H, Tudeau L, Haueter S, Ralvenius WT, Jegen M, Johannssen H, Hosli L, Haenraets K, Ghanem A, Conzelmann KK, Bosl M, Zeilhofer HU: Targeted ablation, silencing, and activation establish glycinergic dorsal horn neurons as key components of a spinal gate for pain and itch. Neuron 2015;85:1289–1304.
22 Ross SE, Mardinly AR, McCord AE, Zurawski J, Cohen S, Jung C, Hu L, Mok SI, Shah A, Savner EM, Tolias C, Corfas R, Chen S, Inquimbert P, Xu Y, McInnes RR, Rice FL, Corfas G, Ma Q, Woolf CJ, Greenberg ME: Loss of inhibitory interneurons in the dorsal spinal cord and elevated itch in Bhlhb5 mutant mice. Neuron 2010;65:886–898.
23 Kardon AP, Polgár E, Hachisuka J, Snyder LM, Cameron D, Savage S, Cai X, Karnup S, Fan CR, Hemenway GM, Bernard CS, Schwartz ES, Nagase H, Schwarzer C, Watanabe M, Furuta T, Kaneko T, Koerber HR, Todd AJ, Ross SE: Dynorphin acts as a neuromodulator to inhibit itch in the dorsal horn of the spinal cord. Neuron 2014;82:573–586.
24 Akiyama T, Carstens MI, Piecha D, Steppan S, Carstens E: Nalfurafine suppresses pruritogen- and touch-evoked scratching behavior in models of acute and chronic itch in mice. Acta Derm Venereol 2015;95:147–150.

25 Wikström B, Gellert R, Ladefoged SD, Danda Y, Akai M, Ide K, Ogasawara M, Kawashima Y, Ueno K, Mori A, Ueno Y: Kappa-opioid system in uremic pruritus: multicenter, randomized, double-blind, placebo-controlled clinical studies. J Am Soc Nephrol 2005;16:3742–3747.
26 Braz JM, Juarez-Salinas D, Ross SE, Basbaum AI: Transplant restoration of spinal cord inhibitory controls ameliorates neuropathic itch. J Clin Invest 2014;124:3612–3616.
27 Davidson S, Zhang X, Khasabov SG, Moser HR, Honda CN, Simone DA, Giesler GJ Jr: Pruriceptive spinothalamic tract neurons: physiological properties and projection targets in the primate. J Neurophysiol 2012;108:1711–1723.
28 Johanek LM, Meyer RA, Hartke T, Hobelmann JG, Maine DN, LaMotte RH, Ringkamp M: Psychophysical and physiological evidence for parallel afferent pathways mediating the sensation of itch. J Neurosci 2007;27:7490–7497.
29 Moser HR, Giesler GJ Jr: Characterization of pruriceptive trigeminothalamic tract neurons in rats. J Neurophysiol 2014;111:1574–1589.
30 Jansen NA, Giesler GJ Jr: Response characteristics of pruriceptive and nociceptive trigeminoparabrachial tract neurons in the rat. J Neurophysiol 2014;113:58–70.
31 Akiyama T, Curtis E, Nguyen T, Carstens MI, Carstens E: Anatomical evidence of pruriceptive trigeminothalamic and trigeminoparabrachial projection neurons in mice. J Comp Neurol 2015;524:244–256.
32 Gotoh Y, Andoh T, Kuraishi Y: Noradrenergic regulation of itch transmission in the spinal cord mediated by alpha-adrenoceptors. Neuropharmacology 2011;61:825–831.
33 Zhao ZQ, Liu XY, Jeffry J, Karunarathne WK, Li JL, Munanairi A, Zhou XY, Li H, Sun YG, Wan L, Wu ZY, Kim S, Huo FQ, Mo P, Barry DM, Zhang CK, Kim JY, Gautam N, Renner KJ, Li YQ, Chen ZF: Descending control of itch transmission by the serotonergic system via 5-HT1A-facilitated GRP-GRPR signaling. Neuron 2014;84:821–834.
34 Mochizuki H, Kakigi R: Central mechanisms of itch. Clin Neurophysiol 2015;126:1650–1660.

35 Papoiu AD, Wang H, Coghill RC, Chan YH, Yosipovitch G: Contagious itch in humans: a study of visual 'transmission' of itch in atopic dermatitis and healthy subjects. Br J Dermatol 2011;164:1299–1303.

36 Feneran AN, O'Donnell R, Press A, Yosipovitch G, Cline M, Dugan G, Papoiu AD, Nattkemper LA, Chan YH, Shively CA: Monkey see, monkey do: contagious itch in nonhuman primates. Acta Derm Venereol 2013;93:27–29.

37 Holle H, Warne K, Seth AK, Critchley HD, Ward J: Neural basis of contagious itch and why some people are more prone to it. Proc Natl Acad Sci USA 2012;109:19816–19821.

38 Akiyama T, Carstens MI, Carstens E: Enhanced scratching evoked by PAR-2 agonist and 5-HT but not histamine in a mouse model of chronic dry skin itch. Pain 2010;151:378–383.

39 Akiyama T, Nguyen T, Curtis E, Nishida K, Devireddy J, Carstens MI, Carstens E: A central role for spinal dorsal horn neurons that express neurokinin-1 receptors in chronic itch. Pain 2015;156:1240–1246.

40 Fu K, Qu L, Shimada SG, Nie H, LaMotte RH: Enhanced scratching elicited by a pruritogen and an algogen in a mouse model of contact hypersensitivity. Neurosci Lett 2014;579:190–194.

41 Akiyama T, Carstens MI, Carstens E: Enhanced responses of lumbar superficial dorsal horn neurons to intradermal PAR-2 agonist but not histamine in a mouse hindpaw dry skin itch model. J Neurophysiol 2011;105:2811–2817.

42 Papoiu AD, Emerson NM, Patel TS, Kraft RA, Valdes-Rodriguez R, Nattkemper LA, Coghill RC, Yosipovitch G: Voxel-based morphometry and arterial spin labeling fMRI reveal neuropathic and neuroplastic features of brain processing of itch in end-stage renal disease. J Neurophysiol 2014;112:1729–1738.

Prof. Earl Carstens
Department of Neurobiology, Physiology and Behavior
University of California, Davis
1 Shields Avenue, Davis, CA 95616 (USA)
E-Mail eecarstens@ucdavis.edu

Dr. Tasuku Akiyama
Temple Itch Center, Departments of Dermatology and Anatomy and Cell Biology, Temple University
3500 N. Broad Street MERB452, Philadelphia, PA 19140 (USA)
E-Mail tasuku.akiyama@temple.edu

Szepietowski JC, Weisshaar E (eds): Itch – Management in Clinical Practice.
Curr Probl Dermatol. Basel, Karger, 2016, vol 50, pp 18–23 (DOI: 10.1159/000446012)

Peripheral Mechanisms of Itch

Ehsan Azimi[a] · Jimmy Xia[b] · Ethan A. Lerner[a]

[a]Cutaneous Biology Research Center, Department of Dermatology, Massachusetts General Hospital and Harvard Medical School,
Charlestown, Mass., and [b]Brown University, Providence, R.I., USA

Abstract

A multitude of exogenous environmental stimuli and endogenous molecular and cellular components interface directly or indirectly with the free nerve endings of sensory nerves in the skin. Environmental stimuli include substances derived from the microbiome and materials, such as allergens, that otherwise come in contact with the skin. Endogenous stimuli include components of or mediators derived from the epidermal barrier, keratinocytes, mast cells, and additional resident and skin-homing immune cells. The sensation of itch is ultimately provoked by mediators that interact with and activate pruriceptors on the sensory nerve fibers. These peripheral fibers convey signals from the skin to the dorsal root and trigeminal ganglia and on to the spinal cord and brain where central processing of the itch sensation occurs. A discussion of the nature and sources of itch stimuli and receptors in the periphery form the basis of this chapter. The development of drugs that target these processes is in the process of revolutionizing therapeutic approaches to itch.

© 2016 S. Karger AG, Basel

A simple view of peripheral itch is that a stimulus generates an action potential in a sensory nerve fiber that the brain interprets as the sensation of itch. This view, while convenient, does not reflect the remarkable complexity and redundancy in mechanisms that contribute to itch. Here, we address the panoply that contributes to peripheral itch. Our focus is on aspects that are most relevant to the practicing clinician so that mechanisms are appreciated while ongoing advances in therapies can be placed within an approachable context.

A multitude of exogenous environmental stimuli and endogenous molecular and cellular components interface directly or indirectly with sensory nerves in the skin. Environmental stimuli include substances derived from the microbiome, temperature, humidity, and materials that otherwise come in contact with the skin. Endogenous components include the epidermal barrier, pH, keratinocytes, and resident and skin-homing immune cells. It is now appreciated that communication between nerves, stimuli, and cutaneous components, including the dermal milieu of vessels and stroma, which provide a scaffold, is bi- or multidirectional such that each may serve to modulate the sensation of itch.

Nerve Fibers and Itch

Itch is sensed by nerve fibers called pruriceptors. Fibers that transmit pain and other noxious stimuli are called nociceptors. These are all afferent fibers that convey signals from the periphery to the dorsal root and trigeminal ganglia and on to the spinal cord where they synapse with second-order neurons. Signals are then transmitted to the brain for interpretation as itch and then back to the skin via motor neurons instructing us to scratch, in an effort to relieve this sensation. Complex neurocircuitry at the level of the spinal cord, as discussed in the previous chapter, can serve to not only activate, but also to inhibit itch signaling.

The sensation of itch, but not pain, requires at least a portion of the epidermis. It was demonstrated more than 50 years ago that free nerve endings can be found in the epidermis [1]. It is likely that these free nerve endings are innate sensors probing the environment and communicating with adjacent skin cells. These sensory fibers are characterized and distinguished by a number of features. Two distinct types of fibers that transmit itch are recognized: A-fibers and C-fibers [2]. A-fibers are myelinated, rapidly conduct nerve impulses, and are divided further into Aδ- and Aβ-fibers. Aδ-fibers can function as pruriceptors and nociceptors. Aβ-fibers do not [2].

Being unmyelinated, C-fibers conduct impulses slowly. They are of smaller diameter as compared to A-fibers. There are two populations of C-fibers. One population can respond to mechanical stimulation and heat, and is thus referred to as CM or CMH fibers. The other class is insensitive to such stimulation and is referred to as CMi fibers. CMi fibers respond to histamine and, upon stimulation, release the neuropeptides substance P and calcitonin gene-related peptide. Substance P and calcitonin gene-related peptide participate in vascular flare and the activation of mast cells. CMH fibers do not respond to histamine, but they do respond to cowhage [3]. Cowhage refers to a tropical bean plant, the pods of which are covered with small needles, also called cowhage. Contact with the skin allows the active component, a protease, to interact with a receptor on sensory fibers to provoke itch, pricking, and stinging sensations, akin to many clinical itches, including that of atopic dermatitis [4]. While we may ask a patient if he or she itches, or they tell us that they itch, further questioning often reveals the presence of additional, but less intense, sensations of pricking or stinging. It is likely that most itches are mediated by CMH fibers.

It is not clear whether humans have fibers that specifically sense itch as opposed to pain, although such a distinction has been shown in mice. There are theories that can account for the differentiation between itch and pain. For our purposes, the stimulation of overlapping populations of cutaneous sensory fibers combined with interpretation of signals in the spinal cord and brain result in the sensation of itch.

Acute versus Chronic Itch

Acute itches are those that last anywhere from an instant to 6 weeks. Examples range from a spontaneous itch that necessitates a simple scratch, to the itch, scratch, and dermatographism occurring in some people while changing into pajamas at night or the itch from poison ivy that lasts approximately 3 weeks. These are self-limited itches although treatment is often indicated.

Chronic itch is that which persists for 6 weeks or longer. Chronic itches associated with inflammation include atopic dermatitis, psoriasis, or the persistence of contact with an unknown allergen. Systemic diseases are also associated with chronic itch but may not include apparent inflammation. Examples include chronic kidney disease and the itch of cholestasis. Neurogenic and neuropathic chronic itches include notalgia paresthetica and postherpetic neuralgia.

Itch mediators that turn on pruriceptors in the skin may be present in both acute and chronic itches. Blocking the mediators, treatment of the inflammation, or a kidney transplant in a patient with renal itch may ameliorate these itches. However, both the peripheral and central nervous systems can become sensitized over time. When this happens, the neural architecture is altered such that despite removal of the initial itch stimulus, itch may persist. We do not yet understand the role of mediators and pruriceptors in these situations, nor do we know how to reverse the effect of sensitization.

Sources of Mediators of Itch

As noted in the Introduction, exogenous environmental stimuli and endogenous molecular and cellular components interface in a direct or indirect manner with sensory nerves in the skin to provoke itch (fig. 1). Direct stimuli include mediators, such as proteases, released by members of the microbiome. These stimuli and how they work are discussed in more detail below. An indirect stimulus could be a contact allergen that generates an allergic response leading to the release, from immune cells, of itch mediators which then stimulate sensory nerves. Using atopic dermatitis as another example, there is a complex interplay between bacteria, the epidermal barrier, keratinocytes, immune cells, and sensory nerves, which together leads to itch, inflammation, and the itch-scratch cycle. This interplay is being teased apart as manifest by the development of new therapeutics for atopic dermatitis. Ironically, with the exception of some urticarias associated with histamine, there is not a single clinical situation in which the mediators of itch are defined.

Receptors, Channels, and Mediators of Itch

There are three classes of *receptors* that can be activated by itch mediators. These include members of the G protein-coupled receptor (GPCR), Toll-like receptor (TLR), and cytokine families, respectively. There is one class of *channels* broadly associated with itch. This is the transient receptor potential (TRP) channel family. Generation of an action potential and transmission of an itch signal ultimately depends upon activation of sodium channels.

G Protein-Coupled Receptors

Histamine and the H_1 receptor remain the most widely known mediator and receptor in itch, but they are no longer considered the most important. Their diminished importance arises from the clinical observation that antihistamines are not effective in most itches, including atopic dermatitis. Histamine is important in some urticarias. A number of other mediators and their cognate receptors are in the process of replacing the classic view of the importance of histamine and the H_1 receptor in itch. There are four histamine receptors. One of these, H_4, is also involved in itch [5]. H_4 antagonists are helpful in itch, but side effects have limited their use for now [5].

Most of the currently known endogenous and exogenous pruritogens activate GPCRs. GPCR activation does not lead directly to the generation of an action potential. GPCR activation is coupled via intracellular signaling pathways to TRP channels, the activation of which allows for sufficient current influx to generate action potentials. As a general rule, histamine and activation of the histamine receptor is linked to TRPV1 sensitization and activation, whereas histamine-independent itch works through other GPCRs and is linked to TRPA1 [6, 7].

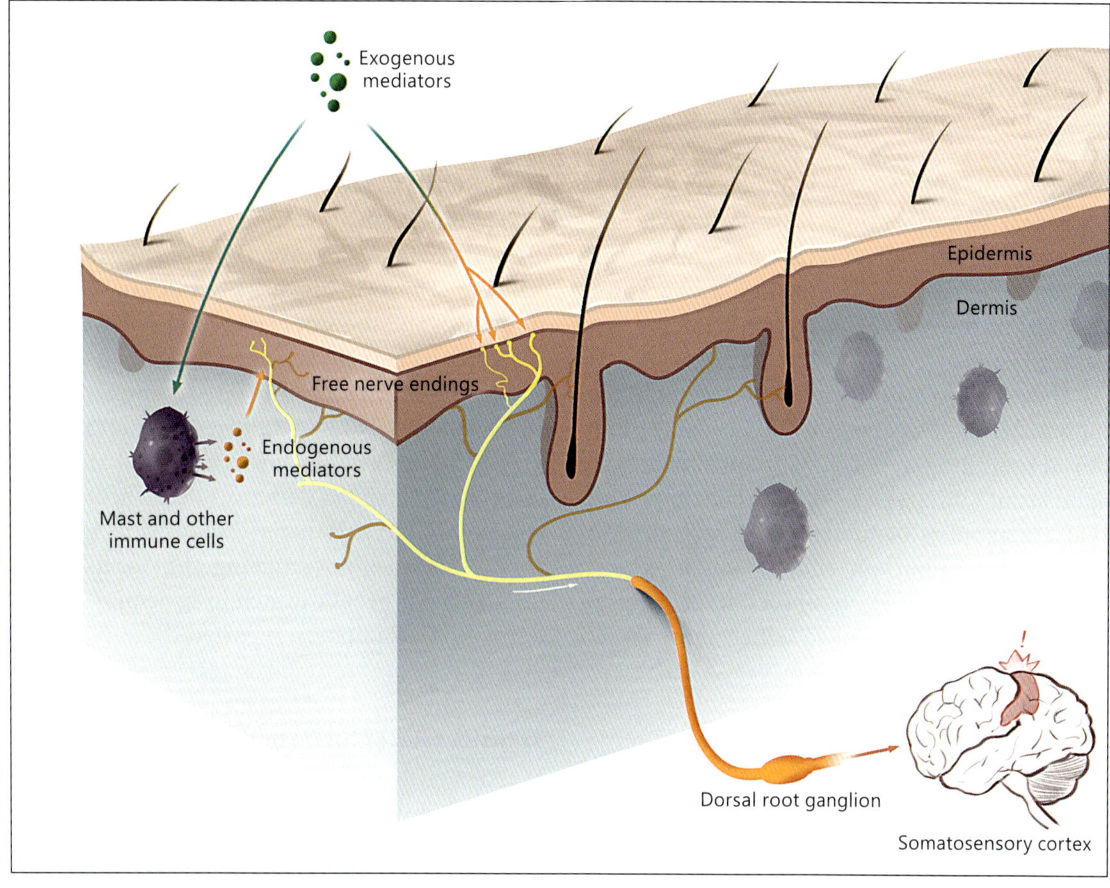

Fig. 1. Itch is provoked by the interaction of exogenous and endogenous stimuli with free nerve endings in the epidermis. Itch-selective free nerve endings reach all layers of the epidermis and are depicted in yellow. Pain-selective free nerve endings are depicted in a darker color. The pain and itch nerve endings may be part of the same sensory nerve with cell bodies in dorsal root ganglia (figure generated by Jimmy Xia).

Nonhistamine receptors of importance in itch include protease-activated receptors, Mas-related G protein-coupled receptors, the neurokinin 1 receptor, and those for serotonin, endothelin, and lysophatidic acid. Protease-activated receptors are activated by proteases, including tryptase from mast cells and kallikreins and cathepsin S from keratinocytes. Mas-related G protein-coupled receptors are activated by some proteases but also by many other substances, including antimicrobial peptides [8, 9]. Substance P, a neuro-peptide associated with neurogenic inflammation and atopic dermatitis, activates both Mas-related G protein-coupled receptors and the neurokinin 1 receptor [10]. Drugs that the target neurokinin 1 receptor are in clinical trials for itch. Autotaxin is the enzyme responsible for the production of lysophosphatidic acid. Autotaxin and the lyso-phosphatidic acid family of receptors may be involved with cholestatic itch [11].

Prostaglandins and leukotrienes can induce itch in human skin and can signal through

GPCRs. However, it appears that their function is to potentiate itch rather than evoke it directly. Gastrin-releasing peptide and its receptor as well as brain natriuretic peptide and its receptor are important in itch, but these seem to be primarily in the spinal cord, not the skin [12, 13]. Morphine and other opiates cause itch via activation of certain opiate receptors. These itches are not relieved by scratching and the receptors are thus in the central, not peripheral, nervous system.

There is also a protective side to GPCR signaling. Activation of certain GPCRs has the benefit of inhibiting itch. Cannabinoids, which are agonists of CB_1 and CB_2 receptors, compounds that are agonists of the κ-opioid receptors including dynorphin, an endogenous κ-agonist, and stimulation of H_3 receptors all can inhibit itch [14, 15]. The extent to which these effects are peripheral, central, or a mix is an active area of investigation.

Toll-Like Receptors

TLRs function as innate sensors in the immune system. They may have a similar role in the nervous system but this possibility has not been demonstrated conclusively. TLR3, TLR7, and potentially TLR4 are expressed on small-sized primary sensory neurons. Direct activation of TLRs by any of the classic pruritogens has not been demonstrated. TLRs can thus facilitate itch transmission, but a direct role in itch has not yet been elucidated [16].

Cytokine Receptors: Interleukin-31 and Thymic Stromal Lymphopoietin

Interleukin (IL)-31 is produced by Th2 cells, each of which has been identified as having a role in atopic dermatitis [17]. The receptor for IL-31 is expressed on various cell types, including sensory neurons [18]. Although these observations suggest a role for this receptor in itch, the slow onset of pruritus following injection are consistent with IL-31 being primarily an indirect mediator of itch [19]. Antibodies to the receptor are in development for the treatment of itch.

Thymic stromal lymphopoietin (TSLP) is an IL-7-like cytokine produced primarily by epithelial cells. This cytokine has been linked to atopic dermatitis and the atopic march to asthma. TSLP mediates its effects via a receptor composed of a TSLP receptor chain and an IL-7 receptor α-chain. Itch evoked by TSLP is via its receptor on a subset of sensory nerves [20]. A monoclonal antibody directed to TSLP has demonstrated efficacy in allergen-induced asthmatic responses in humans [21]. Whether or not targeting TSLP or its receptor will be of benefit in itch in general or atopic dermatitis has not been reported.

Transient Receptor Potential Channels

Although a direct role for TRPs in itch remains elusive, TRPs facilitate itch transduction. More than 25 TRP family members have been described and these are broken down further into subfamilies. TRPs are distributed broadly across tissues. TRPs relevant to itch are TRPV1, TRPV3, TRPV4, TRPA1, and TRPM8 [22]. TRPV1 is best known as the receptor for capsaicin, but is also a heat sensor. TRPA1 is a chemosensor that is activated by allyl isothiocyanate, cinnamaldehyde, and allicin, the pungent compounds found in mustard, cinnamon, and garlic extracts, respectively. TRPM8 is a cold sensor and is activated by menthol. Extremes of heat and cold, via activation of TRPV1 and TRPM8, can distract from the sensation of itch. Although TRPV1 and TRPA1 may not be directly associated with most clinical itches, their threshold for activation is modulated by signaling following pruritogen activation of GPCRs.

Conclusions and Future Expectations

Many receptors, channels, and mediators are linked to itch. The importance of each of these in clinical conditions is being deciphered. The possibility of treating itch by targeting the nervous system, not just the immune system, is on the horizon. Drugs directed to some of these targets will be available within the next several years and will usher in a targeted approach for the treatment of many itches.

References

1 Shelley WB, Arthur RP: The neurohistology and neurophysiology of the itch sensation in man. AMA Arch Derm 1957;76:296–323.
2 LaMotte RH, Dong X, Ringkamp M: Sensory neurons and circuits mediating itch. Nat Rev Neurosci 2014;15:19–31.
3 Namer B, Carr R, Johanek LM, Schmelz M, Handwerker HO, Ringkamp M: Separate peripheral pathways for pruritus in man. J Neurophysiol 2008;100:2062–2069.
4 Reddy VB, Iuga AO, Shimada SG, LaMotte RH, Lerner EA: Cowhage-evoked itch is mediated by a novel cysteine protease: a ligand of protease-activated receptors. J Neurosci 2008;28:4331–4335.
5 Thurmond RL, Kazerouni K, Chaplan SR, Greenspan AJ: Antihistamines and itch. Handb Exp Pharmacol 2015;226:257–290.
6 Shim WS, Tak MH, Lee MH, Kim M, Kim M, Koo JY, et al: TRPV1 mediates histamine-induced itching via the activation of phospholipase A2 and 12-lipoxygenase. J Neurosci 2007;27:2331–2337.
7 Wilson SR, Gerhold KA, Bifolck-Fisher A, Liu Q, Patel KN, Dong X, et al: TRPA1 is required for histamine-independent, Mas-related G protein-coupled receptor-mediated itch. Nat Neurosci 2011;14:595–602.
8 Reddy VB, Sun S, Azimi E, Elmariah SB, Dong X, Lerner EA: Redefining the concept of protease-activated receptors: cathepsin S evokes itch via activation of Mrgprs. Nat Commun 2015;6:7864.
9 Subramanian H, Gupta K, Guo Q, Price R, Ali H: Mas-related gene X2 (MrgX2) is a novel G protein-coupled receptor for the antimicrobial peptide LL-37 in human mast cells: resistance to receptor phosphorylation, desensitization, and internalization. J Biol Chem 2011;286:44739–44749.
10 McNeil BD, Pundir P, Meeker S, Han L, Undem BJ, Kulka M, et al: Identification of a mast-cell-specific receptor crucial for pseudo-allergic drug reactions. Nature 2015;519:237–241.
11 Oude Elferink RP, Kremer AE, Martens JJ, Beuers UH: The molecular mechanism of cholestatic pruritus. Dig Dis 2011;29:66–71.
12 Sun YG, Chen ZF: A gastrin-releasing peptide receptor mediates the itch sensation in the spinal cord. Nature 2007;448:700–703.
13 Mishra SK, Hoon MA: The cells and circuitry for itch responses in mice. Science 2013;340:968–971.
14 Kardon AP, Polgar E, Hachisuka J, Snyder LM, Cameron D, Savage S, et al: Dynorphin acts as a neuromodulator to inhibit itch in the dorsal horn of the spinal cord. Neuron 2014;82:573–586.
15 Haruna T, Soga M, Morioka Y, Hikita I, Imura K, Furue Y, et al: S-777469, a novel cannabinoid type 2 receptor agonist, suppresses itch-associated scratching behavior in rodents through inhibition of itch signal transmission. Pharmacology 2015;95:95–103.
16 Taves S, Ji RR: Itch control by Toll-like receptors. Handb Exp Pharmacol 2015;226:135–150.
17 Sonkoly E, Muller A, Lauerma AI, Pivarcsi A, Soto H, Kemeny L, et al: IL-31: a new link between T cells and pruritus in atopic skin inflammation. J Allergy Clin Immunol 2006;117:411–417.
18 Cevikbas F, Wang X, Akiyama T, Kempkes C, Savinko T, Antal A, et al: A sensory neuron-expressed IL-31 receptor mediates T helper cell-dependent itch: involvement of TRPV1 and TRPA1. J Allergy Clin Immunol 2014;133:448–460.
19 Hawro T, Saluja R, Weller K, Altrichter S, Metz M, Maurer M: Interleukin-31 does not induce immediate itch in atopic dermatitis patients and healthy controls after skin challenge. Allergy 2014;69:113–117.
20 Wilson SR, The L, Batia LM, Beattie K, Katibah GE, McClain SP, et al: The epithelial cell-derived atopic dermatitis cytokine TSLP activates neurons to induce itch. Cell 2013;155:285–295.
21 Gauvreau GM, O'Byrne PM, Boulet LP, Wang Y, Cockcroft D, Bigler J, et al: Effects of an anti-TSLP antibody on allergen-induced asthmatic responses. N Engl J Med 2014;370:2102–2110.
22 Lucaciu OC, Connell GP: Itch sensation through transient receptor potential channels: a systematic review and relevance to manual therapy. J Manipulative Physiol Ther 2013;36:385–393.

Ethan A. Lerner, MD, PhD
Cutaneous Biology Research Center, Department of Dermatology
Massachusetts General Hospital and Harvard Medical School
149, 13th Street, Charlestown, MA 02129 (USA)
E-Mail elerner@mgh.harvard.edu

Szepietowski JC, Weisshaar E (eds): Itch – Management in Clinical Practice.
Curr Probl Dermatol. Basel, Karger, 2016, vol 50, pp 24–28 (DOI: 10.1159/000446013)

Diagnostic Procedures of Itch

Adam Reich · Jacek C. Szepietowski

Department of Dermatology, Venereology and Allergology, Wrocław Medical University, Wrocław, Poland

Abstract

A complex and multifactorial pathogenesis of itch makes the proper diagnosis of underlying disease a difficult and challenging clinical problem. The examination of every patient with itch should be started by gathering an accurate history. During the anamnesis it is important to obtain data about the beginning of the appearance of symptoms, its location, diurnal variation, and the factors influencing itch perception. After careful anamnesis the patient should undergo a detailed physical examination, with particular attention to the skin in order to look for any signs of skin lesions. Special attention should be paid to distinguish the primary lesion from the changes resulting from scratching. In patients in whom the etiology of the itch cannot be identified on the basis of the medical examination, a panel of primary screen laboratory examination may be required, and if necessary, depending on the results of basic laboratory results and data from medical history, additional diagnostic tests should be considered. In patients in whom an organic cause of itching has not been established, itch is most likely of undetermined origin; however, psychogenic causes should also be suspected and ruled out. In conclusion, it could be stated that itch is a common symptom of many skin diseases, systemic of neurological diseases. Despite the complex etiology of the disease, an exact cause of itch should be searched for in each patient, as successful therapy is largely dependent on the determination of the cause of the itching. © 2016 S. Karger AG, Basel

Complex and multifactorial pathogenesis of itch makes the proper diagnosis of underlying disease a difficult and challenging clinical problem. Importantly, every patient with itch should be treated individually, as itch can be a symptom of a wide spectrum of often disparate diseases characterized by different courses and prognoses.

An examination of every patient with itch should be started by gathering an accurate history about all concomitant diseases, drug use, foreign travels, the presence of itch among close family members, housing conditions and place of work, the presence of recent skin lesions (which does not necessarily have to be visible at the time of patient examination), and contact with animals or other potential allergens. During the anamnesis it is also important to obtain data about the beginning of the appearance of symptoms, its lo-

Table 1. Basic laboratory examinations which should be performed in patients with chronic itch of unknown etiology

---

Basic assessments (should be done in all subjects)
Blood smear
C-reactive protein level or erythrocyte sedimentation rate
Serum urea and creatinine level
Assessment of liver function: total and free bilirubin, serum activity of aminotransferases and alkaline phosphatase
Serum iron level (in patients with anemia), ferritin level
Serum glucose level
Assessment of thyroid gland function (TSH, fT_3, fT_4)
Stool assessment for parasites

Additional assessments (done in selected patients based on anamnesis, physical examination, and results of basic assessments)
Hormonal examinations: parathormone
Immunoelectrophoresis of serum proteins
Serum lipid levels (triglycerides, total cholesterol)
Detection of hepatitis viruses
Skin biopsy with direct immunofluorescence/immunohistochemistry (e.g. to exclude pemphigoid, mastocytosis, mycosis fungoides)
Detection of occult blood in the stool

---

cation, diurnal variation, and the factors influencing itch perception. Sudden onset of itch is generally unusual for itch caused by systemic diseases, but more often is observed in drug-induced reactions, parasitic infections, and allergic skin reactions. The increased severity of itch after a bath is typical for eczematous lesions with excessive dryness, for polycythemia vera, or in patients who have been exposed to hydroxyethyl starch. Intensification of itch at night is recorded in almost all itch forms, but it is particularly characteristic of scabies.

After careful anamnesis the patient should undergo a detailed physical examination, with particular attention to the skin in order to look for any signs of skin lesions. Special attention should be paid to distinguish the primary lesion from the changes resulting from scratching. Physical examination should also include palpation of the lymph nodes, thyroid gland, and abdomen. In addition, evaluation of hair and nails can provide additional tips on skin or systemic diseases.

In patients in whom the etiology of itch cannot be identified on the basis of the medical ex-amination, a panel of primary screen laboratory examination may be required (table 1), and if necessary, depending on the basic laboratory results and data from medical history, additional diagnostic tests should be considered [1]. Unfortunately, there are no clear cutoffs for laboratory results that can prove the causative role of an internal disease in chronic itch, so it is frequently hard to say when abnormal levels of creatinine or bile salt acids can be attributed to observed itch.

In some patients, especially with a localized itch, a neurological background might be suspected and they may require some diagnostic imaging. In notalgia paresthetica (localized itch in the periscapular area) often some pathology of the spinal nerves is observed at the level of T2–T6, while in brachioradial itch changes may affect the nervous system at the C5–C8 level. Itch can also be a manifestation of brain tumors, stroke or multiple sclerosis, which can be diagnosed on the basis of imaging of the central nervous system. In some patients, for example those with suspected hematological malignancies, a need to perform a

Table 2. Diagnostic criteria of psychogenic itch (based on Misery et al. [2])

Criteria	Definition
Compulsory criteria (all must be present)	Localized or generalized itch of unknown origin (without primary skin lesion) Chronic itch (>6 weeks) No somatic cause of itch
Optional criteria (3 out of 7 must be present)	A chronological relationship of itch with one or several life events that could have psychological repercussions Variations in itch intensity associated with stress Nocturnal variations of itch Predominance during rest or inaction Associated psychological disorder Itch that could be improved by psychotropic drugs Itch that could be improved by psychotherapies

more detailed diagnosis may occur, far beyond a screening performed routinely.

If the medical examination and the results of additional tests do not allow the determination of the cause of itch, it is worth considering whether this symptom is perhaps a side effect of drugs taken by the patients. The list of drugs that potentially can cause itch is very long; however, epidemiological data on this itch subtype are rather limited. In addition, the pathogenesis of drug-induced itch is largely dependent on the drug that caused this symptom: liver damage extending from cholestasis, excessive dryness of the skin, accumulation of the drug or its metabolites in the skin or nerve tissue, phototoxicity, or neurological abnormalities may be possible causes of drug-induced itch. Thus, at present it is difficult to clearly advise diagnostic procedures which might be helpful in defining this itch subtype. If drug-induced itch is suspected in patients with chronic itch, then the accused drug should be discontinued for at least 4–6 weeks to clearly determine whether the perceived problem is indeed caused by the medicinal preparation.

In patients in whom an organic cause of itching has not been established, the itch is most likely of undetermined origin; however, psychogenic causes should also be suspected and ruled out. If the patient does not present any other symptoms suggestive of mental illness or personality disorders, the diagnosis of psychogenic itch can be quite difficult as the diagnosis of psychogenic itch is almost always a diagnosis of exclusion. The diagnostic criteria for psychogenic itch developed by Misery et al. [2, 3] can be helpful in the diagnosis of psychogenic itch; however, it is still not well established whether these criteria are sufficiently sensitive and specific (table 2). Therefore, it is advisable not to diagnose a solely psychogenic cause of itch without a psychiatric evaluation.

However, it must also be underlined that many patients with chronic itch may demonstrate a multifactorial origin of this symptom and the prevalence of itch of mixed origin increases with age. It is also worth mentioning that in a number of patients the underlying cause of itch cannot be established, resulting in it being classified as itch of undetermined origin, although this also depends on how intense and detailed the diagnostic procedures were. Proposal of tests to be done in particular selected diseases is demonstrated in table 3.

Table 3. Proposal of diagnostic tests to be performed in suspicion of different pruritic conditions [4]

Disease	Basic assessments	Additional tests
Atopic dermatitis	Prick tests and atopy patch tests to detect allergens exacerbating the disease	Total serum IgE level Allergen-specific IgE levels Skin biopsy (to exclude other, clinically similar, dermatologic conditions)
Psoriasis	Diagnosis is made based on clinical examination	Skin biopsy in doubtful cases
Urticaria	Physical tests (exposure to pressure, cold, heat, UV light, physical activity, water): induction of wheals after exposure to causative factor Prick tests with specific allergens (aeroallergens, food allergens, medications)	Exposure to drugs (e.g. acetylsalicylic acid) Stool microscopy for detection of parasite eggs Presence of antinuclear antibodies Skin biopsy to exclude urticarial vasculitis
Scabies	Microscopy of skin scrapings to detect mites or their eggs	
Lichen planus	Skin biopsy of the skin lesion	Serologic test exclude hepatitis B or C viruses
Dermatitis herpetiformis	Detection of antibodies to gliadin, reticulin, endomysium, and tissue transglutaminase	Direct immunofluorescence of skin biopsy showing granular deposits of IgA in the dermal papillae Presence of subepidermal blisters that have papillary microabscesses at their periphery in skin biopsy
Bullous pemphigoid	Direct immunofluorescence of skin biopsy detecting deposits of IgA, IgG and complement at the dermoepidermal junction	Indirect immunofluorescence detecting circulating anti-BP1 and anti-BP2 antibodies Subepidermal blisters with perivascular infiltrates in skin biopsy Blood smear: eosinophilia (>400 eosinophils/µl)
Postherpetic itch	Diagnosis is clinical	
Postburn itch	Diagnosis is clinical	
Cholestatic itch	Total bilirubin	Direct bilirubin Serum bile acid level Serum activity of liver enzymes
Chronic renal failure	Plasma creatinine level	Creatinine clearance Level of urea Serum level of phosphorus Total plasma calcium level
Thyroid dysfunction	TSH level	fT_3, fT_4 levels Sonography of thyroid gland
Diabetes (neuropathy)	Diagnosis is clinical	Nerve conduction tests ENG/EMG
Drug-induced itch	Diagnosis is clinical	
Hodgkin's lymphoma	Biopsy of lymph nodes showing features of Hodgkin's disease	Sonography: hepatomegaly, splenomegaly, enlargement of lymph nodes

Table 3 (continued)

Disease	Basic assessments	Additional tests
Polycythemia vera	Blood smear with high number of erythrocytes, leucocytes or platelets Anisocytosis and poikilocytosis of erythrocytes	Bone marrow assessment Genetic examination – presence of Jak Mutation
HIV infection	Serologic tests to identify anti-HIV antibodies	Virus load Number of CD4+
Brain tumor/stroke	MRI	Computed tomography
Brachioradial itch	X-ray of vertebral column (cervical part)	MRI of vertebral column (cervical part): abnormalities in C5–C8 region Neurological examination
Notalgia paresthetica	X-ray of vertebral column (thoracic part)	MRI of vertebral column (thoracic part): abnormalities in the T2–T6 region
Somatoform itch (psychogenic itch)	Diagnosis is clinical (after exclusion of other causes)	
Persistent delusional disorder	Microscopy of skin scrapings shows absence of mites or their eggs	

In conclusion, it can be stated that itch is a common symptom of many skin diseases, systemic of neurological diseases. Due to the subjective nature of itch, its comprehensive assessment is an important clinical problem. Despite the complex etiology of the disease, an exact cause of itch should be searched for in each patient, as successful therapy is largely dependent on the determination of the cause of the itch.

References

1 Weisshaar E, Szepietowski JC, Darsow U, Misery L, Wallengren J, Mettang T, Gieler U, Lotti T, Lambert J, Maisel P, Streit M, Greaves MW, Carmichael AJ, Tschachler E, Ring J, Ständer S: European guideline on chronic itch. Acta Derm Venereol 2012;92:563–581.

2 Misery L, Alexandre S, Dutray S, Chastaing M, Consoli SG, Audra H, Bauer D, Bertolus S, Callot V, Cardinaud F, Corrin E, Feton-Danou N, Malet R, Touboul S, Consoli SM: Functional itch disorder or psychogenic itch: suggested diagnosis criteria from the French psychodermatology group. Acta Derm Venereol 2007; 87:341–344.

3 Misery L, Wallengren J, Weisshaar E, Zalewska A; French Psychodermatology Group: Validation of diagnosis criteria of functional itch disorder or psychogenic itch. Acta Derm Venereol 2008;88: 503–504.

4 Szepietowski JC, Reich A: Evaluation of itch. Epocrates Online. https://online. epocrates.com/u/2911612/ Evaluation+of+itch.

Prof. Jacek C. Szepietowski, MD, PhD
Department of Dermatology, Venereology and Allergology, Wrocław Medical University
Ul. Chałubińskiego 1
PL–50-368 Wrocław (Poland)
E-Mail jacek.szepietowski@umed.wroc.pl

Szepietowski JC, Weisshaar E (eds): Itch – Management in Clinical Practice.
Curr Probl Dermatol. Basel, Karger, 2016, vol 50, pp 29–34 (DOI: 10.1159/000446014)

Measurement of Itch Intensity

Adam Reich · Jacek C. Szepietowski

Department of Dermatology, Venereology and Allergology, Wrocław Medical University, Wrocław, Poland

Abstract

Measurement of itch intensity is essential to properly evaluate pruritic disease severity, to understand the patients' needs and burden, and especially to assess treatment efficacy, particularly in clinical trials. However, measurement of itch remains a challenge, as, per definition, it is a subjective sensation and assessment of this symptom represents significant difficulty. Intensity of itch must be considered in relation to its duration, localization, course of symptoms, presence and type of scratch lesions, response to antipruritic treatment, and quality of life impairment. Importantly, perception of itch may also be confounded by different cofactors including but not limited to patient general condition and other coexisting ailments. In the current chapter we characterize the major methods of itch assessments that are used in daily clinical life and as research tools. Different methods of itch assessment have been developed; however, so far none is without limitations and any data on itch intensity should always be interpreted with caution. Despite these limitations, it is strongly recommended to implement itch measurement tools in routine daily practice, as it would help in proper assessment of patient clinical status. In order to improve evaluation of itch in research studies, it is recommended to use at least two independent methods, as such an approach should increase the validity of achieved results.

Measurement of itch remains a challenge. By definition, itch is a subjective sensation and assessment of this symptom represents significant difficulty. It can only be measured subjectively; however, we can try to objectively measure the reactions to itch, like scratching. Itch may also be perceived by patients in different ways, as many additional descriptive terms like prickling, stinging, tickling, tingling, etc., are used in relation to itch, suggesting that 'one person's itch' may not be the same sensation as 'another person's itch'. Importantly, itch may be an isolated medical problem, but in many patients it is a symptom of other conditions. Therefore, perception of itch may also be confounded by the general condition of the patient and concomitant ailments related to the underlying disease which causes itch. Intensity of itch must also be considered in relation to its duration, localization (localized versus generalized), course of symptoms, presence and type of scratch lesions, response to antipruritic treatment, and quality of life impairment [1, 2].

Despite all these difficulties, a valid measurement of itch is of crucial importance for several reasons. It is necessary to properly assess disease severity, especially for such entities like urticaria, (the questionnaire has to be useful as an outcome measure and should be able to detect changes in itch severity over time) [16]. It has been proposed that such a questionnaire should contain questions about localization, duration, frequency and intensity of itch, sensory qualities, scratch response, data about itch origin and aggravating and relieving factors of itch, affective problems, disability, itch cognition, coping and quality of life impairment in patients with itch, and data about response to current and previous antipruritic treatment modalities.

Questionnaires may also be used to assess patient-relevant benefits achieved during the treatment. This novel concept is based on the idea that various patients may have different expectations regarding the treatment and that they should personally indicate the most relevant treatment goals before the treatment is initiated. Some years ago, researchers from the CVderm – German Center for Health Services Research in Dermatology (Institute for Health Services Research in Dermatology, Hamburg, Germany) developed the Patient Benefit Index – Itch (PBI-P) [17]. PBI-P is an instrument consisting of two parts – the Patient Needs Questionnaire and the Patient Benefit Questionnaire. With the Patient Needs Questionnaire, patients have to assess how important different predefined treatment aims are to them, while with the Patient Benefit Questionnaire, which is applied after treatment completion, they have to articulate how the antipruritic therapy helped them to achieve these treatment goals using a 5-point Likert scale with the answers ranging from 'not at all' (0 points) to 'very' (4 points). Based on the achieved results, the PBI is calculated providing the final result ranging from 0 (i.e. no benefit was achieved) to 4 (maximum benefit was achieved). The weighted algorithm used to calculate PBI places more emphasis on the objectives which were indicated by the patients as being more important, so that these objectives have greater impact on the final PBI values [17].

Measurement of Sensory Threshold

It has been suggested that some patients may suffer from chronic itch because of increased nerve density in the skin and subsequent lowering of the threshold for itchy stimuli. Furthermore, it seems that at least some patients with chronic itch may demonstrate a small nerve fiber dysfunction and measurement of the electric sensory threshold might be a valuable and promising adjunct diagnostic method for assessment of such patients. If this hypothesis is true, measurement of the threshold for different sensations might be of help in assessment of patients with chronic itch, as having a lower sensory threshold should be linked with greater itch.

One of the methods to measure the sensory threshold is to expose tested patients to different current types of different frequencies depending on the nerves which need to be stimulated and to instruct them to indicate the moment of the first current perception. According to our recent data, it could be suggested that indeed measurement of sensory threshold may be of some value in the assessment of itchy patients; however, further studies are needed to better establish their real usefulness. While studying patients with atopic dermatitis and psoriasis, we observed significant correlations between sensory threshold for 5-Hz alternate current and itch intensity [18]. It is believed that the alternate current of 5 Hz mostly stimulates sensory C-fibers, which are thought to be the most important nerves for conduction of itch stimuli [19]. Thus, it could be that with a 5-Hz current we should be able to test the excitation threshold of cutaneous C-fibers. However, it should be underlined that a great variability of the sensory threshold between patients may hinder the proper interpretation of such measurements and limit their clinical application. Therefore, any reference ranges for sensory thresholds must be established with great caution.

Measurement of Scratching Activity

As itch is defined as an unpleasant sensation which provokes a desire to scratch, measurement of scratching should provide further data on itch intensity as logically patients with more severe itch should scratch more intensively compared to those subjects with less severe itch. However, again, significant interindividual differences have been observed regarding the scratch response to itch stimuli. Furthermore, in some types of severe itch (e.g. itch after hydroxyethyl starch infusion) patients even try to avoid scratching as such behavior may aggravate itch. Importantly, scratching may also be influenced by several external factors, which further impedes the proper interpretation of scratching assessment in relation to itch severity. Despite all of these limitations, a lot of efforts have been made to adequately measure scratching behavior in animals and human beings [20, 21]. The following methods have been used so far:

- Observations or counting of excoriations/lichenification areas
- Measurement of hand and feet motions (measurement of muscle potentials from forearms, monitoring of wrist activity, use of pressure sensors or electromagnetic movement detector)
- Infrared video recording of scratch episodes
- Acoustic evaluation of scratching
- Use of a fingernail vibration transducer or pruritometer

One of the most frequently used methods to assess scratching activity is probably wrist movement counting using different devices called accelerometers. They may measure movements of extremities during sleeping. Although this seems to be promising, several factors limit its application. To date, there are very few studies validating this type of assessment in itch studies [20, 22–25]. Murray and Rees [22] observed 117 patients with atopic dermatitis, psoriasis, cholestasis, and idiopathic itch, and found no correlation between VAS scoring and actigraphy measurements. Also, Bringhurst et al. [20] did not find any relationships between VAS and actigraphy results. Similarly, in our recent study we observed only a very weak correlation between wrist movement activity and itch intensity assessed with the VAS and Itch Questionnaire [24]. Even more importantly, change in wrist movement activity correlated much less with the improvement of the patient's quality of life compared to other methods of itch evaluation. In another study with 336 children with eczema (aged 6 months to 16 years) conducted by Wootton et al. [25], actigraphy did not correlate well with disease severity or quality of life when used as an objective outcome measure, and was not responsive to change over time. These authors noticed significant difficulties in distinguishing between eczema-related and eczema-nonrelated movements (so-called 'restless movements') which could be related to other factors like nightmares, anxiety, concomitant diseases, or temperature in the room at night. Therefore, further studies are needed to validate accelerometers in itch studies and to improve data analysis achieved during patient monitoring.

In conclusion, proper assessment of itch still remains a challenge. Different methods have been developed; however, none is without limitations and any data on itch intensity should always be interpreted with some caution. Despite these limitations, it is strongly recommended to implement itch measurement tools in routine daily practice, as it is still of value and would help in proper assessment of the patient's clinical status. We suggest using at least the NRS or VAS in daily practice as they are rapid and reliable methods of itch intensity measurement. However, in order to improve evaluation of itch in research studies, it is recommended to use at least two independent methods, as such an approach should increase the validity of achieved results.

References

1 Ständer S, Augustin M, Reich A, Blome C, Ebata T, Phan NQ, Szepietowski JC; International Forum for the Study of Itch Special Interest Group Scoring Itch in Clinical Trials: Itch assessment in clinical trials: consensus recommendations from the International Forum for the Study of Itch (IFSI) Special Interest Group Scoring Itch in Clinical Trials. Acta Derm Venereol 2013;93:509–514.

2 Ständer S, Blome C, Breil B, Bruland P, Darsow U, Dugas M, Evers A, Fritz F, Metz M, Phan NQ, Raap U, Reich A, Schneider G, Stench S, Szepietowski J, Weisshaar E, Augustin M: Assessment of itch – current standards and implications for clinical practice: consensus paper of the Action Group Itch Parameter of the International Working Group on Itch Research (AGP) (in German). Hautarzt 2012;63:521–522, 524–531.

3 Reich A, Hrehorów E, Szepietowski JC: Itch is an important factor negatively influencing the well-being of psoriatic patients. Acta Derm Venereol 2010;90: 257–263.

4 Phan NQ, Blome C, Fritz F, Gerss J, Reich A, Ebata T, Augustin M, Szepietowski JC, Ständer S: Assessment of itch intensity: prospective study on validity and reliability of the visual analogue scale, numerical rating scale and verbal rating scale in 471 patients with chronic itch. Acta Derm Venereol 2012; 92:502–507.

5 Reich A, Heisig M, Phan NQ, Taneda K, Takamori K, Takeuchi S, Furue M, Blome C, Augustin M, Ständer S, Szepietowski JC: Visual analogue scale: evaluation of the instrument for the assessment of itch. Acta Derm Venereol 2012; 92.497–501.

6 Furue M, Ebata T, Ikoma A, Takeuchi S, Kataoka Y, Takamori K, Satoh T, Saeki H, Augustin M, Reich A, Szepietowski J, Fleischer A, Blome C, Phan NQ, Weisshaar E, Yosipovitch G, Ständer S: Verbalizing extremes of the visual analogue scale for itch: a consensus statement. Acta Derm Venereol 2013;93:214–215.

7 Kido-Nakahara M, Katoh N, Saeki H, Mizutani H, Hagihara A, Takeuchi S, Nakahara T, Masuda K, Tamagawa-Mineoka R, Nakagawa H, Omoto Y, Matsubara K, Furue M: Comparative cut-off value setting of itch intensity in visual analogue scale and verbal rating scale. Acta Derm Venereol 2015;95:345–346.

8 Reich A, Chatzigeorkidis E, Zeidler C, Osada N, Mędrek K, Szepietowski JC, Ständer S: Cut-off values of the visual analogue scale (VAS) and numeric rating scale (NRS) in itch assessment. Acta Derm Venereol 2015;95:889.

9 Reich A, Riepe C, Anastasiadou Z, Mędrek K, Augustin M, Szepietowski J, Ständer S: Itch assessment with visual analogue scale (VAS) and numeric rating scale (NRS): determination of minimal clinically important difference (MCID) in chronic itch. Acta Derm Venereol 2016, Epub ahead of print.

10 van Laarhoven AI, van der Sman-Mauriks IM, Donders AR, Pronk MC, van de Kerkhof PC, Evers AW: Placebo effects on itch: a meta-analysis of clinical trials of patients with dermatological conditions. J Invest Dermatol 2015;135:1234–1243.

11 Majeski CJ, Johnson JA, Davison SN, Lauzon CJ: Itch Severity Scale: a self-report instrument for the measurement of itch severity. Br J Dermatol 2007;156: 667–673.

12 Elman S, Hynan LS, Gabriel V, Mayo MJ: The 5-D Itch Scale: a new measure of itch. Br J Dermatol 2010;162:587–593.

13 Reich A, Mędrek K, Szepietowski JC: Four-item itch questionnaire – validation of questionnaire. Przegl Dermatol 2012;99:600–604.

14 Darsow U, Mautner VF, Bromm B, Scharein E, Ring J: The Eppendorf Pruritus Questionnaire (in German). Hautarzt 1997;48:730–733.

15 Darsow U, Scharein E, Simon D, Walter G, Bromm B, Ring J: New aspects of itch pathophysiology: component analysis of atopic itch using the 'Eppendorf Itch Questionnaire'. Int Arch Allergy Immunol 2001;124:326–331.

16 Weisshaar E, Gieler U, Kupfer J, Furue M, Saeki H, Yosipovitch G; International Forum on the Study of Itch: Questionnaires to assess chronic itch: a consensus paper of the special interest group of the International Forum on the Study of Itch. Acta Derm Venereol 2012;92:493–496.

17 Blome C, Augustin M, Siepmann D, Phan NQ, Rustenbach SJ, Ständer S: Measuring patient-relevant benefits in itch treatment: development and validation of a specific outcomes tool. Br J Dermatol 2009;161:1143–1148.

18 Krzyżanowska M, Muszer K, Chabowski K, Reich A: Assessment of the sensory threshold in patients with atopic dermatitis and psoriasis. Postepy Dermatol Alergol 2015;32:94–100.

19 Koga K, Furue H, Rashid MH, Takaki A, Katafuchi T, Yoshimura M: Selective activation of primary afferent fibers evaluated by sine-wave electrical stimulation. Mol Pain 2005;1:13.

20 Bringhurst C, Waterston K, Schofield O, et al: Measurement of itch using actigraphy in pediatric and adult populations. J Am Acad Dermatol 2004;51:893–898.

21 Yngman-Uhlin P, Johansson A, Fernström A, et al: Fragmented sleep: an unrevealed problem in peritoneal dialysis patients. Scand J Urol Nephrol 2011; 45:206–215.

22 Murray CS, Rees JL: Are subjective accounts of itch to be relied on? The lack of relation between visual analogue itch scores and actigraphic measures of scratch. Acta Derm Venereol 2011;91: 18–23.

23 Bender BG, Ballard R, Canono B, et al: Disease severity, scratching, and sleep quality in patients with atopic dermatitis. J Am Acad Dermatol 2008;58:415–420.

24 Domagała A, Reich A: Antihistamines in the treatment of psoriatic itch: a double-blind placebo-controlled pilot study. Acta Derm Venereol 2015;95:885.

25 Wootton CI, Koller K, Lawton S, et al: Are accelerometers a useful tool for measuring disease activity in children with eczema? Validity, responsiveness to change, and acceptability of use in a clinical trial setting. Br J Dermatol 2012; 167:1131–1137.

Prof. Jacek C. Szepietowski, MD, PhD
Department of Dermatology, Venereology and Allergology, Wrocław Medical University
Ul. Chałubińskiego 1
PL–50-368 Wrocław (Poland)
E-Mail jacek.szepietowski@umed.wroc.pl

Szepietowski JC, Weisshaar E (eds): Itch – Management in Clinical Practice.
Curr Probl Dermatol. Basel, Karger, 2016, vol 50, pp 35–39 (DOI: 10.1159/000446039)

Itch Management: General Principles

Laurent Misery

Department of Dermatology, University Hospital of Brest, and Laboratory of Neurosciences of Brest, University of
Western Brittany, Brest, France

Abstract

Like pain, itch is a challenging condition that needs to be
managed. Within this setting, the first principle of itch
management is to get an appropriate diagnosis to perform an etiology-oriented therapy. In several cases it is
not possible to treat the cause, the etiology is undetermined, there are several causes, or the etiological treatment is not effective enough to alleviate itch completely.
This is also why there is need for symptomatic treatment.
In all patients, psychological support and associated
pragmatic measures might be helpful. General principles
and guidelines are required, yet patient-centered individual care remains fundamental.

© 2016 S. Karger AG, Basel

Suffering from a chronic or acute itch can largely
modify the life of patients with important effects
on sleep as well as social, sexual, and mental life,
and has an impact on each moment of the day [1].
The Global Burden of Diseases Study showed that
skin conditions were the fourth leading cause of
nonfatal disease burden and that the symptom
'itch' played a major part [2]. More recently, a
large epidemiological study on the burden of
common skin conditions in dermatological patients across Europe was performed with 4,995
participants [3]. It showed that patients reporting
itch compared to those not reporting it constitut-
ed a larger proportion when assessed by the Dermatology Life Quality Index: 60 versus 25%. Doc-
tors sometimes believe that itch is not so important for patients suffering from diseases like
psoriasis; however, it has recently been demonstrated that itch is the most bothersome symptom
for these patients [4].

Like pain, itch is a challenging condition that
needs to be managed. Within this setting, the first
principle of itch management is to get an appropriate diagnosis to suggest a therapeutic alternative according to the cause of the pruritus. In
several cases, it is not possible to treat the cause,
the cause is undetermined, there are several causes, or the etiological treatment is not effective
enough to alleviate itch completely. There is always a need for symptomatic treatment in any
stage of itch. In all patients, psychological support might be helpful. General recommendations
for subjects suffering from chronic itch are given
in table 1.

Table 1. General recommendations for itch management

Keep the body cool
Maintain a cool ambient environment that is not too dry
Take tepid showers and baths
Avoid alcohol and hot and/or spicy food and drinks
Wear light cool clothes with natural materials
Keep nails short
Use dermocosmetics with a pH of 5.5

Etiological Treatment

The diagnostic procedures and specific managements are detailed in other chapters of this book, but it is important to underline that etiological treatment is the first therapeutic option. The European guidelines [5] have inventoried specific treatments according to the bibliographical data and some consensus experts. As a consequence of the diversity of possible underlying diseases, no single therapy concept can be recommended, and each form of pruritus has to be considered individually [5]. In particular, some adaptations are necessary in specific populations like the elderly, pregnant women, children, or people with kidney or liver insufficiency.

Symptomatic Treatment

There is a significant lack of randomized controlled trials, which can be explained by the diversity and complexity of this symptom, the multifactorial etiologies of pruritus, and the lack of well-defined outcome measures [5], and results are sometimes conflicting.

To complicate matters, the placebo (and nocebo) effect can be huge in studies of itch treatments. Hence, a meta-analysis demonstrated that placebo treatment significantly decreased itch (1.3 out of 10, 95% CI: 1.02–1.61) compared with baseline itch (effect size 0.55), indicating that placebo effects play a considerable role in these patients' treatment [6]. As with pain treatments [7], it is probable that there will be increasing placebo (and nocebo) responses over time, and it is necessary to better understand these facts. A role for individual psychological characteristics and personality traits regarding negative outcome expectancies has been evidenced [8], but there are probably numerous other predictive factors.

Topical Therapy
Local anesthetics, like benzocaine, lidocaine, and pramoxine, as well as a mixture of prilocaine and lidocaine, can be used but have only a short-term effect. Polidocanol, menthol, and their derivatives may have more prolonged effects.

Glucocorticosteroids should not be used as long-term treatment or in the absence of a primary rash. They are not a symptomatic treatment of pruritus. Moreover, the repeated application of glucocorticosteroids exacerbates pruritus [9].

In contrast, topical calcineurin inhibitors, like tacrolimus and pimecrolimus, might be used as symptomatic treatments. Indeed, their effects are not restricted to specific immunological effects, but are also mediated through their neuronal properties [10]. Tacrolimus and pimecrolimus are effective in localized forms of pruritus in immunological diseases like atopic dermatitis and in other conditions like uremic pruritus [5], but they have to be used with caution due to their putative side effects.

Topical application of capsaicin, a transient receptor potential cation channel V1 antagonist, activates sensory C fibers to release neurotransmitters inducing dose-dependent erythema and burning. After repeated applications of capsaicin, the burning fades due to tachyphylaxis and retraction of epidermal nerve fibers [11]. Capsaicin can be effective in localized forms of chronic pruritus, but patient compliance due to side effects can restrict usage [5]. The use of capsaicin is especially interesting for neuropathic pruritus [12].

The tricyclic antidepressant doxepin showed antipruritic effects when applied as a 5% cream in double-blind studies, but the increased risk of contact allergy restricted its use [5]. Menthol and camphor have also been shown to have interesting effects on pruritus, but have putative allergic effects. Topical cannabinoid receptor agonists could also be used in the symptomatic treatment of pruritus, but there are few convincing clinical trials at the moment. Due to the lack of studies, topical acetylsalicylic acid can currently not be recommended.

Other topicals may be effective in itch patients, but clinical trials are frequently poorly documented, and it is difficult to separate their effects from placebo effects. Nevertheless, they may not be ineffective and can be very helpful in some patients (see chapter by Metz and Staubach [this vol., pp. 40–45]).

Systemic Therapy
This important part of the treatment is detailed in the chapter by Pongcharoen and Fleischer [this vol., pp. 46–53]. Antihistamines are the most widely used systemic antipruritic drugs in dermatology. Nonetheless, they cannot be considered as a symptomatic treatment of itch in conditions where itch is not histamine dependent. Itch is not related to histamine in the majority of itchy conditions, and this is why antihistamines are only indicated in treating itch in urticaria [5]. Sedating antihistamines might be recommended to be applied during the nighttime to improve sleep [5], and the associated anticholinergic effect might be interesting in a few conditions. Glucocorticosteroids are not a symptomatic treatment of itch either. There are no studies investigating the efficacy of the exclusive use of systemic glucocorticosteroids in pruritus [5]. Systemic corticosteroids can be used as short-term treatment in severe cases but should not be used for more than 2 weeks

[5] because they induce side effects in almost all patients.

Opioid μ-receptor antagonists or κ-receptor agonists may be effective, especially in uremic pruritus [13]. Gabapentin and pregabalin can be recommended in the treatment of uremic pruritus and neuropathic pruritus [5]. Antidepressants might be used due to their psychotropic effects but also putative pharmacological effects on pruritus through the serotonin and acetylcholine pathways. They can be recommended for the treatment of somatoform, paraneoplastic, or cholestatic pruritus [5]. Other drugs, like serotonin receptor antagonists, thalidomide, leukotriene receptor antagonists, aprepitant, or cyclosporine, are sometimes used.

Physical Approach
UV therapy [5] can be considered as an etiological but also as a symptomatic treatment because of the deleterious effects of UV light on nerve endings. A meta-analysis showed that acupuncture therapy was effective to alleviate itch compared with placebo acupuncture and a no-treatment group [14]. The effects of spa treatments are not proven, but some patients have reported dramatic improvements. More details are given in the chapter by Chan and Murrell [this vol., pp. 54–63].

Associated Measures

The patient should be informed about general pruritus-relieving measures [5]. These are helpful to improve itch and to prevent its exacerbation.

Exposure to heat is known to enhance itch whereas cold or luke-warm temperatures are soothing. It is better to take showers than baths, to avoid detergents and all irritant substances or even soaps, and to choose syndets. Emollients are appreciated by patients: they repair the skin barrier, ameliorate skin perceptions, and their use may cut the vicious cycle of itch and scratching.

Concerning clothes, cotton is better than wool, and loose clothes are better than tight clothing. Stimulants such as alcohol, coffee, tea, and spices should be avoided. To prevent scratch marks, the nails should be cut short.

Psychological Support

Psychogenic itch is a rare condition, but a psychological component of itch is almost a compulsory criterion [15], and psychological consequences of itch are frequently severe (see chapters by Evers et al. [this vol., 64–70] and Szepietowski and Reich [this vol., pp. 102–110]). Psychological support has to be considered as an important part of the management of itch.

The vicious itch-scratch cycle has to be taken into account when a patient is treated for pruritus. In addition to causal and symptomatic therapy, behavioral therapy to avoid scratching should be considered, such as conscious suppression of the reflex by intense concentration, distraction, or alternative techniques against scratching like habit reversal [5].

Relaxation techniques and education programs are useful as a complementary treatment for managing chronic pruritus, especially in atopic dermatitis [5].

In patients with coexisting depression, psychotherapy in combination with psychotropic medication can be helpful even to treat pruritus of a different etiology [5, 16]. This should be done interdisciplinarily with a psychiatrist/psychosomatic physician. The psychiatric consequences of itch have to be managed, too. There is a need to treat depression, anxiety, sleep disorders, and sexual disorders by psychotherapeutic and/or pharmacological interventions.

Conclusion

The management of itch is frequently difficult. As a consequence of the multifactorial origin of chronic pruritus, its management implies all medical disciplines that work with patients suffering from chronic itch. Due to the many different conditions evoking pruritus and the diversity of the patients, there is a need for general principles and guidelines; however, patient-centered care remains fundamental.

References

1 Misery L, Ständer S: Pruritus. London, Springer, 2010.
2 Hay RJ, Johns NE, Williams HC, Bolliger IW, Dellavalle RP, Margolis DJ, Marks R, Naldi L, Weinstock MA, Wulf SK, Michaud C, Murray C, Naghavi M: The global burden of skin disease in 2010: an analysis of the prevalence and impact of skin conditions. J Invest Dermatol 2014; 134:1527–1534.
3 Dalgard FJ, Gieler U, Tomas-Aragones L, Lien L, Poot F, Jemec GB, Misery L, Szabo C, Linder D, Sampogna F, Evers AW, Halvorsen JA, Balieva F, Szepietowski J, Romanov D, Marron SE, Altunay IK, Finlay AY, Salek SS, Kupfer J: The psychological burden of skin diseases: a cross-sectional multicenter study among dermatological out-patients in 13 European countries. J Invest Dermatol 2015;135:984–991.
4 Lebwohl MG, Bachelez H, Barker J, Girolomoni G, Kavanaugh A, Langley RG, Paul CF, Puig L, Reich K, van de Kerkhof PC: Patient perspectives in the management of psoriasis: results from the population-based Multinational Assessment of Psoriasis and Psoriatic Arthritis Survey. J Am Acad Dermatol 2014;70: 871–881.
5 Weisshaar E, Szepietowski JC, Darsow U, Misery L, Wallengren J, Mettang T, Gieler U, Lotti T, Lambert J, Maisel P, Streit M, Greaves MW, Carmichael AJ, Tschachler E, Ring J, Ständer S: European guideline on chronic pruritus. Acta Derm Venereol 2012;92:563–581.
6 Van Laarhoven AI, van der Sman-Mauriks IM, Donders AR, Pronk MC, van de Kerkhof PC, Evers AW: Placebo effects on itch: a meta-analysis of clinical trials of patients with dermatological conditions. J Invest Dermatol 2015;135:1234–1243.
7 Tuttle AH, Tohyama S, Ramsay T, Kimmelman J, Schweinhardt P, Bennett GJ, Mogil JS: Increasing placebo responses over time in US clinical trials of neuropathic pain. Pain 2015;156: 2616–2626.

8   Bartels DJ, van Laarhoven AI, van de Kerkhof PC, Evers AW: Placebo and nocebo effects on itch: effects, mechanisms and predictors. Eur J Pain 2016; 20:8–13.

9   Yamaura K, Doi R, Suwa E, Ueno K: Repeated application of glucosteroids exacerbates pruritus via inhibition of prostaglandin D_2 production of mast cells in a murine model of allergic contact dermatitis. J Toxicol Sci 2012;37: 1127–1134.

10 Pereira U, Boulais N, Lebonvallet N, Pennec JP, Dorange G, Misery L: Mechanisms of the sensory effects of tacrolimus on the skin. Br J Dermatol 2010; 163:70–77.

11 Szolcsanyi J: Forty years in capsaicin research for sensory pharmacology and physiology. Neuropeptides 2004;38: 377–384.

12 Misery L, Brenaut E, Le Garrec R, Abasq C, Genestet S, Marcorelles P, Zagnoli F: Neuropathic pruritus. Nat Rev Neurol 2014;10:408–416.

13 Kumagai H, Ebata T, Takamori K, Muramatsu T, Nakamoto H, Suzuki H: Effect of a novel kappa-receptor agonist, nalfurafine hydrochloride, on severe itch in 337 haemodialysis patients: a phase III, randomized, double-blind, placebo-controlled study. Nephrol Dial Transplant 2010; 25:1251–1257.

14 Yu C, Zhang P, Lv ZT, Li JJ, Li HP, Wu CH, Gao F, Yuan XC, Zhang J, He W, Jing XH, Li M: Efficacy of acupuncture in itch: a systematic review and meta-analysis of clinical randomized controlled trials. Evid Based Complement Alternat Med 2015;2015:208690.

15 Misery L, Alexandre S, Dutray S, Chastaing M, Consoli SG, Audra H, Bauer D, Bertolus S, Callot V, Cardinaud F, Corrin E, Feton-Danou N, Malet R, Touboul S, Consoli SM: Functional itch disorder or psychogenic pruritus: suggested diagnosis criteria from the French Psychodermatology Group. Acta Derm Venereol 2007;87:341–344.

16 Schut C, Mollanazar NK, Kupfer J, Gieler U, Yosipovitch G: Psychological interventions in the treatment of chronic itch. Acta Derm Venereol 2016;96:157–161.

Prof. Laurent Misery
Service de dermatologie et de vénéréologie, CHU Brest
2, avenue Foch
FR–29200 Brest (France)
E-Mail laurent.misery@chu-brest.fr

Szepietowski JC, Weisshaar E (eds): Itch – Management in Clinical Practice.
Curr Probl Dermatol. Basel, Karger, 2016, vol 50, pp 40–45 (DOI: 10.1159/000446040)

Itch Management: Topical Agents

Martin Metz[a] · Petra Staubach[b]

[a]Department of Dermatology, Venerology and Allergology, Charité – Universitätsmedizin Berlin, Berlin, and
[b]Department of Dermatology, University Medical Center Mainz, Mainz, Germany

Abstract

Chronic pruritus is a common problem in patients with inflammatory skin diseases as well as in subjects with dry or sensitive skin. Regardless of the underlying cause of the pruritus, a topical therapy is not only useful but most often necessary to achieve symptom control. A good topical therapy should fulfill different functions. An optimal basic therapy based on the condition of the skin is important to repair epithelial barrier defects and to rehydrate the skin. An adequate disease-specific topical therapy is crucial for inflamed skin, e.g. anti-inflammatory topical therapy is an important part in the treatment of atopic dermatitis. Finally, the use of specific antipruritic substances can help to improve pruritus in patients irrespective of the underlying disease. Here, we summarize topical agents used in the treatment of chronic pruritus.

© 2016 S. Karger AG, Basel

Topical therapy is an important part in the treatment of chronic pruritus for a variety of reasons: (1) patients with chronic pruritus often suffer from dry or very dry skin and/or disruption of the epithelial barrier, (2) except for some antihistamines that are licensed for the treatment of pruritus in urticaria, no systemic treatment is licensed for itch, and (3) systemic drugs can induce considerable side effects that are avoided if these substances are directly applied to the relevant organ, i.e. the skin. Topical therapy in chronic pruritus can therefore fulfill different functions. As the mandatory basic therapy in patients with dry skin and/or epithelial barrier defects, it can help break the itch-scratch cycle and help reduce topical steroid use or systemic treatment. Topical agents can also be employed for specific therapy of skin diseases which can ultimately result in the improvement of chronic pruritus. Finally, antipruritic substances can be used in topical treatment to directly improve pruritus in patients. Here, we discuss commonly used topical agents in chronic pruritus.

Basic Therapy

An effective and continuous basic therapy is crucial for patients with chronic pruritus. Even if the skin is not considered to be the main cause of the chronic pruritus, basic therapy can help maintain or restore barrier function and prevent additional itch induction due to dry skin. Patients already presenting with dry skin or with defects in the epithelial barrier require basic therapy as a very important part of their treatment, even in symptom-free intervals, in order to interrupt the itch-scratch cycle [1].

An effective basic therapy can lead to the improvement of quality of life in patients and indirectly to the reduction of the socioeconomic costs. Furthermore, it can result in the reduction of the use of topical steroids and thus to a reduction of potential side effects. Unfortunately, an effective basic therapy is often a substantial financial burden for the patient, as patients with chronic pruritus, regardless of the potential underlying disease, usually have to pay for the topical therapy themselves. A topical treatment in adults requires up to 60 g for the whole body, which adds up to more than 3 kg per month if used twice daily. Because of this high financial burden for the patient, there is a high risk of not using the therapy enough and for not using it as often as needed, resulting in flare-ups or worsening of the symptoms [1].

What Is the Best Basic Therapy?
The type of basic therapy should be chosen based on the condition of the skin and the potential underlying skin disease. In general, the drier the skin is, the higher the lipid content should be in any basic therapy. Nonetheless, a well-balanced combination of lipids, water, and humectants is important for an optimal treatment [2]. For example, complete or almost complete water-free systems, despite having a high lipid content, can result in worsening of pruritus also in patients with very dry skin because of the occlusive effect. In most patients with chronic pruritus, lipophilic bases such as hydrophobic basic cream containing high amounts of water and glycerin are recommended. However, the optimal basic therapy should be identified individually in every patient depending on the body region affected, the condition of the skin, the use of active ingredients, the presence of an underlying disease, and the individual preferences of the patient [2]. To be comfortable with the basic therapy is a very important aspect, especially in patients with pruritus and very dry skin, as it is mandatory for the patient to use the therapy on a regular basis.

Common Active Ingredients in Basic Therapy
In chronic pruritus, it is recommended to use topical agents that contain urea, glycerin, or sodium chloride to enhance the beneficial effects of the basic therapy.

Urea is a substance that has been used in dermatology for many decades. Endogenous urea is part of the natural moisturizing factor [3] and is of importance for the hydrating effect in the skin. As the production of the natural moisturizing factor is reduced in many skin conditions, especially in dry skin [4], the addition of exogenous urea can help to increase skin hydration. Urea is generally recommended to be used in concentrations of 5–10%; in patients with inflamed skin, lower concentrations may be necessary as the urea can lead to irritation and a burning sensation; in particular, children with atopic dermatitis often describe a stinging effect of urea.

Sodium chloride is also able to increase the hydration of the skin. Especially to avoid irritations due to high urea concentrations, urea and sodium chloride can be combined in basic therapy.

Glycerin can be used in concentrations of 5–10%, especially in oil-in-water creams. Glycerin can increase the degradation of desmosomes by reducing desmoglein-1 and is especially helpful in patients with ichthyosis [5, 6]. Overall, the hydrating effect is not as potent as similar concentrations of urea [1].

While all of these agents do not directly reduce or suppress pruritus, they can be important in maintaining or restoring the epithelial barrier and can help to break the itch-scratch cycle.

Disease-Specific Topical Therapy

Skin diseases are often associated with chronic pruritus: 40–50% of patients presenting with skin disorders report chronic pruritus [7, 8], and this is considered to be a severe itch in roughly every fourth patient [7]. In chronic inflammatory skin diseases such as atopic dermatitis, psoriasis, lichen planus, and many others, the majority of patients suffer severely from chronic pruritus, often making this symptom the most important factor affecting the quality of life in these patients [9–11]. Thus, effective topical therapy of any known underlying dermatological disease is absolutely necessary and can be the most effective treatment for chronic pruritus in these patients. The topical agents used for the treatment of pruritus in specific underlying dermatoses vary depending on the disease and range from anti-inflammatory therapy or vitamin A or D analogs to antiseptic or antifungal agents. In some patients the treatment of the skin disease will lead to improvement of the visible skin lesions but fail in relieving the pruritus, requiring a specific topical or systemic antipruritic treatment.

As inflamed skin is often associated with chronic pruritus, anti-inflammatory therapy with topical corticosteroids (TCS) or calcineurin inhibitors (TCI) is commonly used in these patients as antipruritic therapy. While the direct antipruritic effect of TCS and TCI in chronic pruritus is negligible, the efficacy of these substances in reducing itch in inflamed skin conditions is well documented. In many clinical trials and larger case series the effects of TCS or TCI on itch in inflamed skin have been investigated. It has been shown for example that methylprednisolone aceponate can reduce itch in patients with atopic eczema [12, 13] and in allergic contact dermatitis [14]. It has also been demonstrated that the TCI pimecrolimus and tacrolimus relieve pruritus in atopic eczema patients [15, 16].

As chronic inflammatory skin conditions usually require a prolonged or repeated steroid treatment, it is recommended to use TCS with a favorable therapeutic index such as fluticasone propionate, methylprednisolone aceponate, or mometasone furoate [17]. It is important to note, however, that TCS and TCI are able to help improve pruritus in inflamed skin, but they might not be sufficient to completely inhibit the itch [18]. In general, TCS or TCI should only be used for the treatment of chronic pruritus associated with inflamed skin and should not be used as an antipruritic therapy in noninflamed skin.

Pruritus-Specific Topical Therapy

Currently, there is no topical therapy licensed for the treatment of pruritus. Nevertheless, there is some evidence for a direct antipruritic effect of certain active ingredients in the topical therapy of patients with chronic pruritus. Randomized controlled trials on the efficacy of these antipruritic active ingredients are still missing and the efficacy of these topical agents can therefore not be appreciated in full.

Capsaicin
Capsaicin is a substance derived from hot pepper and induces initially a burning and warming sensation if topically applied. Capsaicin activates the vanilloid receptor transient receptor potential cation channel V1 (TRPV1) which is expressed on keratinocytes and sensory nerve fibers in the skin and leads to the release of neuropeptides such as substance P from sensory nerves [19, 20]. Capsaicin is usually used in a concentration of 0.025–0.1%, and, if used continuously, the burning sensation as well as pain and itch are reduced after several days. Controlled trials have shown the efficacy of this treatment in chronic pruritus, especially in localized forms of itch [21]. The major disadvantage of this treatment option is the poor compliance of patients because of the initial and sometimes intense burning sensation and the necessity of an application of up to 5–6 times per

day. A different approach is the use of an 8% capsaicin patch in localized neuropathic pruritus. Recently, various case reports and case series have reported a very effective treatment of neuropathic pruritus with a single application of a high-dose capsaicin patch [22–24].

Topical Anesthetics
Local anesthetics can act through various types of receptors in the skin and can have different properties with respect to effects on pain or pruritus. Various agents such as pramoxine or lidocaine or benzocaine have been shown to be effective in the treatment of chronic pruritus [25–27]. The effect of these substances is often only short lasting, can be associated with a numb feeling of the skin, and it is not possible to use them on larger skin areas.

Polidocanol (laureth-9) is commonly used as an antipruritic agent in basic therapy and was originally described as a local anesthetic, but this was not confirmed in later studies [28]. In experimentally induced histamine-independent and PAR-2-dependent pruritus, polidocanol, but not placebo, was able to effectively reduce itch responses in the individuals tested [28].

Menthol, Camphor
Menthol and camphor are naturally occurring substances of plant origin, which are often used as antipruritic substances and are mentioned in guidelines for the management of chronic pruritus [29, 30]. Both substances act through TRP channels: menthol via the cold receptor TRPM8 and camphor via the warm receptor TRPV3 [31]. Concentrations of menthol 1–3% and camphor 2% have been reported to result in good short-term relief of pruritus [2].

Cannabinoid Receptor Agonists
Endocannabinoids can have anti-inflammatory and antinociceptive effects in the skin by acting on cannabinoid receptors on keratinocytes, mast cells, and sensory nerves [32, 33]. N-palmitoylethanolamide, an agonist of the cannabinoid receptor CB2, has been described in a large noncontrolled study to be effective in treating pruritus [34].

Experimental Topical Agents
It is surprising that up to now only few substances have been tested for their efficacy in reducing pruritus. In patients whose pruritus originates from the skin, a topical treatment is a logical approach, especially as systemic side effects can largely be avoided. Topical application of antagonists of neuropeptide receptors including neurokinin-1-receptor antagonists seem to be a suitable approach; however, recent reports have failed to show efficacy [35]. Randomized controlled trials in appropriate formulations will have to be performed to provide a final answer. Recently, a topical TrkA kinase inhibitor has been shown to be effective in the treatment of pruritus in a randomized controlled trial in patients with psoriasis [36]. The authors of this trial speculate that the substance could be a first-in-class treatment for chronic pruritus patients. Finally, apremilast, an oral inhibitor of phosphodiesterase-4 has recently been shown to effectively reduce itch in psoriasis patients [37]. Currently, topical phosphodiesterase-4 inhibitors are being tested for their efficacy in relieving itch in atopic dermatitis patients.

References

1 Staubach P, Lunter DJ: Basic or maintenance therapy in dermatology. Appropriate vehicles, possibilities and limitations (in German). Hautarzt 2014;65: 63–72; quiz 73–74.
2 Staubach P, Metz M: Magistral formulations and pruritus therapy – what is established, what is confirmed, what is new? J Dtsch Dermatol Ges 2013;11: 1049–1055.
3 Harding CR, Watkinson A, Rawlings AV, Scott IR: Dry skin, moisturization and corneodesmolysis. Int J Cosmet Sci 2000;22:21–52.

4 Feng L, Chandar P, Lu N, Vincent C, Bajor J, McGuiness H: Characteristic differences in barrier and hygroscopic properties between normal and cosmetic dry skin. II. Depth profile of natural moisturizing factor and cohesivity. Int J Cosmet Sci 2014;36:231–238.

5 Blanchet-Bardon C, Tadini G, Machado Matos M, Delarue A: Association of glycerol and paraffin in the treatment of ichthyosis in children: an international, multicentric, randomized, controlled, double-blind study. J Eur Acad Dermatol Venereol 2012;26:1014–1019.

6 Rawlings A, Harding C, Watkinson A, Banks J, Ackerman C, Sabin R: The effect of glycerol and humidity on desmosome degradation in stratum corneum. Arch Dermatol Res 1995;287:457–464.

7 Verhoeven EW, Kraaimaat FW, van de Kerkhof PC, van Weel C, Duller P, van der Valk PG, van den Hoogen HJ, Bor JH, Schers HJ, Evers AW: Prevalence of physical symptoms of itch, pain and fatigue in patients with skin diseases in general practice. Br J Dermatol 2007; 156:1346–1349.

8 Wolkenstein P, Grob JJ, Bastuji-Garin S, Ruszczynski S, Roujeau JC, Revuz J; Société Française de Dermotologie: French people and skin diseases: results of a survey using a representative sample. Arch Dermatol 2003;139:1614–1619; discussion 1619.

9 Blume-Peytavi U, Metz M: Atopic dermatitis in children: management of pruritus. J Eur Acad Dermatol Venereol 2012;26(suppl 6):2–8.

10 Wright A, Wijeratne A, Hung T, Gao W, Whittaker S, Morris S, Scarisbrick J, Beynon T: Prevalence and severity of pruritus and quality of life in patients with cutaneous T-cell lymphoma. J Pain Symptom Manage 2013;45:114–119.

11 Yosipovitch G, Goon A, Wee J, Chan YH, Goh CL: The prevalence and clinical characteristics of pruritus among patients with extensive psoriasis. Br J Dermatol 2000;143:969–973.

12 Bieber T, Vick K, Folster-Holst R, Belloni-Fortina A, Stadtler G, Worm M, Arcangeli F: Efficacy and safety of methylprednisolone aceponate ointment 0.1% compared to tacrolimus 0.03% in children and adolescents with an acute flare of severe atopic dermatitis. Allergy 2007; 62:184–189.

13 Peserico A, Stadtler G, Sebastian M, Fernandez RS, Vick K, Bieber T: Reduction of relapses of atopic dermatitis with methylprednisolone aceponate cream twice weekly in addition to maintenance treatment with emollient: a multicentre, randomized, double-blind, controlled study. Br J Dermatol 2008;158:801–807.

14 Curto L, Carnero L, Lopez-Aventin D, Traveria G, Roura G, Gimenez-Arnau AM: Fast itch relief in an experimental model for methylprednisolone aceponate topical corticosteroid activity, based on allergic contact eczema to nickel sulphate. J Eur Acad Dermatol Venereol 2014;28:1356–1362.

15 Eichenfield LF, Tom WL, Berger TG, Krol A, Paller AS, Schwarzenberger K, Bergman JN, Chamlin SL, Cohen DE, Cooper KD, Cordoro KM, Davis DM, Feldman SR, Hanifin JM, Margolis DJ, Silverman RA, Simpson EL, Williams HC, Elmets CA, Block J, Harrod CG, Smith Begolka W, Sidbury R: Guidelines of care for the management of atopic dermatitis: section 2. Management and treatment of atopic dermatitis with topical therapies. J Am Acad Dermatol 2014; 71:116–132.

16 Sigurgeirsson B, Boznanski A, Todd G, Vertruyen A, Schuttelaar ML, Zhu X, Schauer U, Qaqundah P, Poulin Y, Kristjansson S, von Berg A, Nieto A, Boguniewicz M, Paller AS, Dakovic R, Ring J, Luger T: Safety and efficacy of pimecrolimus in atopic dermatitis: a 5-year randomized trial. Pediatrics 2015;135:597–606.

17 Luger T, Loske KD, Elsner P, Kapp A, Kerscher M, Korting HC, Krutmann J, Niedner R, Rocken M, Ruzicka T, Schwarz T: Topical skin therapy with glucocorticoids – therapeutic index. J Dtsch Dermatol Ges 2004;2:629–634.

18 Kawashima M, Tango T, Noguchi T, Inagi M, Nakagawa H, Harada S: Addition of fexofenadine to a topical corticosteroid reduces the pruritus associated with atopic dermatitis in a 1-week randomized, multicentre, double-blind, placebo-controlled, parallel-group study. Br J Dermatol 2003;148:1212–1221.

19 Caterina MJ: Transient receptor potential ion channels as participants in thermosensation and thermoregulation. Am J Physiol Regul Integr Comp Physiol 2007;292:R64–R76.

20 Patel T, Yosipovitch G: Therapy of pruritus. Expert Opin Pharmacother 2010; 11:1673–1682.

21 Hautkappe M, Roizen MF, Toledano A, Roth S, Jeffries JA, Ostermeier AM: Review of the effectiveness of capsaicin for painful cutaneous disorders and neural dysfunction. Clin J Pain 1998;14:97–106.

22 Metz M, Krause K, Maurer M, Magerl M: Treatment of notalgia paraesthetica with an 8% capsaicin patch. Br J Dermatol 2011;165:1359–1361.

23 Misery L, Erfan N, Castela E, Brenaut E, Lanteri-Minet M, Lacour JP, Passeron T: Successful treatment of refractory neuropathic pruritus with capsaicin 8% patch: a bicentric retrospective study with long-term follow-up. Acta Derm Venereol 2015;95:864–865.

24 Zeidler C, Luling H, Dieckhofer A, Osada N, Schedel F, Steinke S, Augustin M, Stander S: Capsaicin 8% cutaneous patch: a promising treatment for brachioradial pruritus? Br J Dermatol 2015; 172:1669–1671.

25 Bauer M, Schwameis R, Scherzer T, Lang-Zwosta I, Nishino K, Zeitlinger M: A double-blind, randomized clinical study to determine the efficacy of benzocaine 10% on histamine-induced pruritus and UVB-light induced slight sunburn pain. J Dermatolog Treat 2015;26: 367–372.

26 Shuttleworth D, Hill S, Marks R, Connelly DM: Relief of experimentally induced pruritus with a novel eutectic mixture of local anaesthetic agents. Br J Dermatol 1988;119:535–540.

27 Young TA, Patel TS, Camacho F, Clark A, Freedman BI, Kaur M, Fountain J, Williams LL, Yosipovitch G, Fleischer AB Jr: A pramoxine-based anti-itch lotion is more effective than a control lotion for the treatment of uremic pruritus in adult hemodialysis patients. J Dermatolog Treat 2009;20:76–81.

28 Hawro T, Fluhr JW, Mengeaud V, Redoules D, Church MK, Maurer M, Metz M: Polidocanol inhibits cowhage – but not histamine-induced itch in humans. Exp Dermatol 2014;23:922–923.

29 Stander S, Darsow U, Mettang T, Gieler U, Maurer M, Stander H, Beuers U, Niemeier V, Gollnick H, Vogelgsang M, Weisshaar E: S2k guideline – chronic pruritus (in German). J Dtsch Dermatol Ges 2012;10(suppl 4):S1–S27.

30 Weisshaar E, Szepietowski JC, Darsow U, Misery L, Wallengren J, Mettang T, Gieler U, Lotti T, Lambert J, Maisel P, Streit M, Greaves MW, Carmichael AJ, Tschachler E, Ring J, Ständer S: European guideline on chronic pruritus. Acta Derm Venereol 2012;92:563–581.

31 Patel T, Ishiuji Y, Yosipovitch G: Menthol: a refreshing look at this ancient compound. J Am Acad Dermatol 2007; 57:873–878.

32 Ständer S, Weisshaar E, Luger TA: Neurophysiological and neurochemical basis of modern pruritus treatment. Exp Dermatol 2008;17:161–169.

33 Sugawara K, Biro T, Tsuruta D, Toth BI, Kromminga A, Zakany N, Zimmer A, Funk W, Gibbs BF, Zimmer A, Paus R: Endocannabinoids limit excessive mast cell maturation and activation in human skin. J Allergy Clin Immunol 2012;129: 726–738.e8.

34 Eberlein B, Eicke C, Reinhardt HW, Ring J: Adjuvant treatment of atopic eczema: assessment of an emollient containing N-palmitoylethanolamine (ATOPA study). J Eur Acad Dermatol Venereol 2008;22:73–82.

35 Wallengren J, Edvinsson L: Topical nonpeptide antagonists of sensory neurotransmitters substance P and CGRP do not modify patch test and prick test reactions: a vehicle-controlled, double-blind pilot study. Arch Dermatol Res 2014;306:505–509.

36 Roblin D, Yosipovitch G, Boyce B, Robinson J, Sandy J, Mainero V, Wickramasinghe R, Anand U, Anand P: Topical TrkA kinase inhibitor CT327 is an effective, novel therapy for the treatment of pruritus due to psoriasis: results from experimental studies, and efficacy and safety of CT327 in a phase 2b clinical trial in patients with psoriasis. Acta Derm Venereol 2015;95:542–548.

37 Paul C, Cather J, Gooderham M, Poulin Y, Mrowietz U, Ferrandiz C, Crowley J, Hu C, Stevens RM, Shah K, Day RM, Girolomoni G, Gottlieb AB: Efficacy and safety of apremilast, an oral phosphodiesterase 4 inhibitor, in patients with moderate-to-severe plaque psoriasis over 52 weeks: a phase III, randomized controlled trial (ESTEEM 2). Br J Dermatol 2015;173:1387–1399.

Martin Metz, MD
Department of Dermatology, Venerology and Allergology
Charité – Universitätsmedizin Berlin
Charitéplatz 1, DE–10117 Berlin (Germany)
E-Mail martin.metz@charite.de

Table 3. Systemic agents for paraneoplastic itch

Medications	Dose	Adverse effects	Notes
SSRIs			
Paroxetine	10–40 mg/day orally	nausea, dizziness, dry mouth, weight	
Fluvoxamine	25–150 mg/day orally	gain/loss, agitation, insomnia	
SNRIs			
Mirtazapine	15–30 mg/day orally at night	dry mouth, sedation, weight gain	
Thalidomide	50–400 mg/day orally at night	teratogenicity, peripheral neuropathy, risk of thromboembolism, somnolence, constipation, dizziness	pregnancy category X, expensive
Aprepitant	80 mg/day orally	nausea, vertigo, drowsiness	expensive

SSRIs = Selective serotonin reuptake Inhibitors; SNRIs = serotonin-norepinephrine reuptake inhibitors.

Table 4. Systemic agents for neuropathic itch, e.g. notalgia paresthetica, brachioradial pruritus, and postherpetic neuralgia

Medications	Dose	Adverse effects	Notes
Neuroleptics			
Gabapentin	300–3,600 mg/day orally	drowsiness, dizziness, nausea,	gradually dosage titration
Pregabalin	50–300 mg/day orally	vomiting, leg swelling	and when discontinuing, taper gradually
Tricyclic antidepressants			
Amitriptyline	25–150 mg/day orally	drowsiness, hypotension,	do not use concurrently with
Trimipramine	25–100 mg/day orally	hyponatremia, dry mouth, urinary retention, palpitation	monoamine oxidase; avoid in patients with glaucoma and prostatism
Aprepitant	80 mg/day orally	nausea, vertigo, drowsiness	expensive

μ-Opioid Receptor Antagonists

Acute opioid-induced itch, for example after epidural or intrathecal morphine, is quickly reversed by use of μ-opioid antagonists [2]. These μ-opioid antagonists have also been demonstrated to have anti-itch effects in other types of itch.

Naltrexone is an orally active, long-acting, competitive μ-opioid antagonist. Three RCTs have shown anti-itch effects of oral naltrexone in patients with cholestatic itch and atopic eczema [3–5]. However, the results of 2 RCTs with naltrexone in uremic itch are still conflicting [6, 7]. Single-arm studies and case series have reported variable responses in the other types of itch such as psoriasis vulgaris, prurigo nodularis, and cutaneous lymphoma.

Nalmefene is a potent, orally active μ-, κ-, and δ-opioid antagonist, which has longer plasma concentrations and greater oral bioavailability than naltrexone. One small RCT and one small open-label trial have shown that nalmefene orally can ameliorate itch in patients with cholestasis [8, 9].

Naloxone has low oral bioavailability and requires parenteral administration. Additionally, its duration of action is short, precluding its use as a long-term therapy for itch. A few RCTs in cholestatic itch patients have shown that intravenous infusions of naloxone are associated with a decrease in the subjectively perception of itch and decrease in scratching activity [10, 11].

The common adverse effects of μ-opioid antagonists are insomnia, dizziness, nausea, vomiting, headache, and abdominal cramps. They do not cause physical dependence and have no abuse potential. However, transient symptoms of opioid withdrawal-like reaction have been reported to occur. These symptoms usually resolve spontaneously within a few days. The opioid withdrawal-like reaction is more prominent with nalmefene than other agents.

κ-Opioid Receptor Agonists

Nalfurafine hydrochloride is a selective κ-opioid receptor agonist. Two large-scale RCTs and one open-label study showed that nalfurafine had an anti-itch effect in hemodialysis patients with intractable uremic itch [12–14]. The main adverse effects were insomnia, vertigo, headache, nausea, and vomiting, which transiently and spontaneously resolved. Neither opioid addiction nor withdrawal symptoms were noted in the trials.

On the basis of these data, nalfurafine appears effective and safe for treatment of uremic itch resistant to conventional treatments in hemodialysis patients. Note that the magnitude of the observed benefit is relatively small. Nalfurafine is not currently available in the United States, but is approved for this indication in Japan.

κ-Opioid Receptor Agonists and μ-Opioid Receptor Antagonists

Intranasal butorphanol has been reported to reduce itch in a case series of 5 patients who had intractable itch associated with various etiologies [15]. However, prospective controlled studies are needed to validate the anti-itch effect of butorphanol.

Neuroleptics

Gabapentin and pregabalin are very similar regarding their structure and mechanism of action. They are structural analogs of the neurotransmitter γ-aminobutyric acid (GABA). Pregabalin seems to have an advantage over gabapentin in terms of its more rapid response of actions.

Gabapentin has been established as an effective and safe therapeutic option in uremic itch through 2 RCTs at a dose of 300–400 mg after hemodialysis sessions [16, 17]. By contrast, an RCT showed that gabapentin was not beneficial in patients with cholestatic itch and furthermore produced several adverse events [18]. Gabapentin has been reported to be effective in several types of itch through case series and uncontrolled studies such as brachioradial pruritus, notalgia paresthetica, pruritus of unknown origins, senile pruritus, and pruritus associated with cutaneous lymphoma. In summary, a low dose of gabapentin had benefit and was well tolerated in patients with uremic itch, but was not found to be efficacious for cholestatic itch. The higher doses of gabapentin may have benefit in a variety of itch conditions, especially neuropathic itch.

Pregabalin was investigated in 2 RCTs and found to reduce uremic itch in dialysis patients. Moreover, pregabalin and gabapentin were found to be equally effective in the treatment of uremic pruritus in hemodialysis patients [19, 20].

The frequent adverse effects are drowsiness, fatigue, vertigo, nausea, vomiting, and leg swelling. The careful titration of the dose is required to obtain an optimal response and minimize the possible adverse effects.

Antidepressants

Selective Serotonin Reuptake Inhibitors

Sertraline has been shown to be an effective treatment for cholestatic itch in 1 small RCT and a retrospective case series of the patients with primary biliary cirrhosis [21, 22]. These data suggest that sertraline would be effective for cholestatic itch. An open-labeled small-scale study also showed it might be useful for the treatment of uremic pruritus in hemodialysis patients [23].

Paroxetine was found to reduce itch in patients with various nondermatological conditions in a small RCT [24]. In an open-label study in which 72 patients with severe, chronic pruritus were treated with paroxetine or fluvoxamine, 68% of patients responded to treatment [25].

In general, selective serotonin reuptake inhibitors have much lower cardiovascular side effects and better tolerability when compared with tricyclic antidepressants. Adverse effects to be considered are nausea, dry mouth, dizziness, agitation, sexual dysfunction, weight gain/loss, and insomnia.

Serotonin-Norepinephrine Reuptake Inhibitors
Mirtazapine has been reported to relieve itch in patients with advanced cancers, chronic kidney disease, and cholestasis, as well as be useful for the treatment of nocturnal itch [26]. However, mirtazapine has not been studied in an RCT. Mirtazapine is a relatively safe medication without serious adverse effects. The most common reported adverse effects are dry mouth, significant sedation, and weight gain.

Tricyclic Antidepressants
Amitriptyline, nortriptyline, and trimipramine were reported to be useful in itch, especially when it is of neuropathic origin [27]. However, these medications have not been studied for itch treatment in an RCT.

Doxepin is a tricyclic antidepressant with potent antipruritic properties resulting from its antihistaminic activity both with H_1- and H_2-receptor-binding affinity. One small RCT found an anti-itch effect of doxepin in patients with renal itch [28]. Doxepin may be a useful agent in chronic urticaria and HIV-induced pruritus [29].

The main side effects of tricyclic antidepressants are drowsiness, hypotension, hyponatremia, dry mouth, urinary retention, and palpitation. Because of anticholinergic side effects, the drug should be avoided in those with a history of prostatic hypertrophy and glaucoma. It should not be prescribed concurrently with a monoamine oxidase inhibitor. Because of their adverse effects and no large controlled studies, tricyclic antidepressants should be considered as a second- or third-line therapy for itch.

Rifampin

Rifampin has been suggested as a beneficial agent for cholestasis-induced itch in patients with primary biliary cirrhosis by 3 small RCTs [30–32]. However, 1 small RCT found that rifampin was not effective in relieving pruritus in a variety of chronic liver diseases [33]. The mechanism of action of rifampin in pruritus is unclear. It has been hypothesized to reduce the hepatic uptake or alter the metabolism of bile salts and other pruritogens. Worsened hepatic function, unconjugated hyperbilirubinemia, renal tubular damage, and thrombocytopenia have been noted in case reports. Long-term trials involving a large number of patients will further enhance the safety and efficacy profile of rifampin.

Bile Acid Sequestrants

Bile-acid-binding agents may reduce itch by binding to bile acids and other pruritogens in the intestinal lumen and enhancing their elimination in feces.

Cholestyramine showed some benefit in patients with cholestatic itch in 2 RCTs [34, 35]. However, the interpretations of its efficacy were limited by small sample size.

Colesevelam is an anion-exchange resin with a 7-fold higher bile-acid-binding capacity and fewer side effects than cholestyramine. One RCT showed that colesevelam had no advantage over placebo in cholestatic itch, although colesevelam significantly decreased the serum bile acid level [36].

Guar gum is a gel-forming dietary fiber. One RCT found that oral guar gum is beneficial in relieving itch in patients with intrahepatic cholestasis of pregnancy [37].

Bile-acid-binding agents are commonly used agents for cholestatic itch treatment because of their safety and inexpensive medications. The common adverse effects are nausea, bloating, mild constipation, and diarrhea.

Ursodeoxycholic Acid

Ursodeoxycholic acid is a hydrophilic bile acid that is used for the treatment of various cholestatic liver diseases. It was concluded from a meta-analysis of 7 RCTs that ursodeoxycholic acid is safe and improved maternal itch in intrahepatic cholestasis of pregnancy, although the size of the benefit is small [38].

Neurokinin Receptor 1 Antagonist

Aprepitant is a highly selective neurokinin receptor 1 antagonist. It could alleviate itch by inhibiting the receptor of substance P via the neurokinin receptor 1 antagonist. In recent case reports and case series, aprepitant demonstrated a significant antipruritic effect in acute and chronic intractable pruritus [39]. Aprepitant had a strong anti-itch effect and had a rapid onset as early as a few days after initiating treatment. Its side effects were mild such as nausea, vertigo, and drowsiness. However, the data from RCTs are not available and a major limitation for its use is its high cost.

Thalidomide

The antipruritic action of thalidomide may be secondary to inhibition of tumor necrosis factor. A crossover RCT of thalidomide for the treatment of refractory uremic pruritus demonstrated improvements in itch scores [40]. In recent case reports and case series, thalidomide demonstrated a significant antipruritic effect in paraneoplastic pruritus and prurigo nodularis [41].

The most severe toxicity of thalidomide is teratogenicity. Peripheral neuropathy is another major side effect and can be slow to resolve or even irreversible. Thromboembolic complications are mostly associated with thalidomide's use in the cancer setting. Other common side effects are somnolence, constipation, nonspecific rash, and dizziness. Due to its side effects, thalidomide is not considered as a first-line treatment for itch, but should be considered when the underlying conditions are disabling and recalcitrant to other treatments.

Other Agents

Various systemic agents have been studied in hemodialysis patients with uremic itch, including cromolyn sodium [42], montelukast [43], zinc sulfate [44], omega-3 fatty acids [45], activated charcoal [46], and erythropoietin [47]. However, the roles of these agents remain unclear and need to be confirmed by further large RCTs.

Ondansetron is a serotonin type 3-receptor antagonist. The results from the individual RCTs and a meta-analysis showed that ondansetron had no significant effect on itch reduction [48]. Therefore, ondansetron cannot be recommended for treatment of itch.

Conclusion

This review describes the evidence-based usefulness of the systemic medications in the treatment of itch of different etiologies. Limitations of this study are profound, in as much as the number and quality of studies are limited. Well-designed RCTs are needed to verify the effectiveness or noneffectiveness of systemic anti-itch agents currently being used. Certainly, the development of novel targeted therapies would be a welcome addition to our current anti-itch agents.

References

1 O'Donoghue M, Tharp MD: Antihistamines and their role as antipruritics. Dermatol Ther 2005;18:333–340.
2 Friedman JD, Dello Buono FA: Opioid antagonists in the treatment of opioid-induced constipation and pruritus. Ann Pharmacother 2001;35:85–91.
3 Wolfhagen FH, Sternieri E, Hop WC, Vitale G, Bertolotti M, Van Buuren HR: Oral naltrexone treatment for cholestatic pruritus: a double-blind, placebo-controlled study. Gastroenterology 1997; 113:1264–1269.
4 Terg R, Coronel E, Sordá, J, Muñoz AE, Findor J: Efficacy and safety of oral naltrexone treatment for pruritus of cholestasis, a crossover, double blind, placebo-controlled study. J Hepatol 2002;37: 717–722.
5 Malekzad F, Arbabi M, Mohtasham N, Toosi P, Jaberian M, Mohajer M, Mohammadi MR, Roodsari MR, Nasiri S: Efficacy of oral naltrexone on pruritus in atopic eczema: a double-blind, placebo-controlled study. J Eur Acad Dermatol Venereol 2009;23:948–950.
6 Pauli-Magnus C, Mikus G, Alscher DM, Kirschner T, Nagel W, Gugeler N, Risler T, Berger ED, Kuhlmann U, Mettang T: Naltrexone does not relieve uremic pruritus: results of a randomized, double blind, placebo controlled crossover study. J Am Soc Nephrol 2000;11:514–519.
7 Peer G, Kivity S, Agami O, Fireman E, Silverberg D, Blum M, Iaina A: Randomized crossover trial of naltrexone in uraemic pruritus. Lancet 1996;348: 1552–1554.
8 Bergasa NV, Alling DW, Talbot TL, Wells MC, Jones EA: Oral nalmefene therapy reduces scratching activity due to the pruritus of cholestasis: a controlled study. J Am Acad Dermatol 1999; 41:431–434.
9 Bergasa NV, Schmitt JM, Talbot TL, Alling DW, Swain MG, Turner ML, Jenkins JB, Jones EA: Open-label trial of oral nalmefene therapy for the pruritus of cholestasis. Hepatology 1998;27:679–684.
10 Bergasa NV, Talbot TL, Alling DW, Schmitt JM, Walker EC, Baker BL, Korenman JC, Park Y, Hoofnagle JH, Jones EA: A controlled trial of naloxone infusions for the pruritus of chronic cholestasis. Gastroenterology 1992;102: 544–549.
11 Bergasa NV, Alling DW, Talbot TL, Swain MG, Yurdaydin C, Turner ML, Schmitt JM, Walker EC, Jones EA: Effects of naloxone infusions in patients with the pruritus of cholestasis: a double-blind randomized controlled trial. Ann Intern Med 1995;123:161–167.
12 Wikström B, Gellert R, Ladefoged SD, Danda Y, Akai M, Ide K, Ogasawara M, Kawashima Y, Ueno K, Mori A, Ueno Y: Kappa-opioid system in uremic pruritus: multicenter, randomized, double-blind, placebo-controlled clinical studies. J Am Soc Nephrol 2005;16:3742–3747.
13 Kumagai H, Ebata T, Takamori K, Muramatsu T, Nakamoto H, Suzuki H: Effect of a novel kappa-receptor agonist, nalfurafine hydrochloride, on severe itch in 337 haemodialysis patients: a phase III, randomized, double-blind, placebo-controlled study. Nephrol Dial Transplant 2010;25:1251–1257.
14 Kumagai H, Ebata T, Takamori K, Miyasato K, Muramatsu T, Nakamoto H, Kurihara M, Yanagita T, Suzuki H: Efficacy and safety of a novel κ-agonist for managing intractable pruritus in dialysis patients. Am J Nephrol 2012;36:175–183.
15 Dawn AG, Yosipovitch G: Butorphanol for treatment of intractable pruritus. J Am Acad Dermatol 2006;54:527–531.
16 Gunal AI, Ozalp G, Yoldas TK, Gunal SY, Kirciman E, Celiker H: Gabapentin therapy for pruritus in haemodialysis patients: a randomized, placebo-controlled, double-blind trial. Nephrol Dial Transplant 2004;19:3137–3139.
17 Naini AE, Harandi AA, Khanbabapour S, Shahidi S, Seirafiyan S, Mohseni M: Gabapentin: a promising drug for the treatment of uremic pruritus. Saudi J Kidney Dis Transpl 2007;18:378–381.
18 Nora VB, Monnie MG, Iona HG, Danielle E: Gabapentin in patients with the pruritus of cholestasis: a double-blind, randomized, placebo-controlled trial. Hepatology 2006;44:1317–1323.
19 Ji Y, Shoufeng J, Yangfei X, Wei R, Tingbao Z, Jianzhong M: Comparison of pregabalin with ondansetron in treatment of uraemic pruritus in dialysis patients: a prospective, randomized, double-blind study. Int Urol Nephrol 2015;47:161–167.
20 Solak Y, Biyik Z, Atalay H, Gaipov A, Guney F, Turk S, Covic A, Goldsmith D, Kanbay M: Pregabalin versus gabapentin in the treatment of neuropathic pruritus in maintenance haemodialysis patients: a prospective, crossover study. Nephrology (Carlton) 2012;17:710–717.
21 Mayo MJ, Handem I, Saldana S, Jacobe H, Getachew Y, Rush AJ: Sertraline as a first-line treatment for cholestatic pruritus. Hepatology 2007;45:666–674.
22 Browning J, Combes B, Mayo MJ: Long-term efficacy of sertraline as a treatment for cholestatic pruritus in patients with primary biliary cirrhosis. Am J Gastroenterol 2003;98:2736–2741.
23 Shakiba M, Sanadgol H, Azmoude HR, Mashhadi MA, Sharifi H: Effect of sertraline on uremic pruritus improvement in ESRD patients. Int J Nephrol 2012; 2012:363901.

24 Zylicz Z, Krajnik M, Sorge AA, Constantini M: Paroxetine in the treatment of severe non-dermatological pruritus: a randomized, controlled trial. J Pain Symptom Manage 2003;26:1105–1112.

25 Ständer S, Böckenholt B, Schürmeyer-Horst F, Weishaupt C, Heuft G, Luger TA, Schneider G: Treatment of chronic pruritus with the selective serotonin re-uptake inhibitors paroxetine and fluvoxamine: results of an open-labelled, two-arm proof-of-concept study. Acta Derm Venereol 2009;89:45–51.

26 Davis MP, Frandsen JL, Walsh D, Andresen S, Taylor S: Mirtazapine for pruritus. J Pain Symptom Manage 2003;25:288–291.

27 Gupta MA, Guptat AK: The use of antidepressant drugs in dermatology. J Eur Acad Dermatol Venereol 2001;15:512–518.

28 Pour-Reza-Gholi F, Nasrollahi A, Firouzan A, Nasli Esfahani E, Farrokhi F: Low-dose doxepin for treatment of pruritus in patients on hemodialysis. Iran J Kidney Dis 2007;1:34–37.

29 Greene SL, Reed CE, Schroeter AL: Double-blind crossover study comparing doxepin with diphenhydramine for the treatment of chronic urticaria. J Am Acad Dermatol 1985;12:669–675.

30 Podesta A, Lopez P, Terg R, Villamil F, Flores D, Mastai R, Udaondo CB, Companc JP: Treatment of pruritus of primary biliary cirrhosis with rifampin. Dig Dis Sci 1991;36:216–220.

31 Ghent CN, Carruthers SG: Treatment of pruritus in primary biliary cirrhosis with rifampin: results of a double-blind, crossover, randomized trial. Gastroenterology 1988;94:488–493.

32 Bachs L, Pares A, Elena M, Piera C, Rodes J: Comparison of rifampicin with phenobarbitone for treatment of pruritus in biliary cirrhosis. Lancet 1989;1:574–576.

33 Woolf GM, Reynolds TB: Failure of rifampin to relieve pruritus in chronic liver disease. J Clin Gastroenterol 1990;12:174–177.

34 Duncan JS, Kennedy HJ, Triger DR: Treatment of pruritus due to chronic obstructive liver disease. Br Med J 1984;289:22.

35 Di Padova C, Tritapepe R, Rovagnati P, Rossetti S: Double-blind placebo-controlled clinical trial of microporous cholestyramine in the treatment of intra- and extra-hepatic cholestasis: relationship between itching and serum bile acids. Methods Find Exp Clin Pharmacol 1984;6:773–776.

36 Kuiper EM, Van Erpecum KJ, Beuers U, Hansen BE, Ansen BE, Thio HB, De Man RA, Janssen HLA, Van Buuren HR: The potent bile acid sequestrant colesevelam is not effective in cholestatic pruritus: results of a double-blind, randomized, placebo-controlled trial. Hepatology 2010;52:1334–1340.

37 Riikonen S, Savonius H, Gylling H, Nikkila K, Tuomi AM, Miettinen TA: Oral guar gum, a gel-forming dietary fiber relieves pruritus in intrahepatic cholestasis of pregnancy. Acta Obstet Gynecol Scand 2000;79:260–264.

38 Gurung V, Stokes M, Middleton P, Milan SJ, Hague W, Thornton JG: Interventions for treating cholestasis in pregnancy. Cochrane Database Syst Rev 2013;6:CD000493.

39 Sonja S, Dorothee S, Ilka H, Cord S, Thomas AL: Targeting the neurokinin receptor 1 with aprepitant: a novel antipruritic strategy. PLoS One DOI: 10.1371/journal.pone.0010968.

40 Silva SR, Viana PC, Lugon NV, Hoette M, Ruzany F, Lugon JR: Thalidomide for the treatment of uremic pruritus: a crossover randomized double-blind trial. Nephron 1994;67:270–273.

41 Doherty SD, Hsu S: A case series of 48 patients treated with thalidomide. J Drugs Dermatol 2008;7:769–773.

42 Vessal G, Sagheb MM, Shilian S, Jafari P, Samani SM: Effect of oral cromolyn sodium on CKD-associated pruritus and serum tryptase level: a double-blind placebo-controlled study. Nephrol Dial Transplant 2010;25:1541–1547.

43 Nasrollahi A, Miladipour A, Ghanei E, Yavari P, Haghverdi F: Montelukast for treatment of refractory pruritus in patients on hemodialysis. Iran J Kidney Dis 2007;1:73–77.

44 Najafabadi MM, Faghihi G, Emami A, Monghad M, Moeenzadeh F, Sharif N, Davarpanah Jazi AH: Zinc sulfate for relief of pruritus in patients on maintenance hemodialysis. Ther Apher Dial 2012;16:142–145.

45 Ghanei E, Zeinali J, Borghei M, Homayouni M: Efficacy of omega-3 fatty acids supplementation in treatment of uremic pruritus in hemodialysis patients: a double-blind randomized controlled trial. Iran Red Crescent Med J 2012;14:515–522.

46 Pederson JA, Matter BJ, Czerwinski AW, Llach F: Relief of idiopathic generalized pruritus in dialysis patients treated with activated oral charcoal. Ann Intern Med 1980;93:446–448.

47 De Marchi S, Cecchin E, Villalta D, Sepiacci G, Santini G, Bartoli E: Relief of pruritus and decreases in plasma histamine concentrations during erythropoietin therapy in patients with uremia. N Engl J Med 1992;326:969–974.

48 Pongcharoen P, Fleischer AB Jr: An evidence-based review of systemic treatments for itch. Eur J Pain 2016;20:24–31.

Padcha Pongcharoen, MD
Dermatology Unit, Department of Internal Medicine, Thammasat University
95 Phaholyothin road
Bangkok, 12120 (Thailand)
E-Mail padchapreme@gmail.com

Szepietowski JC, Weisshaar E (eds): Itch – Management in Clinical Practice.
Curr Probl Dermatol. Basel, Karger, 2016, vol 50, pp 54–63 (DOI: 10.1159/000446044)

Itch Management: Physical Approaches (UV Phototherapy, Acupuncture)

Isaac H.Y. Chan · Dedee F. Murrell

Department of Dermatology, St. George Hospital, and Faculty of Medicine, University of New South Wales, Sydney, N.S.W., Australia

Abstract

Background: Physical therapies refer to non-medical treatment strategies, including surgery, cryotherapy, UV phototherapy, and acupuncture. Most physical approaches are inappropriate in the context of itch. UV phototherapy and acupuncture may be effective in the management of itch. ***Methods:*** A literature search was performed using MEDLINE and EMBASE. Bibliographies were reviewed for relevant articles. ***Results:*** Narrowband UVB (311–313 nm) and UVA1 (340–400 nm) are equally effective in managing atopic dermatitis and associated itch. The efficacy of broadband UVB in reducing uraemic itch has been demonstrated in a series of randomised controlled trials, but more recent studies have failed to reproduce these results. Non-randomised, uncontrolled studies and case series suggest that UV is effective in managing itch associated with cholestasis, chronic urticaria, prurigo, cutaneous T-cell lymphoma, aquagenic itch, and scleroderma. UV phototherapy is well tolerated, and no significant relationship between UVB therapy and skin cancer has been found. Experimentally, acupuncture has been shown to reduce allergen-related itch, although this finding has been limited by the small number of studies, inconsistency in agreement on acupuncture sites and study design, small sample sizes, and limited follow-up. ***Conclusions:*** UV phototherapy is an effective treatment for itch associated with atopic dermatitis. UVB may be effective in managing itch associated with end-stage kidney disease, cholestasis, chronic urticaria, prurigo, cutaneous T-cell lymphoma, aquagenic itch, and scleroderma. Phototherapy should be combined with standard first-line therapies. Insufficient evidence exists to justify acupuncture as a physical therapy for itch. Further well-designed studies are required to establish the effectiveness of physical therapies in managing itch.

© 2016 S. Karger AG, Basel

Physical therapies refer to non-medical treatment strategies, including surgery, cryotherapy, UV phototherapy, and acupuncture. Most physical approaches are inappropriate in the context of itch, but UV phototherapy and acupuncture may be effective. UV phototherapy is a physical approach to managing itch which exposes patients to controlled quantities of UV light in order to induce changes in the skin that reduce itch sensation, while acupuncture is a complementary therapy that involves the insertion of needles into acupuncture points, which may reduce allergen-induced itch sensation. The exact mechanism by which UV reduces itch in patients with atopic dermatitis, psoriasis, end-stage kidney disease, biliary obstruction, and chronic urticaria is not yet fully understood, but is thought to be related to its immunosuppressive effects. This chapter seeks to assess the evidence behind the use of physical therapies in itch involving normal-looking and diseased skin, and clarify their clinical application. It should be noted that studies investigating the antipruritic effects of UV phototherapy in diseased skin rarely use itch as a primary study outcome. Rather, they focus on itch as a component of the overall disease state.

History of the Development of UV Delivery Devices

While the therapeutic potential of sunlight was already noted in Ancient Egypt and during the Islamic Golden Age, modern phototherapy involving sophisticated UV delivery devices able to control wavelength and dosage did not exist until the 20th century [1, 2]. Experiments with PUVA (psoralen + UVA) in 1974 and broadband (BB) UVB throughout the 20th century found UV phototherapy to be effective treatments for psoriasis and associated itch [3]. These techniques were refined, leading to the finding that narrowband (NB) UVB is more effective than BB-UVB at treating psoriasis [2, 4]. The efficacy of UV phototherapy as a treatment modality for psoriasis and the observation that atopic dermatitis improved during summer, possibly because of increased sunlight exposure, led to trials investigating the possible role of UV as a treatment for atopic dermatitis, first with BB-UVB, and later

with NB-UVB and UVA1 [5, 6]. These studies demonstrated the effectiveness of UV phototherapy as a second-line treatment for atopic dermatitis and associated itch. UV phototherapy has also been shown to be an effective treatment for itch in diseased and normal-looking skin, as discussed later in this chapter.

Currently Available UV Devices

UV phototherapy can include BB-UVB (280–315 nm), BB-UVA (315–400 nm), NB-UVB (311–313 nm), UVA1 (340–400 nm), and PUVA. Longer wavelengths (UVA) are capable of penetrating deeper into the skin, and may work via a different mechanism to UVB. Full body machines cost approximately USD 40,000, while 'hand and foot' machines cost approximately USD 10,000.

UVB (Narrowband and Broadband)

BB-UVB refers to UV light with a wavelength of between 280 and 315 nm. BB-UVB combined with coal tar was first shown in 1925 by Goeckerman as an effective treatment for psoriasis [7]. However, the popularity of BB-UVB has declined in recent years, as NB-UVB has been found to be more effective and less carcinogenic at clinically effective doses [8–10].

While medical UVB units only emit UV along a specific wavelength spectrum, at a specific level of irradiance, tanning booths emit an inconsistent proportion of UVA and UVB wavelengths, at an irradiance level up to 10–15 times stronger than the midday Mediterranean sun [11]. No significant link between medical UVB and skin cancer has been established, but sunbed use is associated with a significant increase in melanoma risk, especially when initial usage begins at a young age (<35 years) [11–13]. However, long-term follow-up of medical UVB use is required because of the potential for carcinogenicity [14, 15].

Broadband UVA and UVA1

BB-UVA refers to wavelengths between 315 and 400 nm. Clinically, BB-UVA is often combined with psoralen (a photosensitising agent) as PUVA, or photochemotherapy, for the treatment of psoriasis [16]. However, NB-UVB is preferred as a first-line treatment for psoriasis, as it does not lead to the systemic photosensitivity of the eyes and liver, or the increased skin cancer risk associated with PUVA [17]. A limited number of studies suggest that BB-UVA is effective in reducing the severity of atopic dermatitis, but is less effective than BB-UVB and NB-UVB in reducing itch [18, 19]. A more comprehensive body of work has established the efficacy of UVA1 (340–400 nm, lower UVA wavelengths filtered out) as a treatment for atopic dermatitis and itch [20–22]. However, UVA1 machines are a rarity in many countries. In this case, NB-UVB can often be used.

Guidelines for Use

Figure 1 shows an example of a BB-UVA/NB-UVB unit. Patients wearing underwear and eye protection stand in the centre of the machine. The machine then closes to expose the patient to BB-UVA or NB-UVB from all directions.

Dosage guidelines vary by UV wavelength, cause of itch, and country. For atopic dermatitis, NB-UVB dosage protocols in studies frequently begin at 70% of the minimum erythema dose (MED) [22, 23], increasing by 10–20% on subsequent visits to a maximum of 1.3–1.5 J/cm^2 [10, 19]. This is less intensive than the UV dosage schedule recommended in psoriasis, but dosage and frequency are not standardised and vary between studies. To determine the MED, a section of the patient's skin is exposed to UV light at intervals and the exposed area is examined after 24–48 h. The section of skin that is erythematous after the shortest period of UV exposure indi-

cates the MED [24]. Modern machines will automatically increase dosage by 10% per session, plateauing after 15 treatments for safety. Dosages should not be increased if patients experience burning, and should be reduced if patients miss sessions. Typically, patients undergo 3 sessions per week, but frequency can range from 2 per week to daily as inpatients. Some clinicians may also opt to follow the psoriasis dosage guidelines [25]. Dosage may vary depending on the Fitzpatrick skin type of the patient, and should always be adjusted to the needs of the individual patient. Treatment courses usually last at least 6 weeks or until a satisfactory outcome is achieved.

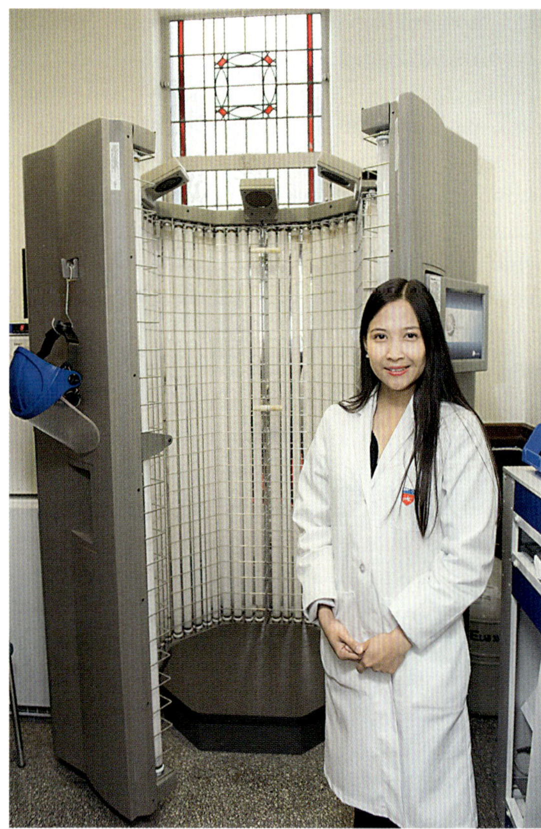

Fig. 1. NB-UVB and BB-UVA unit with alternating bulbs.

Adverse Effects of Phototherapy

Phototherapy is generally well tolerated, and short-term adverse effects are minimal. These include burning, exacerbation of eczema [26, 27], erythema and burns [15, 28, 29], itch [30] sweating [31], and herpes simplex and varicella zoster reactivation [14]. Evidence suggests that there is no significant relationship between UVB therapy and skin cancer, but long-term follow-up is required [12–15]. PUVA in psoriasis patients is, however, linked with a significant increase in the risk of squamous cell carcinoma [32]. UV is safe and effective in paediatric populations when they are mature enough to protect their eyes during treatment, but patients should be monitored for long-term adverse effects not documented in the literature [23, 29].

UV Phototherapy in Itchy Skin Diseases

Atopic Dermatitis

Phototherapy is a second-line treatment modality for atopic dermatitis which can involve NB-UVB, BB-UVB, BB-UVA, UVA1, PUVA, and UVA and UVB simultaneously [25]. Numerous studies have shown UV phototherapy to be effective in treating atopic dermatitis and associated itch [6]. Initial research in this area focused on the efficacy of BB-UVB (280–315 nm) [33]. In recent years, it has been established that NB-UVB is more effective than BB-UVB, without an increased risk of adverse effects [4].

NB-UVB produces clinically significant reductions in atopic dermatitis symptoms, including itch, and improvement is sustained 3 months after treatment (p < 0.0001 at 3 months) [23, 26]. Medium-dose UVA1 and NB-UVB are equally effective in treating atopic dermatitis and associated itch, although lower levels of irradiation are required to produce a similar therapeutic effect with NB-UVB [6, 10, 22]. A 2001 randomised controlled trial by Reynolds et al. [26] noted that NB-UVB was more effective than BB-UVA in reducing itch. High-dose UVA1 and medium-dose UVA1 are similarly effective [34].

Given that NB-UVB is cheaper, more readily available, and requires lower dosages than UVA1 [10], its use may be preferred in clinical practice. The long-term efficacy of phototherapy is difficult to judge, owing to lack of follow-up in trials. A study of medium-dose UVA1 found that symptoms recurred within 3 months [27], and a trial of NB-UVB in children found that beneficial effects are sustained for at least 6 months after treatment (p = 0.0012) [23].

The antipruritic mechanisms of UV phototherapy in atopic dermatitis have not yet been fully elucidated, but it is thought to be related to its immunosuppressive effects, which reduces overall disease activity [35]. UVA1, which penetrates deeper into the skin [36], decreases T_H2-cell-derived IL-5, IL-13, and IL-31 mRNA expression [37]. Similar effects on T_H2 pathways have been observed in NB-UVB [38]. UVA1 and UVB also induce apoptosis of T lymphocytes and antigen-presenting Langerhans cells [39–41], reducing inflammatory infiltrate. UVA and UVB are also able to modulate the activity of ICAM1, the overexpression of which acts as a binding site for inflammatory leukocytes [41–43]. UVB further prevents the degranulation of mast cells [44].

While the literature focuses on UV monotherapy because of the need to study its effects in isolation, phototherapy should be combined with topical corticosteroids and other first-line treatments in clinical practice.

Itch in Psoriasis

Psoriasis is an inflammatory disorder that manifests as scaly erythematous patches, papules, and plaques [45]. While itch may accompany these skin lesions, it is typically not a major complaint. Itch is not included in the Psoriasis Area and Severity Index (PASI), which is used to assess the extent of the disease. Phototherapy, including

NB-UVB or BB-UVB, is a first-line treatment for psoriasis that reduces both overall disease severity and itch [46, 47]. PUVA is an effective treatment, but is not first-line because of risks associated with photosensitivity and skin cancer [17]. Topical PUVA (e.g. with 0.01% oxsoralen cream) may be used for palmoplantar psoriasis, and does not involve the systemic adverse effects of oral psoralen [17, 48, 49]. Further information may be found in the chapter by Szepietowski and Reich [this vol., pp. 102–110].

Itch in Chronic Urticaria
UV light may also be used as an adjunct treatment for symptomatic relief of itch in chronic idiopathic urticaria. A 2012 study found that NB-UVB was effective in clearing or reducing itch compared to baseline in chronic urticaria, although this study was not blinded or randomised [50]. NB-UVB with antihistamine has also been found to be more effective in reducing itch than antihistamine monotherapy [51]. PUVA and NB-UVB are equally effective at reducing itch in chronic urticaria [52]. A retrospective review of NB-UVB in 84 patients with chronic urticaria reported that 85% of subjects experienced clearance or moderate improvement [53]. Overall, studies and evidence in this area are poor, no rigorous randomised controlled trials have been carried out, and phototherapy is not included in the treatment algorithm of major chronic urticaria guidelines [54, 55]. Nevertheless, it may be considered as an adjunct second-line treatment if systemic agents are deemed inappropriate.

Other Indications for UV Phototherapy in Itchy Skin Diseases
Case series have documented the successful use of BB-UVB [56] (monotherapy or supplemented with topical steroids + coal tar [57] or PUVA [58]), NB-UVA + PUVA [59], and UVA1 + topical steroids [60] in reducing itch associated with prurigo nodularis.

Cutaneous T-cell lymphoma (CTCL) may present with itch, and PUVA is an established therapy for early-stage CTCL [61]. BB-UVB, NB-UVB, and UVA1 have also been shown in case series to be effective in patients with CTCL [62–64]. UV phototherapy may reduce itch in these patients by treating the underlying CTCL, but studies of UV in CTCL have not examined the effect of UV on itch directly [65]. Low-dose UVA1, medium-dose UVA1, and NB UVB have been trialled with success in localised scleroderma, but only medium-dose UVA1 significantly reduced itch [66, 67]. UVA1 and PUVA may be effective in systemic scleroderma, but evidence in this area is poor [68, 69].

UV Phototherapy for Itch in Normal-Looking Skin

Uraemic Itch
Itch is commonly associated with renal failure. Gilchrest et al. [70–72] found BB-UVB phototherapy to be more effective than a UVA placebo in treating uraemic itch, with long-lasting relief following treatment for 50% of patients. It appears to have a systemic effect, as half-body exposures to BB-UVB light resulted in whole-body reductions in itch [70]. However, a 1981 double-blind crossover study with 12 subjects failed to confirm these findings [73]. An uncontrolled trial suggested that NB-UVB could be effective in the treatment of uraemic itch [74], but a 2011 randomised controlled trial did not reach significance compared to placebo [75]. A 2003 case report involving a single patient found that BB-UVB, but not NB-UVB, was effective in clearing uraemic itch. Dosage in the Gilchrest studies on which this treatment is based started at 75% of the MED, increasing by 25% of the MED to a maximum of 480 mJ/cm^2 [70].

The mechanisms of phototherapy in treatment uraemic itch are unknown, but its systemic effects are thought to be related to the photoinactivation of an itch-inducing substance produced in renal failure [70, 76]. Other theories include mast cell apoptosis by UVB [77], an UVB-induced reduction in mast cell histamine release [78], and a reduction in skin divalent ion content, particularly phosphorus [79].

Cholestatic Itch
Itch is a common symptom associated with chronic liver disease and cholestasis. The efficacy of phototherapy has only been examined in a small number of unblinded, non-randomised pilot studies and case reports. These studies suggest that BB-UVB is effective in reducing cholestatic itch [80–83]. BB-UVB treatment was further found to reduce itch in 12/13 patients with cholestasis in a 2012 study [84]. Due to the lack of randomised controlled trials investigating the use of UV phototherapy in cholestatic itch, it is not recommended as a treatment modality in major treatment guidelines [85, 86]. Further information can be found in the chapter by Mittal [this vol., pp. 142–148].

Other Indications for UV Phototherapy in Normal-Looking Skin
BB-UVB, NB-UVB, and PUVA have all been reported as being effective in reducing aquagenic itch in case series, but remission appears to be short-lived [87–89].

Acupuncture and Itch

Acupuncture belongs to the traditional Chinese medicine family of complementary therapies, dating as far back as 6000 BC, and formally codified in 'The Yellow Emperor's Classic of Internal Medicine' around 100 BC [90]. Acupuncture involves the insertion of needles (0.25 × 40 mm) 2–3 cm deep into acupuncture points (as defined by traditional literature) for a variable amount of time, ostensibly to influence the flow of 'Qi', or energy, around the body in order to reduce itch sensation [91, 92]. Electroacupuncture is a form of acupuncture that involves passing an electrical current through an inserted needle. As a complementary and alternative therapy, research investigating the role of acupuncture in managing itch is largely insufficient.

Acupoints linked to itch are located on the upper and lower limbs, and preventive electroacupuncture applied before the induction of itch by an allergen at these locations were more effective than placebo and equally effective as oral cetirizine (antihistamine) at reducing the intensity of itch, although these were unable to reduce itch to below the scratch threshold [91, 93]. Abortive acupuncture, where acupuncture and itch induction occur simultaneously, is more effective than both preventive acupuncture and oral cetirizine, reducing itch to below the itch threshold [91, 93]. Electroacupuncture, where an electrical current is passed through the needle, is more effective than acupuncture without electrical stimulation [94].

The antipruritic mechanisms of acupuncture are poorly understood, but are thought to be related to a reduction in sensory nerve fibre density [95], reduced basophil activation [96], and its ability to distract the patient [91]. Acupuncture reduces itch-induced response in the putamen and insular, premotor, and prefrontal cortical areas of the human brain, as measured by changes in cerebral blood flow [97]. Furthermore, referred itch sites appear to have a high degree of correlation with acupuncture meridians [98].

The small sample size and number of trials, as well as lack of follow-up to evaluate long-term effectiveness diminishes the usefulness of acupuncture in a clinical setting [91, 99]. Furthermore, acupuncture regimens are not standardised and clinical trials utilise inconsistent acupoints and protocols, making it difficult to determine the best course of treatment [91, 94]. In addition to inadequate experimental evidence, there are also differences of opinion amongst acupuncture practitioners regarding the locations and therapeutic effects of acupoints [98]. While acupuncture enjoys a good safety profile [100], it remains costly and invasive compared to medical and other physical approaches. Therefore, while acupuncture has demonstrated antipruritic effects in atopic itch under controlled conditions, its use in clinical practice remains questionable. There is also insufficient evidence to justify the use of acupuncture for uraemic itch [101].

Other Physical Approaches

Massage as an adjunct to standard care has been shown to significantly reduce itch in children with atopic dermatitis compared to conventional treatments [102]. The addition of essential oils to the massage regimen does not further reduce itch, suggesting that the physical act of massage plays a role in mediating itch sensation in children [103].

Conclusion

Physical approaches to itch are largely limited to UV phototherapy and acupuncture. Convincing evidence exists for the use of UV phototherapy in itch associated with atopic dermatitis and psoriasis. Evidence supporting the use of UV in itch related to chronic urticaria, end-stage kidney disease, and biliary obstruction is less convincing, but UV phototherapy may be indicated in these conditions when first-line therapies are inappropriate. On the basis of current evidence, acupuncture cannot be recommended as a therapy to treat itch in a clinical setting.

References

1 Roelandts R: The history of phototherapy: something new under the sun? J Am Acad Dermatol 2002;46:926–930.

2 Honigsmann H: History of phototherapy in dermatology. Photochem Photobiol Sci 2013;12:16–21.

3 Parrish JA, Fitzpatrick TB, Tanenbaum L, Pathak MA: Photochemotherapy of psoriasis with oral methoxsalen and longwave ultraviolet light. N Engl J Med 1974;291:1207–1211.

4 An appraisal of narrowband (TL 01) UVB phototherapy. British Photodermatology Group Workshop Report (April 1996). Br J Dermatol 1997;137:327–330.

5 Morison WL, Parrish JA, Fitzpatrick TB: Oral psoralen photochemotherapy of atopic eczema. Br J Dermatol 1978;98:25–30.

6 Garritsen FM, Brouwer MW, Limpens J, Spuls PI: Photo(chemo)therapy in the management of atopic dermatitis: an updated systematic review with implications for practice and research. Br J Dermatol 2014;170:501–513.

7 Gupta R, Debbaneh M, Butler D, Huynh M, Levin E, Leon A, et al: The Goeckerman regimen for the treatment of moderate to severe psoriasis. J Vis Exp 2013;(77):e50509.

8 Van Weelden H, Baart De La Faille H, Young E, Van Der Leun JC: A new development in UVB phototherapy of psoriasis. Br J Dermatol 1988;119:11–19.

9 Coven TR, Burack LH, Gilleaudeau P, Keogh M, Ozawa M, Krueger JG: Narrowband UV-B produces superior clinical and histopathological resolution of moderate-to-severe psoriasis in patients compared with broadband UV-B2. Arch Dermatol 1997;133:1514–1522.

10 Gambichler T, Othlinghaus N, Tomi NS, Holland-Letz T, Boms S, Skrygan M, et al: Medium-dose ultraviolet (UV) A1 vs narrowband UVB phototherapy in atopic eczema: a randomized crossover study. Br J Dermatol 2009;160:652–658.

11 Boniol M, Autier P, Boyle P, Gandini S: Cutaneous melanoma attributable to sunbed use: systematic review and meta-analysis. BMJ 2012;345:e4757.

12 Hearn RM, Kerr AC, Rahim KF, Ferguson J, Dawe RS: Incidence of skin cancers in 3867 patients treated with narrow-band ultraviolet B phototherapy. Br J Dermatol 2008;159:931–935.

13 Lee E, Koo J, Berger T: UVB phototherapy and skin cancer risk: a review of the literature. Int J Dermatol 2005;44:355–360.

14 Jury CS, McHenry P, Burden AD, Lever R, Bilsland D: Narrowband ultraviolet B (UVB) phototherapy in children. Clin Exp Dermatol 2006;31:196–189.

15 Clayton TH, Clark SM, Turner D, Goulden V: The treatment of severe atopic dermatitis in childhood with narrowband ultraviolet B phototherapy. Clin Exp Dermatol 2007;32:28–33.

16 Menter A, Korman NJ, Elmets CA, Feldman SR, Gelfand JM, Gordon KB, et al: Guidelines of care for the management of psoriasis and psoriatic arthritis: section 5. Guidelines of care for the treatment of psoriasis with phototherapy and photochemotherapy. J Am Acad Dermatol 2010;62:114–135.

17 Ling TC, Clayton TH, Crawley J, Exton LS, Goulden V, Ibbotson S, et al: British Association of Dermatologists and British Photodermatology Group guidelines for the safe and effective use of psoralen-ultraviolet A therapy 2015. Br J Dermatol 2016;174:24–55.

18 Jekler J, Larko O: UVA solarium versus UVB phototherapy of atopic dermatitis: a paired-comparison study. Br J Dermatol 1991;125:569–572.

19 Reynolds NJ, Franklin V, Gray JC, Diffey BL, Farr PM: Narrow-band ultraviolet B and broad-band ultraviolet A phototherapy in adult atopic eczema: a randomised controlled trial. Lancet 2001; 357:2012–2016.

20 Krutmann J, Czech W, Diepgen T, Niedner R, Kapp A, Schöpf E: High-dose UVA1 therapy in the treatment of patients with atopic dermatitis. J Am Acad Dermatol 1992;26:225–230.

21 Krutmann J, Diepgen TL, Luger TA, Grabbe S, Meffert H, Sönnichsen N, et al: High-dose UVA1 therapy for atopic dermatitis: results of a multicenter trial. J Am Acad Dermatol 1998;38:589–593.

22 Majoie IM, Oldhoff JM, van Weelden H, Laaper-Ertmann M, Bousema MT, Sigurdsson V, et al: Narrowband ultraviolet B and medium-dose ultraviolet A1 are equally effective in the treatment of moderate to severe atopic dermatitis. J Am Acad Dermatol 2009;60:77–84.

23 Darne S, Leech SN, Taylor AE: Narrow-band ultraviolet B phototherapy in children with moderate-to-severe eczema: a comparative cohort study. Br J Dermatol 2014;170:150–156.

24 Heckman CJ, Chandler R, Kloss JD, Benson A, Rooney D, Munshi T, et al: Minimal erythema dose (MED) testing. J Vis Exp 2013;(75):e50175.

25 Sidbury R, Davis DM, Cohen DE, Cordoro KM, Berger TG, Bergman JN, et al: Guidelines of care for the management of atopic dermatitis. J Am Acad Dermatol 2014;71:327–349.

26 Reynolds NJ, Franklin V, Gray JC, Diffey BL, Farr PM: Narrow-band ultraviolet B and broad-band ultraviolet A phototherapy in adult atopic eczema: a randomised controlled trial. Lancet 2001; 357:2012–2016.

27 Abeck D, Schmidt T, Fesq H, Strom K, Mempel M, Brockow K, et al: Long-term efficacy of medium-dose UVA1 phototherapy in atopic dermatitis. J Am Acad Dermatol 2000;42:254–257.

28 Jekler J, Larkö O: Combined UVA-UVB versus UVB phototherapy for atopic dermatitis: a paired-comparison study. J Am Acad Dermatol 1990;22:49–53.

29 Pavlovsky M, Baum S, Shpiro D, Pavlovsky L, Pavlotsky F: Narrow band UVB: is it effective and safe for paediatric psoriasis and atopic dermatitis? J Eur Acad Dermatol Venereol 2011;25:727–729.

30 von Kobyletzki G, Pieck C, Hoffmann K, Freitag M, Altmeyer P: Medium-dose UVA1 cold-light phototherapy in the treatment of severe atopic dermatitis. J Am Acad Dermatol 1999;41:931–937.

31 Valkova S, Velkova A: UVA/UVB phototherapy for atopic dermatitis revisited. J Dermatolog Treat 2004;15:239–244.

32 Stern RS, Laird N: The carcinogenic risk of treatments for severe psoriasis. Cancer 1994;73:2759–2764.

33 Jekler J, Larko O: Combined UVA-UVB versus UVB phototherapy for atopic dermatitis: a paired-comparison study. J Am Acad Dermatol 1990;22:49–53.

34 Tzaneva S, Seeber A, Schwaiger M, Hönigsmann H, Tanew A: High-dose versus medium-dose UVA1 phototherapy for patients with severe generalized atopic dermatitis. J Am Acad Dermatol 2001;45:503–507.

35 Horio T: Indications and action mechanisms of phototherapy. J Dermatol Sci 2000;23(suppl 1):S17–S21.

36 Godar DE: UVA1 radiation triggers two different final apoptotic pathways. J Invest Dermatol 1999;112:3–12.

37 Gambichler T, Kreuter A, Tomi NS, Othlinghaus N, Altmeyer P, Skrygan M: Gene expression of cytokines in atopic eczema before and after ultraviolet A1 phototherapy. Br J Dermatol 2008;158:1117–1120.

38 Tintle S, Shemer A, Suárez-Fariñas M, Fujita H, Gilleaudeau P, Sullivan-Whalen M, et al: Reversal of atopic dermatitis with narrow-band UVB phototherapy and biomarkers for therapeutic response. J Allergy Clin Immunol 2011; 128:583–93.e4.

39 Dawe RS: Ultraviolet A1 phototherapy. Br J Dermatol 2003;148:626–637.

40 Toews GB, Bergstresser PR, Streilein JW: Epidermal Langerhans cell density determines whether contact hypersensitivity or unresponsiveness follows skin painting with DNFB. J Immunol 1980; 124:445–453.

41 Krutmann J, Morita A: Mechanisms of ultraviolet (UV) B and UVA phototherapy. J Investig Dermatol Symp Proc 1999; 4:70–72.

42 Krutmann J, Czech W, Parlow F, Trefzer U, Kapp A, Schopf E, et al: Ultraviolet radiation effects on human keratinocyte ICAM-1 expression: UV-induced inhibition of cytokine-induced ICAM-1 mRNA expression is transient, differentially restored for IFN gamma versus TNF alpha, and followed by ICAM-1 induction via a TNF alpha-like pathway. J Invest Dermatol 1992;98:923–928.

43 Norris DA, Lyons MB, Middleton MH, Yohn JJ, Kashihara-Sawami M: Ultraviolet radiation can either suppress or induce expression of intercellular adhesion molecule 1 (ICAM-1) on the surface of cultured human keratinocytes. J Invest Dermatol 1990;95:132–138.

44 Danno K, Toda K, Horio T: Ultraviolet-B radiation suppresses mast cell degranulation induced by compound 48/80. J Invest Dermatol 1986;87:775–778.

45 Menter A, Gottlieb A, Feldman SR, Van Voorhees AS, Leonardi CL, Gordon KB, et al: Guidelines of care for the management of psoriasis and psoriatic arthritis. J Am Acad Dermatol 2008;58:826–850.

46 Lapolla W, Yentzer BA, Bagel J, Halvorson CR, Feldman SR: A review of phototherapy protocols for psoriasis treatment. J Am Acad Dermatol 2011;64: 936–949.

47 Gupta G, Long J, Tillman DM: The efficacy of narrowband ultraviolet B phototherapy in psoriasis using objective and subjective outcome measures. Br J Dermatol 1999;140:887–890.

48 Sezer E, Erbil AH, Kurumlu Z, Taştan HB, Etikan I: Comparison of the efficacy of local narrowband ultraviolet B (NB-UVB) phototherapy versus psoralen plus ultraviolet A (PUVA) paint for palmoplantar psoriasis. J Dermatol 2007;34: 435–440.

49 Hawk JL, Le Grice P: The efficacy of localized PUVA therapy for chronic hand and foot dermatoses. Clin Exp Dermatol 1994;19:479–482.

50 Aydogan K, Karadogan SK, Tunali S, Saricaoglu H: Narrowband ultraviolet B (311 nm, TL01) phototherapy in chronic ordinary urticaria. Int J Dermatol 2012; 51:98–103.

51 Engin B, Ozdemir M, Balevi A, Mevlitoglu I: Treatment of chronic urticaria with narrowband ultraviolet B phototherapy: a randomized controlled trial. Acta Derm Venereol 2008;88:247–251.

52 Khafagy NH, Salem SA, Ghaly EG: Comparative study of systemic psoralen and ultraviolet A and narrowband ultraviolet B in treatment of chronic urticaria. Photodermatol Photoimmunol Photomed 2013;29:12–17.

53 Berroeta L, Clark C, Ibbotson SH, Ferguson J, Dawe RS: Narrow-band (TL-01) ultraviolet B phototherapy for chronic urticaria. Clin Exp Dermatol 2004;29:97–98.

54 Zuberbier T, Aseru R, Bindslev-Jensen C, Walter Canonica G, Church MK, Giménez-Arnau AM, et al: EAACI/GA²LEN/EDF/WAO guideline: management of urticaria. Allergy 2009;64:1427–1443.

55 Bernstein JA, Lang DM, Khan DA, Craig T, Dreyfus D, Hsieh F, et al: The diagnosis and management of acute and chronic urticaria: 2014 update. J Allergy Clin Immunol 2014;133:1270–1277.

56 Hann SK, Cho MY, Park Y-K: UV Treatment of generalized prurigo nodularis. Int J Dermatol 1990;29:436–437.

57 Sorenson E, Levin E, Koo J, Berger TG: Successful use of a modified Goeckerman regimen in the treatment of generalized prurigo nodularis. J Am Acad Dermatol 2015;72:e40–e42.

58 Divekar PM, Palmer RA, Keefe M: Phototherapy in nodular prurigo. Clin Exp Dermatol 2003;28:99–100.

59 Hammes S, Hermann J, Roos S, Ockenfels HM: UVB 308-nm excimer light and bath PUVA: combination therapy is very effective in the treatment of prurigo nodularis. J Eur Acad Dermatol Venereol 2011;25:799–803.

60 Levi A, Ingber A, Enk CD: Ultraviolet A1 exposure is crucial in the treatment of prurigo nodulalis using a ultraviolet A1/topical steroid combination regimen. Photodermatol Photoimmunol Photomed 2011;27:55–66.

61 Querfeld C, Rosen ST, Kuzel TM, et al: Long-term follow-up of patients with early-stage cutaneous T-cell lymphoma who achieved complete remission with psoralen plus UV-A monotherapy. Arch Dermatol 2005;141:305–311.

62 Ramsay DL, Lish KM, Yalowitz CB, Soter NA: Ultraviolet-B phototherapy for early-stage cutaneous T-cell lymphoma. Arch Dermatol 1992;128:931–933.

63 Diederen PV, van Weelden H, Sanders CJ, Toonstra J, van Vloten WA: Narrowband UVB and psoralen-UVA in the treatment of early-stage mycosis fungoides: a retrospective study. J Am Acad Dermatol 2003;48:215–219.

64 Plettenberg H, Stege H, Megahed M, Ruzicka T, Hosokawa Y, Tsuji T, et al: Ultraviolet A1 (340–400 nm) phototherapy for cutaneous T-cell lymphoma. J Am Acad Dermatol 1999;41:47–50.

65 Meyer N, Paul C, Misery L: Pruritus in cutaneous T-cell lymphomas: frequent, often severe and difficult to treat. Acta Derm Venereol 2010;90:12–17.

66 Kreuter A, Hyun J, Stucker M, Sommer A, Altmeyer P, Gambichler T: A randomized controlled study of low-dose UVA1, medium-dose UVA1, and narrowband UVB phototherapy in the treatment of localized scleroderma. J Am Acad Dermatol 2006;54:440–447.

67 Kroft EB, Berkhof NJ, van de Kerkhof PC, Gerritsen RM, de Jong EM: Ultraviolet A phototherapy for sclerotic skin diseases: a systematic review. J Am Acad Dermatol 2008;59:1017–1030.

68 Morita A, Kobayashi K, Isomura I, Tsuji T, Krutmann J: Ultraviolet A1 (340–400 nm) phototherapy for scleroderma in systemic sclerosis. J Am Acad Dermatol 2000;43:670–674.

69 Hofer A, Soyer H: Oral psoralen-UV-A for systemic scleroderma. Arch Dermatol 1999;135:603–604.

70 Gilchrest BA, Rowe JW, Brown RS, Steinman TI, Arndt KA: Ultraviolet phototherapy of uremic pruritus. Long-term results and possible mechanism of action. Ann Intern Med 1979;91:17–21.

71 Gilchrest BA: Ultraviolet phototherapy of uremic pruritus. Int J Dermatol 1979;18:741–748.

72 Gilchrest BA, Rowe JW, Brown RS, Steinman TI, Arndt KA: Relief of uremic pruritus with ultraviolet phototherapy. N Engl J Med 1977;297:136–138.

73 Simpson NB, Davison AM: Ultraviolet phototherapy for uraemic pruritus. Lancet 1981;1:781.

74 Ada S, Seckin D, Budakoglu I, Ozdemir FN: Treatment of uremic pruritus with narrowband ultraviolet B phototherapy: an open pilot study. J Am Acad Dermatol 2005;53:149–151.

75 Ko MJ, Yang JY, Wu HY, Hu FC, Chen SI, Tsai PJ, et al: Narrowband ultraviolet B phototherapy for patients with refractory uraemic pruritus: a randomized controlled trial. Br J Dermatol 2011;165:633–639.

76 Schultz BC, Roenigk HH Jr: Uremic pruritus treated with ultraviolet light. JAMA 1980;243:1836–1837.

77 Szepietowski JC, Morita A, Tsuji T: Ultraviolet B induces mast cell apoptosis: a hypothetical mechanism of ultraviolet B treatment for uraemic pruritus. Med Hypotheses 2002;58:167–170.

78 Imazu LE, Tachibana T, Danno K, Tanaka M, Imamura S: Histamine-releasing factor(s) in sera of uraemic pruritus patients in a possible mechanism of UVB therapy. Arch Dermatol Res 1993;285:423–427.

79 Blachley JD, Blankenship DM, Menter A, Parker TF 3rd, Knochel JP: Uremic pruritus: skin divalent ion content and response to ultraviolet phototherapy. Am J Kidney Dis 1985;5:237–241.

80 Hanid MA, Levi AJ: Phototherapy for pruritus in primary biliary cirrhosis. Lancet 1980;2:530.

81 Cerio R, Murphy GM, Sladen GE, MacDonald DM: A combination of phototherapy and cholestyramine for the relief of pruritus in primary biliary cirrhosis. Br J Dermatol 1987;116:265–267.

82 Rosenthal E, Diamond E, Benderly A, Etzioni A: Cholestatic pruritus: effect of phototherapy on pruritus and excretion of bile acids in urine. Acta Paediatr 1994;83:888–891.

83 Perlstein SM: Phototherapy for primary biliary cirrhosis. Arch Dermatol 1981;117:608.

84 Decock S, Roelandts R, Steenbergen WV, Laleman W, Cassiman D, Verslype C, et al: Cholestasis-induced pruritus treated with ultraviolet B phototherapy. an observational case series study. J Hepatol 2012;57:637–641.

85 Lindor KD, Gershwin ME, Poupon R, Kaplan M, Bergasa NV, Heathcote EJ: Primary biliary cirrhosis. Hepatology 2009;50:291–308.

86 European Association for the Study of the Liver: EASL Clinical Practice Guidelines: Management of cholestatic liver diseases. J Hepatol 2009;51:237–267.

87 Steinman HK, Greaves MW: Aquagenic pruritus. J Am Acad Dermatol 1985;13:91–96.

88 Xifra A, Carrascosa JM, Ferrandiz C: Narrow-band ultraviolet B in aquagenic pruritus. Br J Dermatol 2005;153:1233–1234.

89 Menage HD, Norris PG, Hawk JL, Graves MW: The efficacy of psoralen photochemotherapy in the treatment of aquagenic pruritus. Br J Dermatol 1993;129:163–165.

90 White A, Ernst E: A brief history of acupuncture. Rheumatology 2004;43:662–663.

91 Pfab F, Kirchner MT, Huss-Marp J, Schuster T, Schalock PC, Fuqin J, et al: Acupuncture compared with oral antihistamine for type I hypersensitivity itch and skin response in adults with atopic dermatitis – a patient- and examiner-blinded, randomized, placebo-controlled, crossover trial. Allergy 2012;67:566–573.

92 Pfab F, Schalock PC, Napadow V, Athanasiadis GI, Huss-Marp J, Ring J: Acupuncture for allergic disease therapy – the current state of evidence. Expert Rev Clin Immunol 2014;10:831–841.

93 Pfab F, Huss-Marp J, Gatti A, Fuqin J, Athanasiadis GI, Irnich D, et al: Influence of acupuncture on type I hypersensitivity itch and the wheal and flare response in adults with atopic eczema – a blinded, randomized, placebo-controlled, crossover trial. Allergy 2010;65:903–910.

94 Lundeberg T, Bondesson L, Thomas M: Effect of acupuncture on experimentally induced itch. Br J Dermatol 1987;117:771–777.

95 Carlsson CP, Sundler F, Wallengren J: Cutaneous innervation before and after one treatment period of acupuncture. Br J Dermatol 2006;155:970–976.

96 Pfab F, Athanasiadis GI, Huss-Marp J, Fuqin J, Heuser B, Cifuentes L, et al: Effect of acupuncture on allergen-induced basophil activation in patients with atopic eczema: a pilot trial. J Altern Complement Med 2011;17:309–314.

97 Napadow V, Li A, Loggia ML, Kim J, Schalock PC, Lerner E, et al: The brain circuitry mediating antipruritic effects of acupuncture. Cereb Cortex 2014;24:873–882.

98 Silberstein M: Do acupuncture meridians exist? Correlation with referred itch (mitempfindung) stimulus and referral points. Acupunct Med 2012;30:17–20.

99 Lee KC, Keyes A, Hensley JR, Gordon JR, Kwasny MJ, West DP, et al: Effectiveness of acupressure on pruritus and lichenification associated with atopic dermatitis: a pilot trial. Acupunct Med 2012;30:8–11.

100 Yamashita H, Tsukayama H, Hori N, Kimura T, Tanno Y: Incidence of adverse reactions associated with acupuncture. J Altern Complement Med 2000;6:345–350.

101 Kim KH, Lee MS, Choi S-M, Ernst E: Acupuncture for treating uremic pruritus in patients with end-stage renal disease: a systematic review. J Pain Symptom Manage 2010;40:117–125.

102 Schachner L, Field T, Hernandez-Reif M, Duarte AM, Krasnegor J: Atopic dermatitis symptoms decreased in children following massage therapy. Pediatr Dermatol 1998;15:390–395.

103 Anderson C, Lis-Balchin M, Kirk-Smith M: Evaluation of massage with essential oils on childhood atopic eczema. Phytother Res 2000;14:452–456.

Prof. Dedee F. Murrell
Department of Dermatology, St George Hospital
Gray St, Kogarah
Sydney, NSW 2217 (Australia)
E-Mail d.murrell@unsw.edu.au

Szepietowski JC, Weisshaar E (eds): Itch – Management in Clinical Practice.
Curr Probl Dermatol. Basel, Karger, 2016, vol 50, pp 64–70 (DOI: 10.1159/000446045)

Itch Management: Psychotherapeutic Approach

Andrea W.M. Evers[a] · Christina Schut[c] · Uwe Gieler[d] ·
Saskia Spillekom-van Koulil[b] · Sylvia van Beugen[a]

[a]Health, Medical and Neuropsychology Unit, Institute of Psychology, Faculty of Social and Behavioral Sciences, Leiden University, Leiden, and [b]Department of Medical Psychology, Radboud University Medical Center, Nijmegen, The Netherlands; [c]Institute of Medical Psychology, Justus Liebig University Giessen, and [d]Department of Dermatology, University Clinic Giessen, Giessen, Germany

Abstract

A relationship between the intensity of itch and psychological factors like stress, coping, anxiety, and depression has often been shown in patients with skin diseases. Moreover, the biopsychosocial model of chronic itch nicely summarizes how psychological factors can contribute to a worsening or improvement of chronic itch. Thus, it is reasonable to consider psychological interventions in the treatment of chronic itch. In this chapter we focus on itch-scratch problems as well as stress and anxiety/depression as itch-increasing factors. We summarize the evidence of psychological interventions which can reduce these triggering factors. Hereby, we differentiate between unimodal and multimodal interventions, and emphasize that not every single intervention might help for all patients, but that a comprehensive anamnesis is needed in order to determine whether one or several psychological factors trigger itch in the particular patient.

© 2016 S. Karger AG, Basel

Itch and Scratching: Their Relationship with Psychological Factors

More than half of the patients with chronic skin conditions report experiencing itch, making it one of the most frequent complaints in this patient population [1, 2]. Itch by definition is a sensation, which – when strong enough – will lead to scratching or at least the desire to scratch [3]. The strong correlation between itch and scratching is implied by this definition. Frequent scratching, however, can lead to skin damage which can in turn aggravate skin conditions [2]. The substantial subjective impact of itch is underlined by the fact that patients often indicate that 'itch is worse than pain'. Itch is often regarded as unpleasant or annoying [4]. Moreover, itch is a symptom, which in many cases worsens at night [5, 6] and is associated with sleeping problems [5]. This may lead to chronic fatigue, irritability, and concentration problems during the day, which in time can result in mood problems and impairments in everyday activities [7]. Thus, it is not surprising that itch is related to a low quality of life and great psychological burden [e.g. 8–10]. In addition, the scratching behavior, which at first leads to a decrease of itch, has many negative consequences in the long run. Many patients pass through the cycle of itch/scratching and a worsening of the skin condition many times. On an emotional level, patients often feel helplessness, ashamed, and guilty after scratching. These feelings might even increase when significant others comment on the scratching behavior in a negative way.

Accordingly, a relationship between itch, scratching, and psychological factors clearly exists and there are many studies that have linked, for example, stress, anxiety, depression, or extensive scratching, like it occurs under tension, to the intensity of itch [e.g. 11, 12]. The biopsychosocial model of chronic itch nicely summarizes how these psychological factors can contribute to a worsening or improvement of chronic itch [13]. It explains that internal factors (e.g. personality) and external factors (e.g. stress) go along with certain cognitive, behavioral, and social reactions, which then trigger physiological processes that finally alter the itch sensation [13].

The associations between psychological factors and itch are also reasonable from an immunological point of view: under stress certain neurotransmitters are released which cause neurogenic inflammation and a worsening of skin symptoms [14]. Moreover, it is known that the mechanic stimulation of the skin during scratching leads to a release of neurotransmitters [e.g. 15], which then can cause a worsening of itch.

In this chapter we focus on itch-scratch problems as well as stress, anxiety, depression, and compulsive scratching as itch-increasing factors and describe psychological interventions that address these factors. Most of these approaches have been described in detail in previous reviews [16, 17]. We differentiate between multimodal and unimodal approaches, which have been used to treat itch patients. Evidently, it is not reasonable to use a combination of all of these approaches in every patient. Some patients might predominantly suffer from the stress of itch-scratching behavior, while others report symptoms of anxiety, depression, stress, and compulsive scratching at the same time. Therefore, a comprehensive anamnesis needs to be done before a psychological intervention is recommended.

Unimodal Psychological Itch Treatment

In case the clinician identifies one certain psychological factor as predominant for the worsening of itch, he or she may consider offering only one circumscribable intervention to the patient. The kind of approach he recommends certainly depends on the psychological factors: If *stress* is the main underlying psychological factor that exacerbates itch in the patient, relaxation training or mindfulness-based stress reduction can be considered. Two relaxation techniques which have been shown to be beneficial in the treatment of chronic itch patients are progressive muscle relaxation and autogenic training [18, 19]. Progressive muscle relaxation focuses on the tension and relaxation of certain muscle groups, and has been shown to be effective in reducing itch in patients with atopic dermatitis [18]. Autogenic training demands the itch patient be autosuggestive because patients are asked to imagine during this relaxation training that, for example, body parts become heavy or flooded with light. This kind of intervention has also been shown to be effective in patients with atopic dermatitis [19].

In case patients report that they suffer from scratching episodes which they are not able to stop, the most important goals are usually to improve itch and coping techniques, and to decrease the scratching behavior. In order to cope with itch, the focus is usually on optimizing skin care routines (e.g. by regular application of ointments), avoiding stimuli or situations that may trigger itch (e.g. transpiration or certain fabrics), and learn ways to decrease stress and itch (e.g. relaxation exercises). In order to target scratching behavior, a first and important step is to increase awareness of scratching habits. This can be achieved by educating patients and asking them to register their scratching behavior over a period of time. This results in an overall awareness of early signs of skin deterioration, such as increased redness or itching. When patients become more aware of these early signs, they can take appropriate action in order to prevent further skin deterioration by, for example, using ointments or bandages, or focusing on relaxation in their daily lives. Following this increased awareness, patients learn to use different ways to control their scratching behavior. The best known method for controlling scratching is 'habit reversal' in which patients learn to replace scratching with an alternative behavior. Here, patients learn to replace their scratching behavior by an alternative non-skin-damaging behavior like putting their hands on their thighs or making a fist [20]. The foundation of these itch-scratching interventions lies in increasing patients' autonomy and ability to cope with itching and scratching. When patients experience very severe itching, these types of interventions may be augmented with pharmacological treatment, such as low-dose antidepressants or antihistamines.

Multimodal Psychological Approaches to Cope with Itch-Triggering Factors

In case not just *one* psychological triggering factor is identified, but the patient suffers from, for instance, stress, anxiety, depression, and impulsive scratching at the same time, which often is the case, multimodal approaches should be considered. There are some cognitive behavioral training programs which have been developed es-

pecially for patients with chronic itch [21, 22]. Other, more general psychological interventions have also been shown to be effective in the treatment of chronic itch [23, 24]. These interventions comprise a broader range of different methods and often include psychoeducation, habit-reversal techniques, relaxation trainings, and cognitive restructuring.

Multimodal Treatments for Itch-Scratching Problems

In multimodal treatments for itch-scratching problems, several of the unimodal techniques described above (e.g. habit reversal and optimizing skin care routines) are combined with other techniques to offer a comprehensive treatment program. Several multimodal interventions have been shown to be effective in scientific studies, such as in reducing itching, scratching, and/or disease activity, as well as in increasing the effects of dermatological treatments in patients with atopic dermatitis, psoriasis, or other skin conditions [19, 22, 25–27]. An example of a multimodal treatment that has been effective in reducing disease severity in patients with chronic skin conditions is a 12-session intervention that focuses on self-control techniques and habit reversal to reduce scratching, stress-management techniques, education, communication, and relaxation exercises [19]. Further studies should examine the active mechanisms of these interventions, which have received little attention in research thus far. Habit reversal may be an effective component for scratch-management interventions, considering the positive effects of habit reversal interventions in patients with atopic dermatitis [28]. More research is also needed to determine the optimal dose-response relationship for these interventions. While there is evidence for the effectiveness of treatments including 12 meetings [19], a group-based intervention of only 5 meetings has also shown clinically significant long-term effects [22]. This multidisciplinary training includes a combination of the techniques described above, with the aim to reduce itch-scratching problems, and is led by both a specialized dermatology nurse and a cognitive behavioral therapist.

Multimodal Treatments for Skin-Related Psychosocial Problems

Patients with chronic skin conditions may also benefit from psychological interventions for frequently occurring psychosocial problems that may trigger itch, such as problems with mood and acceptance, social anxiety, perceived stigmatization, and dysfunctional coping methods including avoidance behavior. Cognitive behavioral treatments have been successfully applied in treating these problems [7, 29–31]. Results of a review of randomized controlled trials showed that quality of life improved and disease severity decreased in patients with chronic skin conditions when multidisciplinary patient education interventions including several meetings were applied [32].

Considering the relationship between stress-related factors and chronic skin conditions, interventions including relaxation exercises and stress-management techniques are frequently applied in patients with skin conditions, with the expectation that reducing stress will also reduce inflammatory activity and disease severity. These interventions may include a variety of techniques focused on relaxation, such as progressive relaxation, biofeedback, autogenic training, and visualization. These have been combined with, for example, cognitive restructuring components and exercises to improve problem-solving skills. Beneficial effects of stress-focused relaxation interventions have been found for patients with chronic skin conditions [33], including increased clearance rates after phototherapy in patients with psoriasis [34], and decreased disease severity in patients with atopic dermatitis [19]. For example, a short-term cognitive behavioral group therapy has been successfully applied in patients with psoriasis. This intervention includes cognitive

therapy with a specific focus on disease-related attitudes, perceived stigmatization, and social anxiety. Furthermore, information is provided and stress-management and relaxation techniques are used. This type of intervention may reduce disease-severity, disease-related distress, depression, and anxiety, as was found in a controlled study both after treatment as well as at a 6-month follow-up assessment [26]. Indications that psychological interventions may also influence the cortisol response in patients with atopic dermatitis have also been found. In a recent study, patients with atopic dermatitis who followed a short-term stress management training showed a decreased cortisol response when they were exposed to a psychosocial stressor, compared to a control group [24]. No beneficial effects on disease severity were found in this study, which may have been due to a follow-up that was too short or the small sample size.

Treating Itch and Psychosocial Problems in Children and Adolescents

Multimodal interventions combining cognitive behavioral therapy with relaxation and education have also been developed for children [35]. For example, a standardized group-based psychoeducational intervention consisting of 6 weekly sessions was offered to children with atopic dermatitis and their parents, with separate groups for different age brackets. The sessions were led by a multidisciplinary team including a dermatologist, nurse, psychologist, and dietician [27]. Similar interventions in adults have also shown beneficial effects [32]. Furthermore, improved skin complaints and self-image, and less social constraints, have been reported in children and adolescents with psoriasis following an intervention focused on education, stress-management, and building social skills [36]. To target psychosocial problems in children and adolescents with chronic skin conditions, psychoeducational interventions involving their parents have been used. An example of a multidisciplinary intervention for children with psoriasis and dermatitis and their parents is the Supportive Program for Education, Coping and Training of Parents and Children with Psoriasis and Eczema (SPECTRUM). In this intervention, consisting of 4 group sessions, a dermatologist, clinical psychologist, and nurse worked together to increase the ability of children and parents to cope with the skin condition and associated complaints such as itch [37].

New Developments in Psychological Treatments for Chronic Skin Conditions

In recent years, Internet-delivered (eHealth) self-management and cognitive behavioral interventions for health conditions have been increasingly used, and studies have shown that this may be an effective form of treatment for chronic somatic conditions, with similar effects as face-to-face interventions [38]. Important advantages of these Internet-delivered interventions include increased reach of care and better access to care for patients, as well as reduced time and travel costs and overall greater flexibility for both therapists and patients [39]. The first studies of eHealth treatments specifically for chronic skin conditions underlined the promise of these interventions [40, 41]. Another promising area for interventions may be psychological mindfulness- and acceptance-based interventions, which are also increasingly being used in patients with chronic somatic conditions and have shown beneficial effects in patients with skin conditions [34].

Conclusion

Considering that itch is a prominent complaint in many chronic skin conditions, and psychological factors can contribute to worsening or improvement of chronic itch, psychological approaches should be considered to target itch and its associated triggering factors. In this chapter, we have provided an overview of the scientific evidence of unimodal and multimodal interventions, focusing on itch-scratching problems, as well as on psychosocial aspects such as stress and mood problems as itch-increasing factors. While results of both unimodal and multimodal interventions have been promising thus far, systematic screening and availability of multidisciplinary interventions in clinical practice are still limited [42, 43]. Therefore, it is of great importance that increased attention is paid to the implementation of psychological screening and interventions in the field of dermatology. Furthermore, research should focus on further development and evaluation of psychological interventions for itch- and scratching-related and skin-related psychosocial problems, paying particular attention to working mechanisms and possible interactions between psychological and inflammatory mechanisms, which may provide useful starting points for specific interventions.

References

1 Verhoeven EWM, Kraaimaat FW, van de Kerkhof PCM, van Weel C, Duller P, van der Kalk PGM, van den Hoogen HJM, Bor JHJ, Schers HJ, Evers AWM: Prevalence of physical symptoms of itch, pain and fatigue in patients with skin diseases in general practice. Br J Dermatol 2007;156:1346–1349.

2 Yosipovitch G, Greaves MW, Fleischer Jr AB, McGlone F (eds): Itch: Basic Mechanisms and Therapy. Boca Raton, CRC Press, 2004.

3 Savin J: How should we define itching. J Am Acad Dermatol 1998;39:268–269.

4 Dawn A, Papoiu ADP, Chan YH, Rapp SR, Rassette N, Yosipovitch G: Itch characteristics in atopic dermatitis: results of a web-based questionnaire. Br J Dermatol 2009;160:642–644.

5 Gupta MA, Gupta AK: Sleep-wake disorders and dermatology. Clin Dermatol 2013;31:118–126.

6 Valdes-Rodriguez R, Mollanazar NK, Gonzalez-Muro J, Nattkemper L, Torres-Alvarez B, Lopez-Esqueda FJ, Chan YH, Yosipovitch G: Itch prevalence and characteristics in a Hispanic geriatric population: a comprehensive study using a standardized itch questionnaire. Acta Derm Venereol 2015;95:417–421.

7 Stangier U, Ehlers A: Stress and anxiety in dermatological disorders; in Mostofsky DI, Barlow DH (eds): The Management of Stress and Anxiety in Medical Disorders. Needham Heights, Allyn & Bacon, 2000, pp 304–343.

8 Evers AWM, Lu Y, Duller P, van der Valk PGM, Kraaimaat FW, van de Kerkhof PCM: Common burden of chronic skin diseases? Contributors to psychological distress in adults with psoriasis and atopic dermatitis. Br J Dermatol 2005;152:1275–1281.

9 Marron SE, Tomas-Aragones L, Boira S, Campos-Rodenas R: Quality of life, emotional well-being and family repercussions in dermatological patients experiencing chronic itching: a pilot study. Acta Derm Venereol 2016;96:331–335.

10 Verhoeven EWM, Kraaimaat FW, Van De Kerkhof PCM, van Weel C, Duller P, van der Kalk PGM, van den Hoogen HJM, Bor JHJ, Schers HJ, Evers AWM: Psychosocial well-being of patients with skin diseases in general practice. J Eur Acad Dermatol Venereol 2007;21:662–668.

11 Chrostowska-Plak D, Reich A, Szepietowski JC: Relationship between itch and psychological status of patients with atopic dermatitis. J Eur Acad Dermatol Venereol 2013;27:e239–e242.

12 Schut C, Weik U, Tews N, Gieler U, Deinzer R, Kupfer J: Coping as mediator of the relationship between stress and itch in patients with atopic dermatitis: a regression and mediation analysis. Exp Dermatol 2015;24:148–150.

13 Verhoeven EWM, de Klerk S, Kraaimaat FW, van de Kerkhof PCM, de Jong EMGJ, Evers AWM: Biopsychosocial mechanisms of chronic itch in patients with skin diseases: a review. Acta Derm Venereol 2008;88:211–218.

14 Pavlovic S, Daniltchenko M, Tobin DJ, Hagen E, Hunt SP, Klapp BF, Arck PC, Peters EMJ: Further exploring the brain-skin connection: stress worsens dermatitis via substance P-dependent neurogenic inflammation in mice. J Invest Dermatol 2008;128:434–446.

15 Leung DYM, Boguniewicz M, Howell MD, Nomura I, Hamid QA: New insights into atopic dermatitis. J Clin Invest 2004;113:651–657.

16 Evers AWM, Spillekom-van Koulil S, van Beugen S: Psychological treatments for dermatological conditions; in Nordlind K, Zalewska A (eds): Skin and the Psyche (e-book). Bentham Science Publishers, 2016, pp 168–186.

17 Schut C, Mollananzar NK, Kupfer J, Gieler U, Yosipovitch G: Psychological interventions in the treatment of chronic itch. Acta Derm Venereol 2016;96:157–161.

18 Bae BG, Oh SH, Park CO, Noh S, Noh JY, Kim KR, Lee KH: Progressive muscle relaxation therapy for atopic dermatitis: objective assessment of efficacy. Acta Derm Venereol 2012;92:57–61.

19 Ehlers A, Stangier U, Gieler U: Treatment of atopic dermatitis: a comparison of psychological and dermatological approaches to relapse prevention. J Consult Clin Psychol 1995;62:624–635.

20 Rosenbaum MS, Ayllon T: The behavioral treatment of neurodermatitis through habit-reversal. Behav Res Ther 1981;19:313–318.

21 Bathe A, Matterne U, Dewald M, Grande T, Weisshaar E: Educational multidisciplinary training programme for patients with chronic pruritus. Acta Derm Venereol 2009;89:498–501.

22 Evers AWM, Duller P, de Jong EMGJ, Otero ME, Verhaak CM, van der Valk PGM, van de Kerkhof PCM, Kraaimaat FW: Effectiveness of a multidisciplinary itch-coping training programme in adults with atopic dermatitis. Acta Derm Venereol 2009;89:57–63.

23 Habib S, Morissey S: Stress management for atopic dermatitis. Behav Change 1999;16:226–236.

24 Schut C, Weik U, Tews N, Gieler U, Deinzer R, Kupfer J: Psychophysiological effects of stress management in patients with atopic dermatitis: a randomized controlled trial. Acta Derm Venereol 2013;93:57–61.

25 van Os-Medendorp H, Eland de Kok PC, Ros WJ, Bruijnzeel-Koomen CA, Grypdonck M: The nursing programme 'Coping with Itch': a promising intervention for patients with chronic pruritic skin diseases. J Clin Nurs 2007;16:1238–1246.

26 Fortune DG, Richards HL, Kirby B, Bowcock S, Main CJ, Griffiths CE: A cognitive-behavioural symptom management programme as an adjunct in psoriasis therapy. Br J Dermatol 2002;146:458–465.

27 Staab D, Diepgen TL, Fartasch M, Kupfer J, Lob-Corzilius T, Ring J, Scheewe S, Scheidt R, Schmid-Ott G, Schnopp C, Szczepanski R, Werfel T, Wittenmeier M, Wahn U, Gieler U: Age related, structured educational programmes for the management of atopic dermatitis in children and adolescents: multicentre, randomised controlled trial. Br Med J 2006;332:933–938.

28 Melin L, Frederiksen T, Noren P, Swebilius BG: Behavioural treatment of scratching in patients with atopic dermatitis. Br J Dermatol 1986;115:467–474.

29 Chida Y, Steptoe A, Hirakawa N, Sudo N, Kubo C: The effects of psychological intervention on atopic dermatitis. A systematic review and meta-analysis. Int Arch Allergy Immunol 2007;144:1–9.

30 Koo JYM, Lee CS (eds): Psychocutaneous Medicine. New York, Marcel Dekker, 2003.

31 Lavda AC, Webb TL, Thompson AR: A meta-analysis of the effectiveness of psychological interventions for adults with skin conditions. Br J Dermatol 2012;167:970–979.

32 Bes JD, Legierse CM, Prinsen CAC, de Korte J: Patient education in chronic skin diseases: a systematic review. Acta Derm Venereol 2011;91:12–17.

33 Fordham B, Griffiths CE, Bundy C: Can stress reduction interventions improve psoriasis? A review. Psychol Health Med 2013;18:501–514.

34 Kabat-Zinn J, Wheeler E, Light T, Skillings A, Scharf MJ, Cropley TG, Hosmer D, Bernhard JD: Influence of a mindfulness meditation-based stress reduction intervention on rates of skin clearing in patients with moderate to severe psoriasis undergoing phototherapy (UVB) and photochemotherapy (PUVA). Psychosom Med 1998;60:625–632.

35 Ersser SJ, Cowdell F, Latter S, Gardiner E, Flohr C, Thompson AR, Jackson K, Farasat H, Ware F, Drury A: Psychological and educational interventions for atopic eczema in children. Cochrane Database Syst Rev 2014;1:CD004054.

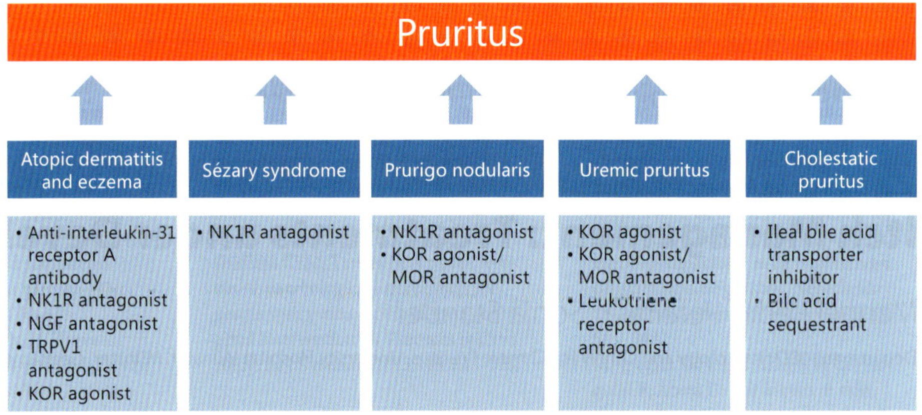

Fig. 1. Novel drugs under development in different conditions causing pruritus. The mechanisms of the drugs being tested in current RCTs are listed separately according to the clinical condition inducing pruritus. NK1R = NK1 receptor; TrkA = tyrosine receptor kinase A; MOR = μ-opioid receptor.

ful in the management of this symptom. The aim of this chapter is to provide an overview of the drugs under development, highlighting the pathophysiological mechanisms they target.

Pruritus: A Symptom of Many Diseases

Dermatological, neurological, and systemic conditions may cause itch. Different pathological mechanisms are involved in each disease and thus pruritus management differs according to its origin [1]. Recent randomized clinical trials (RCTs) have provided important data on novel targets in various conditions causing pruritus. Specifically, novel drugs are being developed for pruritus induced by inflammatory dermatoses (e.g. atopic dermatitis or other types of eczema), systemic conditions (e.g. uremic pruritus, cholestatic pruritus), cutaneous lymphomas (Sézary syndrome), or chronic scratching lesions (prurigo nodularis). Figure 1 illustrates the mechanisms of novel drugs being studied in ongoing RCTs divided by clinical conditions causing itch.

Inflammatory Dermatoses

Antihistamines alone show weak effects in atopic dermatitis. Other drug classes such as topical calcineurin inhibitors, systemic immunosuppressants, anticonvulsants, μ-opioid receptor antagonists, and even antidepressants have shown efficacy in the treatment of pruritus arising from atopic eczema [3, 4]. Recent studies have been able to provide valuable insights into the pathways involved in pruritus processing in inflammatory skin diseases and thus reveal new therapeutic targets.

Anti-Interleukin-31 Receptor A Antibody
Interleukin-31 (IL-31), a cytokine released by CD4+ T cells and Th2 cells, has been shown to play a key role in the processing of pruritus in inflammatory dermatoses, such as atopic dermatitis [5]. In a mouse model of atopic dermatitis, pretreatment with an anti-IL-31 receptor α subunit neutralizing antibody led to suppression of IL-31-induced itch [6]. CIM331, a humanized antihuman IL-31 receptor A antibody showed high antipruritic efficacy in a recently performed phase II RCT [7] (table 1). It will be of interest to see results in a larger popula-

Table 1. Randomized clinical trials

Mechanism	Substance	Route of adminis- tration	Company (clinical trial phase)	Pruritus origin
Anti-interleukin-31 receptor A antibody	CIM331	s.c.	Chugai Pharmaceutical Co. Ltd. (phase II)	atopic dermatitis
NK1R antagonist	aprepitant	p.os.	University of Münster (phase II)	prurigo nodularis
		p.os.	Vanderbilt University (phase IV)	Sézary syndrome
		topical	LEO Pharma (phase II)	prurigo nodularis
	orvepitant	p.os.	NeRRe Therapeutics Ltd. (phase II)	EGFRi-induced rash
	tradipitant	p.os.	Vanda Pharmaceuticals (phase II)	atopic dermatitis
	serlopitant	p.os.	Tigercat Pharma, Inc. (phase II)	prurigo nodularis
		p.os.	Tigercat Pharma Inc. (phase II)	pruritus
		p.os.	Tigercat Pharma Inc. (phase II)	epidermolysis bullosa
NGF antagonist; TrkA kinase inhibitor	CT327	topical	Creabilis SA (phase II)	atopic dermatitis
TRPV1 antagonist	PAC-14028	topical	Amorepacific Corporation (phase II)	eczema
KOR agonist	nalfurafine	i.v.	Toray Industries Inc. (licensed)	uremic pruritus
		p.os.	Mitsubishi Tanabe Pharma Corporation (phase II)	uremic pruritus
	CR845	i.v.	Cara Therapeutics Inc. (phase II)	uremic pruritus
	nalbuphine	p.os.	Trevi (phase II/III)	uremic pruritus
		p.os.	Trevi (phase II/III)	prurigo nodularis
	asimadoline	p.os.	Tioga Pharmaceuticals (phase II)	atopic dermatitis
Leukotriene receptor antagonist	montelukast	p.os.	Shiraz University of Medical Sciences	uremic pruritus
Ileal bile acid transporter inhibitor	LUM001	p.os.	Lumena Pharmaceuticals Inc. (phase II)	progressive familial intrahepatic cholestasis
		p.os.	Lumena Pharmaceuticals Inc. (phase II)	Alagille syndrome
	A4250	p.os.	Sahlgrenska Academy, Sweden (phase II)	primary biliary cirrhosis
	GSK2330672	p.os.	GlaxoSmithKline (phase I)	primary biliary cirrhosis
Bile acid sequestrant	colesevelam	p.os.	Foundation for Liver Research (phase II/III)	cholestatic pruritus
IL-17 inhibitor	secukinumab	s.c.	Novartis Pharmaceuticals (phase III)	psoriasis
Not mentioned	PAC-14028	topical	Ameropacific Corporation (phase II)	skin pruritus
	REGN846 (antibody)	i.v.	Regeneron Pharmaceuticals (phase III)	atopic dermatitis

List of current RCTs performed in patients with pruritus from various origins. Updated and modified from [24]. EGFRi = Epidermal growth factor receptor inhibitor; i.v. = intravenous; NK1R = NK1 receptor; s.c. = subcutaneous; p.os. = per os; TrkA = tyrosine receptor kinase A.

tion and a comparison to the effects of dupilumab, an IL-4/-13 antagonist [8].

Neurokinin 1 Receptor Antagonist
Plasma levels of the neuropeptide substance P are associated with disease activity in atopic dermatitis [9]. Specific sensory nerve terminals distributed throughout the nervous system release substance P and are regulated by neurokinin 1 receptors (NK1R). Consequently, NK1 antagonists induced a reduction in scratching behavior in an atopic dermatitis mouse model [10]. In the clinical setting, off-label use of NK1R antagonists in patients with severe pruritus has shown substantial symptom relief [11]. An ongoing phase II clinical trial is testing the compound tradipitant in patients with atopic dermatitis. Other compounds, aprepitant and serlopitant, are being tested in patients with prurigo nodularis, cutaneous T-cell lymphomas (see Prurigo Nodularis and Cutaneous T-Cell Lymphoma) and epidermolysis bullosa (table 1). In a trial recruiting pa-

tients with chronic pruritus of any type, serlopitant has already proved efficacy [12].

Anti-Nerve Growth Factor Therapy
Increased levels of nerve growth factor (NGF) in the epidermis are associated with increased pruritus in atopic dermatitis [9] and psoriasis. NGF is released, among other agents, by immune system cells including eosinophils, which are present in various inflammatory skin conditions [13]. Supporting the role of this hormone in the transmission of pruritus, anti-NGF antibodies inhibited the development of skin lesions in an atopic dermatitis mouse model [14].

The topical agent CT327, acting as an NGF antagonist by inhibiting the NGF receptor (tyrosine receptor kinase A), is currently being tested in patients with atopic dermatitis and has proven antipruritic effects in psoriasis [15] (table 1). Interestingly, the primary end point (improvement of psoriasis) failed despite the improvement of itch. This points to an important role of NGF in the generation of the symptom over the worsening of the disease. Current trials on psoriasis are investigating both the effect on the disease and on itch with such agents as secukinumab, an IL-17 antagonist.

Other Targets
A topical compound blocking the transient receptor potential cation channel V1 (TRPV1), which also plays a role in pain, itch, and heat transmission, is under development for patients with pruritus arising from eczema, while another RCT is analyzing the effect of oral asimadoline, a κ-opioid receptor (KOR) agonist, on pruritus due to atopic dermatitis.

Cutaneous T-Cell Lymphoma

Paraneoplastic pruritus, for instance pruritus arising from cutaneous T-cell lymphomas, is in most cases resistant to conventional treatments with antidepressants and UV phototherapy [3, 4].

An RCT studying the use of a NK1R antagonist in patients with Sézary syndrome, a form of cutaneous T-cell lymphoma, is underway (table 1).

Prurigo Nodularis

Chronic scratching may lead to secondary lesions of a nodular aspect, which themselves induce severe pruritus [16, 17]. Several topical (calcineurin inhibitors, capsaicin) and systemic therapies (anticonvulsants, antidepressants, μ-opioid receptor antagonists, immunosuppressants) are commonly used to treat this condition [3, 4], often without meaningful outcomes. RCTs with NK1R antagonists are being performed in patients with this condition. Both systemic (aprepitant, serlopitant) and topical (aprepitant) formulations are under development. Additionally, the KOR antagonist nalbuphine is being tested in prurigo nodularis patients (table 1).

Pruritus Induced by Systemic Diseases

KOR Agonists
Pruritus associated with chronic kidney disease is often refractory to the available treatments, such as anticonvulsants, antidepressants, or UV phototherapy [3, 4]. Recently, KOR agonists, acting in the central nervous system, have shown efficacy in the treatment of uremic pruritus. Nalfurafine, which is already licensed in Japan, has shown antipruritic efficacy in previous studies with patients with terminal kidney disease [18, 19] and is currently being tested in RCTs with both its intravenous and oral formulation. Other KOR agonists being developed for uremic pruritus include CR845 and nalbuphine, which additionally acts as a μ-opioid receptor antagonist.

Interestingly, an RCT using the leukotriene receptor antagonist montelukast in patients with uremic pruritus was recently completed (results

are not available yet). A small study has previously shown promising results with this substance
[20].

Cholestatic Pruritus
No antipruritic agents are currently approved for
the treatment of pruritus associated with hepato-
biliary conditions. Antidepressants, both selective serotonin reuptake inhibitors and tetracy-
clics, μ-opioid receptor antagonists, and UV phototherapy have been used in the management of
cholestatic pruritus [3, 4]. Bile acid transporter
inhibitors have now been identified as a possible
new therapeutic option and are being tested for
their antipruritic effects in patients with primary
biliary cirrhosis, as well as in genetic syndromes
causing severe itching (table 1). A previously performed RCT using the compound colesevelam, a
bile acid sequestrant, showed no antipruritic effect [21].

General Considerations and Outlook

Patients with chronic pruritus refractory to approved treatments are highly impaired in their
daily life and experience intense suffering and develop psychiatric comorbidities such as generalized anxiety and chronic depression [22]. The
prescription of off-label medicine may help in
these refractory cases. However, off-label therapies may not be covered by the public health system or by the patients' private insurances, representing a high financial burden to the affected individuals. Furthermore, the use of some drugs,
for instance aprepitant, is only feasible in the hospital environment, and therefore the treatment
with these drugs cannot be continued at home.
RCTs with high-quality standards are thus ur-
gently needed to accelerate the approval of new
drugs for the management of pruritus.

Frequently, chronic pruritus persists after the
underlying cause is treated, which is likely due to
peripheral and central sensitization processes
[23]. Future basic research should address these
chronification mechanisms, while clinical therapeutic studies are essential for the development of
drugs targeting these mechanisms. Here, central
acting drugs may play a pivotal role. However,
these substances are associated with a higher incidence of severe side effects compared to topical
agents. Future research efforts should also focus
on the development of topical compounds, which
can be useful for risk patients such as the elderly,
infants, or patients with multiple systemic comorbidities.

Another aspect to consider is that management of pruritus in specific patient groups, e.g.
children and pregnant or breastfeeding women,
represents a challenge to clinicians since few therapies are approved for these patient groups.
Therefore, future RCTs targeting these specific
groups are needed.

Conclusion

Effective therapies for the various forms of chronic pruritus are still insufficient. Recent research
has provided new insights into pathophysiological mechanisms involved in the transmission of
pruritus arising from different conditions, leading to RCTs testing new compounds directed to
specific targets in pruritus patients due to inflammatory dermatoses, systemic diseases, cutaneous
T-cell lymphoma, and prurigo nodularis. Future
RCTs are needed to broaden the treatment options of acute and chronic pruritus.

References

1 Ständer S, Weisshaar E, Mettang T,
Szepietowski JC, Carstens E, Ikoma A,
Bergasa NV, Gieler U, Misery L, Wallen-
gren J, Darsow U, Streit M, Metze D,
Luger TA, Greaves MW, Schmelz M,
Yosipovitch G, Bernhard JD: Clinical
classification of itch: a position paper of
the International Forum for the Study of
Itch. Acta Derm Venereol 2007;87:291–
294.

2 Pogatzki-Zahn E, Marziniak M, Schneider G, Luger TA, Ständer S: Chronic pruritus: targets, mechanisms and future therapies. Drug News Perspect 2008;21:541–551.
3 Weisshaar E, Szepietowski JC, Darsow U, Misery L, Wallengren J, Mettang T, Gieler U, Lotti T, Lambert J, Maisel P, Streit M, Greaves MW, Carmichael AJ, Tschachler E, Ring J, Ständer S: European guideline on chronic pruritus. Acta Derm Venereol 2012;92:563–581.
4 Ständer S, Darsow U, Mettang T, Gieler U, Maurer M, Stander H, Beuers U, Niemeier V, Gollnick H, Vogelgsang M, Weisshaar E: S2k guideline – chronic pruritus (in German). J Dtsch Dermatol Ges 2012;10(suppl 4):S1–S27.
5 Raap U, Wichmann K, Bruder M, Stander S, Wedi B, Kapp A, Werfel T: Correlation of IL-31 serum levels with severity of atopic dermatitis. J Allergy Clin Immunol 2008;122:421–423.
6 Kasutani K, Fujii E, Ohyama S, Adachi H, Hasegawa M, Kitamura H, Yamashita N: Anti-IL-31 receptor antibody is shown to be a potential therapeutic option for treating itch and dermatitis in mice. Br J Pharmacol 2014;171:5049–5058.
7 Nemoto O, Furue M, Nakagawa H, Shiramoto M, Hanada R, Matsuki S, Imayama S, Kato M, Hasebe I, Taira K, Yamamoto M, Mihara R, Kabashima K, Ruzicka T, Hanifin J, Kumagai Y: The first trial of CIM331, a humanized anti-human IL-31 receptor A antibody, for healthy volunteers and patients with atopic dermatitis to evaluate safety, tolerability and pharmacokinetics of a single dose in a randomised, double-blind, placebo-controlled study. Br J Dermatol 2016;174:296–304.
8 Thaci D, Simpson EL, Beck LA, Bieber T, Blauvelt A, Papp K, Soong W, Worm M, Szepietowski JC, Sofen H, Kawashima M, Wu R, Weinstein SP, Graham NM, Pirozzi G, Teper A, Sutherland ER, Mastey V, Stahl N, Yancopoulos GD, Ardeleanu M: Efficacy and safety of dupilumab in adults with moderate-to-severe atopic dermatitis inadequately controlled by topical treatments: a randomised, placebo-controlled, dose-ranging phase 2b trial. Lancet 2016;387:40–52.
9 Toyoda M, Nakamura M, Makino T, Hino T, Kagoura M, Morohashi M: Nerve growth factor and substance P are useful plasma markers of disease activity in atopic dermatitis. Br J Dermatol 2002;147:71–79.
10 Ohmura T, Hayashi T, Satoh Y, Konomi A, Jung B, Satoh H: Involvement of substance P in scratching behaviour in an atopic dermatitis model. Eur J Pharmacol 2004;491:191–194.
11 Ständer S, Siepmann D, Herrgott I, Sunderkotter C, Luger TA: Targeting the neurokinin receptor 1 with aprepitant: a novel antipruritic strategy. PLoS One 2010;5:e10968.
12 Newswise: Velocity Pharmaceutical Development, Llc and Tigercat Pharma, Inc. announce phase 2 results for Vpd-737 in patients with chronic pruritus. 2014. http://www.newswise.com/articles/velocity-pharmaceutical-development-llc-and-tigercat-pharma-inc-announce-phase-2-results-for-vpd-737-in-patients-with-chronic-pruritus.
13 Liu T, Ji RR: New insights into the mechanisms of itch: are pain and itch controlled by distinct mechanisms? Pflugers Arch 2013;465:1671–1685.
14 Takano N, Sakurai T, Kurachi M: Effects of anti-nerve growth factor antibody on symptoms in the NC/Nga mouse, an atopic dermatitis model. J Pharmacol Sci 2005;99:277–286.
15 Roblin D, Yosipovitch G, Boyce B, Robinson J, Sandy J, Mainero V, Wickramasinghe R, Anand U, Anand P: Topical TrkA kinase inhibitor CT327 is an effective, novel therapy for the treatment of pruritus due to psoriasis: results from experimental studies, and efficacy and safety of CT327 in a phase 2b clinical trial in patients with psoriasis. Acta Derm Venereol 2015;95:542–548.
16 Schedel F, Schürmann C, Metze D, Ständer S: Prurigo. Clinical definition and classification (in German). Hautarzt 2014;65:684–690.
17 Zeidler C, Ständer S: The pathogenesis of prurigo nodularis – 'super-itch' in exploration. Eur J Pain 2016;20:37–40.
18 Inui S: Nalfurafine hydrochloride to treat pruritus: a review. Clin Cosmet Investig Dermatol 2015;8:249–255.
19 Wikstrom B, Gellert R, Ladefoged SD, Danda Y, Akai M, Ide K, Ogasawara M, Kawashima Y, Ueno K, Mori A, Ueno Y: Kappa-opioid system in uremic pruritus: multicenter, randomized, double-blind, placebo-controlled clinical studies. J Am Soc Nephrol 2005;16:3742–3747.
20 Nasrollahi AR, Miladipour A, Ghanei E, Yavari P, Haghverdi F: Montelukast for treatment of refractory pruritus in patients on hemodialysis. Iran J Kidney Dis 2007;1:73–77.
21 Kuiper EM, van Erpecum KJ, Beuers U, Hansen BE, Thio HB, de Man RA, Janssen HL, van Buuren HR: The potent bile acid sequestrant colesevelam is not effective in cholestatic pruritus: results of a double-blind, randomized, placebo-controlled trial. Hepatology 2010;52:1334–1340.
22 Dalgard FJ, Gieler U, Tomas-Aragones L, Lien L, Poot F, Jemec GB, Misery L, Szabo C, Linder D, Sampogna F, Evers AW, Halvorsen JA, Balieva F, Szepietowski J, Romanov D, Marron SE, Altunay IK, Finlay AY, Salek SS, Kupfer J: The psychological burden of skin diseases: a cross-sectional multicenter study among dermatological out-patients in 13 European countries. J Invest Dermatol 2015;135:984–991.
23 Ständer S, Weisshaar E, Luger TA: Neurophysiological and neurochemical basis of modern pruritus treatment. Exp Dermatol 2008;17:161–169.
24 Ständer S, Weisshaar E, Raap U: Emerging drugs for the treatment of pruritus. Expert Opin Emerg Drugs 2015;20:515–521.

Prof. Dr. Dr. Sonja Ständer
Department of Dermatology and Center for Chronic Pruritus
University Hospital Münster, Von-Esmarch-Strasse 58
DE–48149 Münster (Germany)
E-Mail sonja.staender@uni-muenster.de

Szepietowski JC, Weisshaar E (eds): Itch – Management in Clinical Practice.
Curr Probl Dermatol. Basel, Karger, 2016, vol 50, pp 77–85 (DOI: 10.1159/000446047)

Itch in Urticaria Management

Gustavo Deza · Ana M. Giménez-Arnau

Department of Dermatology, Hospital del Mar, Institut Mar d'Investigacions Médiques, Barcelona, Spain

Abstract

Urticaria is a common skin disorder defined by the occurrence of itchy and even painful wheals, angioedema, or both. The lifetime prevalence for its acute and chronic form is 20 and 1%, respectively. The patients' quality of life is impaired because of itch, disfigurement, and high associated comorbidity. To understand the pathophysiology of the wheal in order to ensure a correct therapeutic approach is critical. Mast cells are the primary effector cells in urticaria, which produce and secrete a variety of inflammatory mediators, mainly histamine. Their peripheral effects are responsible for the signs and symptoms of the disease, such as cutaneous swelling and pruritus. Management of itch in urticaria includes both nonpharmacological (avoidance or minimization of aggravating factors) and pharmacological treatments. The main therapeutic objective is to obtain complete relief of signs (hives and angioedema) and symptoms (pruritus) as quickly as possible. Licensed and up-dosed nonsedating H_1-antihistamines are currently the first- and second-line therapies according to the European guidelines. When antihistamines are not enough, other treatments include anti-IgE antibodies, mast cell modulators, mast cell mediator blockers, and immunomodulators. As the knowledge of the pathogenesis of urticaria improves, the development of alternative therapies targeting these pathways may improve the patient's quality of life through the control of the pruritus, its main symptom.

© 2016 S. Karger AG, Basel

Urticaria is a common skin condition defined by the development of wheals, angioedema, or both. A wheal develops rapidly, with central swelling of variable size surrounded by a reflex erythema, and is associated with itching or sometimes a burning sensation. An individual lesion may enlarge, coalesce with other lesions, and typically disappears within 24 h (fig. 1a). Unlike wheals, angioedema involves the lower dermis and subcutis, tends to be painful, and frequently persists for 1–3 days [1, 2] (fig. 1b). Angioedema can be objectified in up to 40–50% of patients with urticaria (wheals) [3], and severe forms of angioedema can be associated with serious complications if the swelling affects the throat or the tongue.

Temporary attacks of urticaria are termed acute, while repeating episodes for longer than 6 weeks are termed chronic. An episode of chronic urticaria can last from 6 months to more than 5

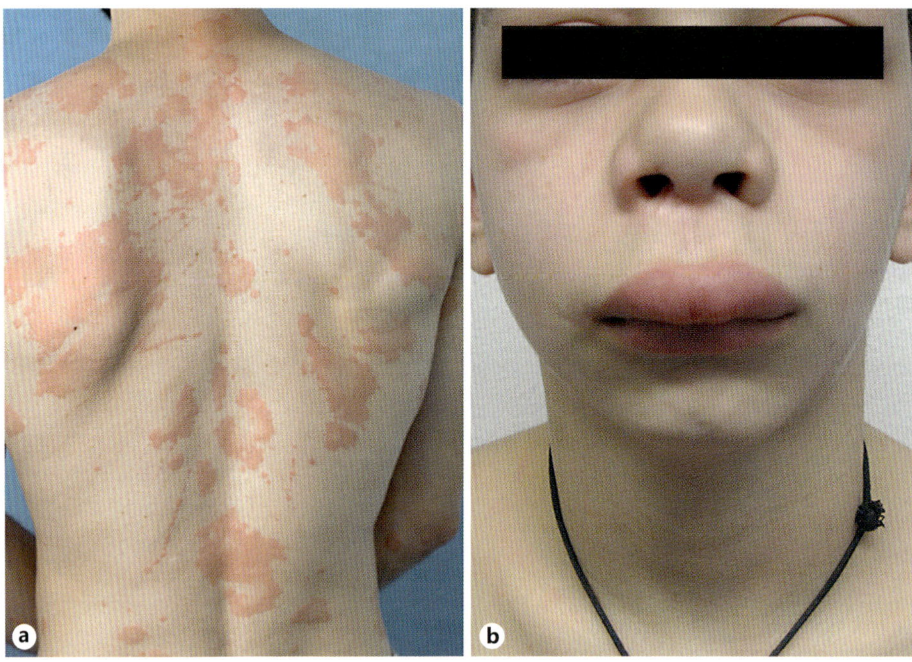

Fig. 1. Clinical appearance of urticaria, presenting as transient pruritic wheals (**a**) or angioedema (**b**).

years. A patient can suffer from more than one episode of acute and chronic urticaria during their life. The overall prevalence of chronic urticaria has been estimated between 1 and 1.5% in the general population, and with a lifetime prevalence of 15–30%, acute spontaneous urticaria represents the most common clinical form [1, 4]. Although urticaria is one of the most frequent skin diseases, very few well-designed studies investigating its prevalence have been reported. Moreover, most of the data are focused on selected patient populations from major European and North American cities with only a few authors attempting to assess prevalence from a global perspective. Notwithstanding, overall prevalence seems to be similar worldwide, although there might be variations in the data due to study methodologies as well as geographical and cultural characteristics [5].

A large number of factors can be responsible for the onset or exacerbation of acute or chronic urticaria episodes. These include mainly drugs, food products, infections, insect stings, physical stimuli (friction, pressure, vibration, cold, heat, and UV light), chemical stimuli (cholinergic, aquagenic, or proteins), and underlying medical diseases [6, 7]. There is not a unique known cause of chronic urticaria for which an autoimmune mechanism has been proposed in a good proportion of patients [8–10]. More than one mechanism can be involved in wheal development simultaneously. At present, chronic spontaneous urticaria of unknown underlying mechanism exists, which demonstrates that a full understanding of the pathogenicity of the disease is still lacking.

Although urticaria is usually not a life-threatening condition and any disfigurement is temporary, its symptoms (cutaneous swelling, itch, and

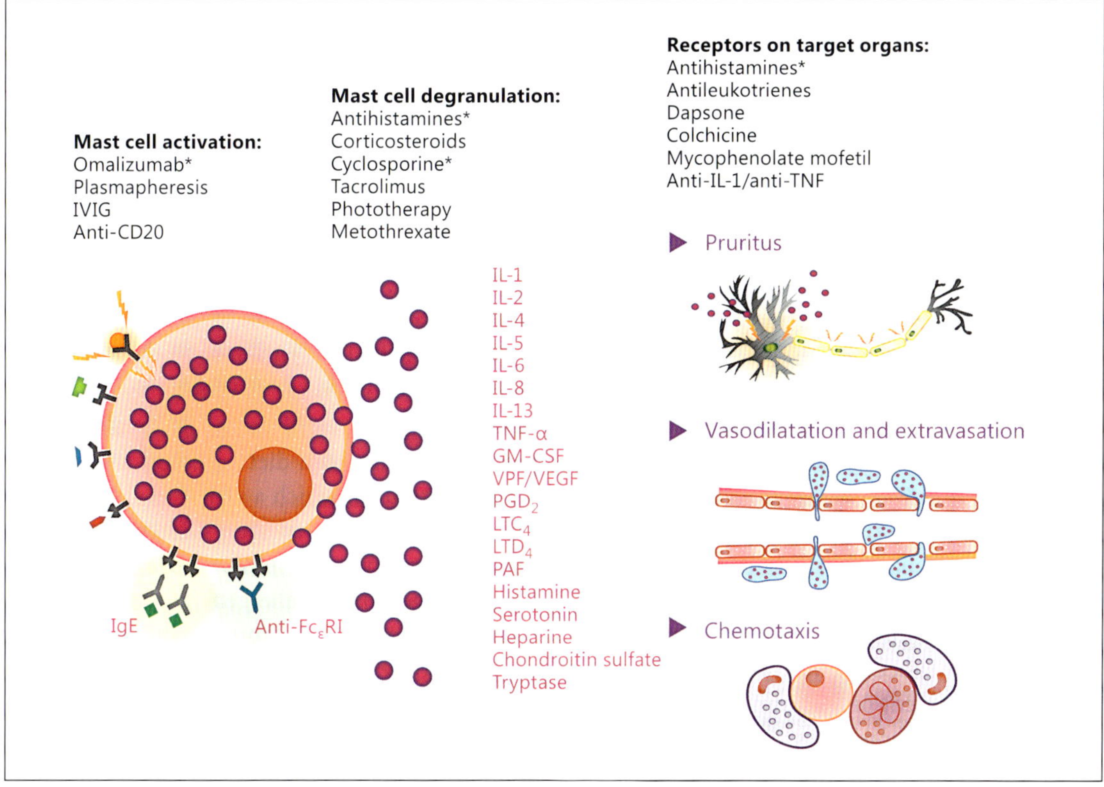

Fig. 2. Pathophysiology of urticaria and mechanism of action of systemic therapies. IVIG = Intravenous immunoglobulin. * Drugs to treat chronic urticaria with a high level of evidence.

pain) may have an impact on various facets of everyday life including home management, personal care, recreation, social interaction, sleep, and work, and health status scores in these patients can be comparable to those reported by patients with coronary artery disease [1, 11].

Pathophysiology of Itch in Urticaria

Mast cells are the main effector cells of urticaria. These cells are distributed throughout the cutaneous surface, but vary in their response to stimuli, and express a multiplicity of cell surface receptors which have the capacity to impact mast cell responses through the regulation of proliferation, migration, and activation. Potential mast cell activators include immunoglobulin E [IgE; the major receptor responsible for regulating mast cell functions is the high-affinity receptor for IgE (FCεRI)] and other nonimmunologic stimuli such as opioids, C5a anaphylatoxin, substance P, enkephalins, and other neuropeptides [7, 12, 13]. The immediate response upon mast cell activation to an appropriate stimulus is degranulation, a process that begins with calcium- and energy-dependent signaling pathways and ends with the fusion of the cytoplasmic granules with the cell membrane, resulting in the release of its contents into the extracellular space (fig. 2). These granules mainly contain histamine, though other preformed and newly synthetized mediators of inally not a life-threatening condition, its symptoms, especially the pruritus, can significantly affect patients' quality of life. While acute urticaria often has an identifiable trigger, chronic urticaria tends to remain idiopathic. First-line treatment is based on the use of nonsedating H_1-antihistamines, whose dose can be increased up to four times the standard dose for achieving symptomatic relief. In nonresponder patients with recalcitrant chronic urticaria, comorbidities and disease characteristics must be assessed individually in order to choose the appropriate alternative treatment. Many aspects in urticaria, especially those concerning the pathophysiology and thus its optimal management, still remain unclear.

References

1 Zuberbier T, Aberer W, Asero R, et al: The EAACI/GA(2) LEN/EDF/WAO guideline for the definition, classification, diagnosis, and management of urticaria: the 2013 revision and update. Allergy 2014;69:868–887.

2 Viegas LP, Ferreira MB, Kaplan AP: The maddening itch: an approach to chronic urticaria. J Investig Allergol Clin Immunol 2014;24:1–5.

3 Soter NA: Acute and chronic urticaria and angioedema. J Am Acad Dermatol 1991;25:146–154.

4 Altman K, Chang C: Pathogenic intracellular and autoimmune mechanisms in urticaria and angioedema. Clin Rev Allergy Immunol 2013;45:47–62.

5 Maurer M, Weller K, Bindslev-Jensen C, et al: Unmet clinical needs in chronic spontaneous urticaria. A GA²LEN task force report. Allergy 2011;66:317–330.

6 Zuberbier T, Iffländer J, Semmler C, Henz BM: Acute urticaria: clinical aspects and therapeutic responsiveness. Acta Derm Venereol 1996;76:295–297.

7 Curto-Barredo L, Silvestre JF, Giménez-Arnau AM: Update on the treatment of chronic urticaria. Actas Dermosifiliogr 2014;105:469–482.

8 Konstantinou GN, Asero R, Maurer M, Sabroe RA, Schmid-Grendelmeier P, Grattan CE: EAACI/GA(2)LEN task force consensus report: the autologous serum skin test in urticaria. Allergy 2009;64:1256–1268.

9 Sabroe RA, Fiebiger E, Francis DM, Maurer D, Seed PT, Grattan CE, Black AK, Stingl G, Greaves MW, Barr RM: Classification of anti-FcepsilonRI and anti-IgE autoantibodies in chronic idiopathic urticaria and correlation with disease severity. J Allergy Clin Immunol 2002;110:492–499.

10 Sabroe RA, Grattan CE, Francis DM, Barr RM, Kobza Black A, Greaves MW: The autologous serum skin test: a screening test for autoantibodies in chronic idiopathic urticaria. Br J Dermatol 1999;140:446–452.

11 O'Donnell BF, Lawlor F, Simpson J, Morgan M, Greaves MW: The impact of chronic urticaria on the quality of life. Br J Dermatol 1997;136:197–201.

12 Thurmond RL, Kazerouni K, Chaplan SR, Greenspan AJ: Antihistamines and itch. Handb Exp Pharmacol 2015;226:257–290.

13 Kikuchi Y, Kaplan AP: A role for C5a in augmenting IgG-dependent histamine release from basophils in chronic urticaria. J Allergy Clin Immunol 2002;109:114–118.

14 Gilfillan AM, Austin SJ, Metcalfe DD: Mast cell biology: introduction and overview. Adv Exp Med Biol 2011;716:2–12.

15 Kaplan AP: Chronic urticaria: pathogenesis and treatment. J Allergy Clin Immunol 2004;114:465–474.

16 Vonakis BM, Saini SS: New concepts in chronic urticaria. Curr Opin Immunol 2008;20:709–716.

17 Khalaf AT, Li W, Jinquan T: Current advances in the management of urticaria. Arch Immunol Ther Exp 2008;56:103–114.

18 Grattan CE: Aspirin sensitivity and urticaria. Clin Exp Dermatol 2003;28:123–127.

19 Murzaku EC, Bronsnick T, Rao BK: Diet in dermatology: part II. Melanoma, chronic urticaria, and psoriasis. J Am Acad Dermatol 2014;71:1053.e1–e16.

20 Bernstein JA, Lang DM, Khan DA, et al: The diagnosis and management of acute and chronic urticaria: 2014 update. J Allergy Clin Immunol 2014;133:1270–1277.

21 Poonawalla T, Kelly B: Urticaria: a review. Am J Clin Dermatol 2009;10:9–21.

22 Epstein S, Rowe RJ: Photoallergy and photocross-sensitivity to phenergan. J Invest Dermatol 1957;29:319–326.

23 Phanuphak P, Schocket AL, Arroyave CM, Kohler PF: Skin histamine in chronic urticaria. J Allergy Clin Immunol 1980;65:371–375.

24 Leurs R, Church MK, Taglialatela M: H_1-antihistamines: inverse agonism, antiinflammatory actions and cardiac effects. Clin Exp Allergy 2002;32:489–498.

25 Jáuregui I, Ferrer M, Montoro J, Dávila I, Bartra J, del Cuvillo A, Mullol J, Sastre J, Valero A: Antihistamines in the treatment of chronic urticaria. J Investig Allergol Clin Immunol 2007;17:41–52.

26 Simons FE: Advances in H_1-antihistamines. N Engl J Med 2004;351:2203–2217.

27 Lee EE, Maibach HI: Treatment of urticaria. An evidence-based evaluation of antihistamines. Am J Clin Dermatol 2001;2:27–32.

28 Kaplan AP: Treatment of chronic spontaneous urticaria. Allergy Asthma Immunol Res 2012;4:326–331.

29 Kaplan AP: Treatment of chronic urticaria: approaches other than antihistamines; in Kaplan A, Greaves M (eds): Urticaria and Angioedema. New York, Informa Healthcare, 2009, pp 365–372.

30 Asero R, Tedeschi A: Usefulness of a short course of oral prednisone in antihistamine-resistant chronic urticaria: a retrospective analysis. J Investig Allergol Clin Immunol 2010;20:386–390.

31 Marsland AM, Soundararajan S, Joseph K, Kaplan AP: Effects of calcineurin inhibitors on an in vitro assay for chronic urticaria. Clin Exp Allergy 2005;35:554–559.

32 Kozel MM, Sabroe RA: Chronic urticaria: aetiology, management and current and future treatment options. Drugs 2004;64:2515–2536.

33 Grattan CE, O'Donnell BF, Francis DM, Niimi N, Barlow RJ, Seed PT, Kobza Black A, Greaves MW: Randomized double-blind study of cyclosporin in chronic 'idiopathic' urticaria. Br J Dermatol 2000;143:365–372.

34 Maxwell DL, Atkinson BA, Spur BW, Lessof MH, Lee TH: Skin responses to intradermal histamine and leukotrienes C_4, D_4, and E_4 in patients with chronic idiopathic urticaria and in normal subjects. J Allergy Clin Immunol 1990;86:759–765.

35 Nettis E, Colanardi MC, Paradiso MT, Ferrannini A: Desloratadine in combination with montelukast in the treatment of chronic urticaria: a randomized, double-blind, placebo-controlled study. Clin Exp Allergy 2004;34:1401–1407.

36 McCormack PL: Omalizumab: a review of its use in patients with chronic spontaneous urticaria. Drugs 2014;74:1693–699.

37 Maurer M, Rosén K, Hsieh HJ, Saini S, Grattan C, Gimenéz-Arnau A, et al: Omalizumab for the treatment of chronic idiopathic or spontaneous urticaria. N Engl J Med 2013;368:924–935.

38 Saini SS, Bindslev-Jensen C, Maurer M, Grob JJ, Bülbül Baskan E, Bradley MS, et al: Efficacy and safety of omalizumab in patients with chronic idiopathic/spontaneous urticaria who remain symptomatic on H_1 antihistamines: a randomized, placebo-controlled study. J Invest Dermatol 2015;135:67–75.

39 Kaplan A, Ledford D, Ashby M, Canvin J, Zazzali JL, Conner E, et al: Omalizumab in patients with symptomatic chronic idiopathic/spontaneous urticaria despite standard combination therapy. J Allergy Clin Immunol 2013;132:101–109.

40 Grattan C, Powell S, Humphreys F, et al: Management and diagnostic guidelines for urticaria and angio-oedema. Br J Dermatol 2001;144:708–714.

Ana M. Giménez-Arnau, MD, PhD
Department of Dermatology
Hospital del Mar – Parc de Salut Mar
Passeig Marítim, 25-29, ES–08003 Barcelona (Spain)
E-Mail anamariagimenezarnau@gmail.com

Szepietowski JC, Weisshaar E (eds): Itch – Management in Clinical Practice.
Curr Probl Dermatol. Basel, Karger, 2016, vol 50, pp 86–93 (DOI: 10.1159/000446048)

Itch in Atopic Dermatitis Management

Yayoi Kamata[a] · Mitsutoshi Tominaga[a] · Kenji Takamori[a, b]

[a]Institute for Environmental and Gender-Specific Medicine, Juntendo University Graduate School of Medicine, and
[b]Department of Dermatology, Juntendo University Urayasu Hospital, Urayasu, Japan

Abstract

Patients with atopic dermatitis (AD) suffer from chronic inflammatory dermatitis and antihistamine-resistant itch. The management of intractable pruritus in AD is important, requiring the development of new therapeutic approaches. At present, the standard treatments for AD include topical anti-inflammatory drugs such as calcineurin inhibitors and corticosteroids. Topical emollient treatment is recommended to moisten the skin and to restore and maintain barrier function. Phototherapy is also effective in reducing the number of epidermal nerve fibers, normalizing imbalances in the levels of expression of axon guidance molecules, and inhibiting pruritus. Systemic treatments such as cyclosporine A and aprepitant are used to treat severe and intractable pruritus in AD. Clinical trials of dupilumab and CIM331 have displayed a significant reduction of pruritus in patients with AD. New antipruritic approaches are targeted to the central nervous system such as spinal interneurons and glial cells. This chapter describes therapeutic approaches for attenuating intractable itch in AD.

Atopic dermatitis (AD) is a common skin disease characterized by dry skin, intense itching, and recurrent eczematous lesions [1]. Generally, intractable itch in patients with AD is resistant to conventional treatments such as H_1-antihistamines [2]. Such intractable itch is a clinical problem that deteriorates the quality of life in AD patients; therefore, development of new antipruritic agents or combinations of agents is needed to reduce intractable itching. Factors involved in histamine-independent itch may include proteases, neuropeptides, cytokines, lipids, and opioids, as well as their cognate receptors, such as protease-activated receptors, Mas-related G protein-coupled receptors, and transient receptor potential channels [2, 3]. In addition, cutaneous hyperinnervation is partly involved in itch sensitization at the periphery [3]. The density of epidermal nerve fibers is higher in skin with epidermal barrier disruption, such as in patients with AD and dry skin, than in healthy skin (fig. 1) [3–5]. This type of epidermal hyperinnervation is mainly caused by an imbalance between nerve elongation factors, including nerve growth factor (NGF), and nerve repulsion factors, such as semaphorin 3A (Sema3A) produced by keratinocytes [3]. Moreover, inflammatory cytokines also play a crucial role in the development of atopic eczema and itch. For example, thymic stromal lymphopoietin was found to promote itch directly by activating cutaneous sensory neurons [6]. Neuropeptides such as substance P, gastrin-releasing peptide, and B-type natriuretic peptide are also involved in AD-associated pruritus [6]. However, the pathological mechanisms of AD-associated pruritus are complex and not fully understood. The simplest treatments of atopic itch are recommended to avoid itch triggers (e.g. dry skin and allergens). Effective treatments include topical and systemic anti-inflammatory agents [7]. This chapter describes the management of atopic itch.

Topical Treatment

Topical agents, including emollients, tacrolimus, and topical corticosteroids, are pivotal in the treatment of atopic itch. They are more successful at reducing atopic itch than systemic treatments [8]. In particular, topical calcineurin inhibitors are the most effective antipruritic agents [8]. Emollients are recommended for mild AD to moisten the skin and to restore and maintain barrier function [6]. Daily application of emollients during the first 32 weeks after birth has been found to reduce the risk of AD in infants [9, 10]. Moreover, using a mouse model of dry skin, topical application of emollients such as heparinoid cream was recently shown to result in greater reductions in epidermal nerve density and epidermal NGF levels than application of petrolatum [4]. In addition, the increase in epidermal nerve fibers was more reduced by the immediate than by the delayed application of emollients to dry

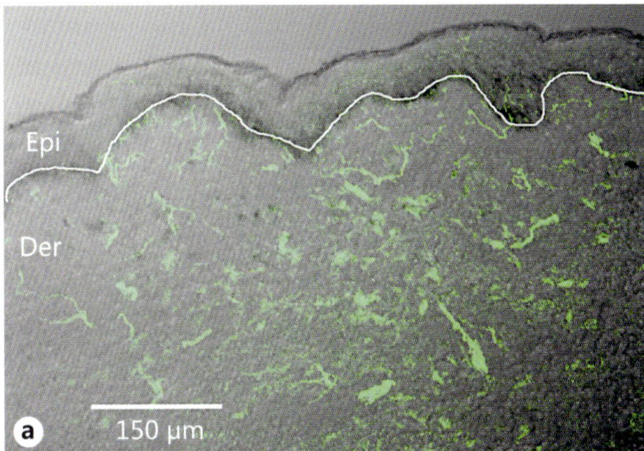

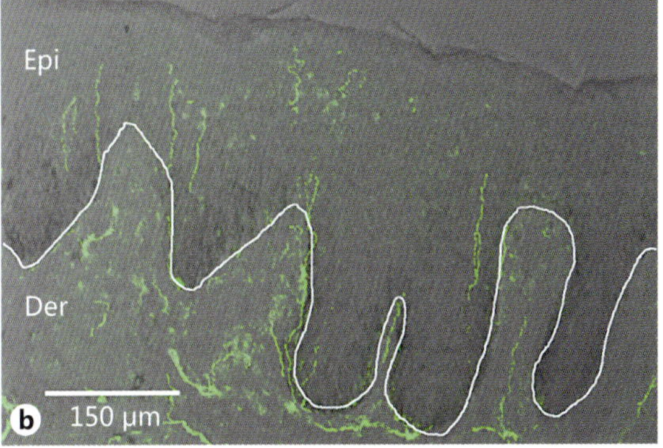

Fig. 1. Distribution of epidermal nerve fibers in normal and atopic skin. Staining of normal healthy skin and lesional skin with AD by antiprotein gene product 9.5 (PGP9.5) antibody. **a** PGP9.5-immunoreactive nerve fibers (green) were mainly distributed in the epidermal-dermal border (white line) of normal healthy skin. **b** Meanwhile, epidermal nerve fibers are present at higher densities in atopic skin.

skin, suggesting that the application of a suitable emollient in the early stage of AD is more effective in normalizing epidermal nerve density. However, heparinoid cream and petrolatum did not improve dermatitis or reduce scratching behavior in AD model mice [11]. Therefore, emollients may be useful preventive agents in the pruritus-associated skin hyperinnervation. Topical calcineurin inhibitors such as tacrolimus and pimecrolimus are nonsteroidal anti-inflammatory drugs available as ointments and creams. Topical calcineurin inhibitors regulate T-cell activation and inhibit release of various inflammatory cytokines [12], as well as reduce pruritus and inflammation in AD [6, 13, 14]. Topical corticosteroids have anti-inflammatory activities rather than acting as direct antipruritics. Randomized controlled trials have shown that topical corticosteroids reduced inflammation and pruritus [6]. These agents may inhibit the action of cytokines and reduce local inflammation, resulting in an indirect control of itch [12].

Systemic Treatment

Evidence for the antipruritic efficacy of H_1-antihismitanes in AD patients is weak worldwide, except in only a few cases [15, 16]. As stated in the European Guideline on AD [17] and the European Guideline on Chronic Pruritus [18], first-generation sedative H_1-antihistamines may be used at the beginning of therapy since they have been reported to be beneficial to patients by improving sleep. Second-generation H_1-antihistamines provide only a weak effect if any [17–21]. Several immunosuppressants, including cyclosporine A (CyA), methotrexate, and azathioprine, have been used to treat pruritus in patients with AD. CyA is currently recommended as a first-line short-term treatment option for patients with moderate-to-severe atopic itch [6, 22]. CyA inhibits T-cell activation and proliferation by blocking nuclear factors associated with cytokine production by activated T cells, including the production of interleukin (IL)-2 and IL-4 [23]. In a mouse model of AD, CyA reduced the number of scratching bouts and epidermal nerve density, and improved dermatitis [24]. Continuous treatment of AD patients with CyA reduced itch severity and then improved dermatitis (fig. 2) [6, 25]. Oral administration of aprepitant, a neurokinin 1 receptor antagonist, has been found to reduce pruritus associated with skin diseases such as AD and prurigo nodularis [26]. Neurotrophin (NTP) is a nonprotein extract isolated from the inflamed skin of rabbits inoculated with vaccinia virus [27]. Clinically, NTP has been shown to have antipruritic effects in patients undergoing hemodialysis [28]. NTP was also reported to reduce intraepidermal nerve growth and to increase epidermal Sema3A mRNA in dry skin model mice [29]. These results suggest that NTP may reduce epidermal nerve density by inducing the expression of Sema3A in the epidermis, resulting in the suppression of pruritus.

Phototherapy

Phototherapy is useful in the treatment of severe AD and associated pruritus [30, 31]. Ultraviolet (UV) A and narrowband (NB)-UVB are effective treatments for the reduction of clinical symptoms [31]. Psoralen UVA (PUVA), bath PUVA, and balneophototherapy have also been shown to have efficacy equal to UVA1 and NB-UVB. It has been reported that these also exert immunosuppressive effects including alteration of cytokine production and both Langerhans cell and eosinophil functions in AD patients [30]. In addition to an anti-inflammatory effect, PUVA and NB-UVB irradiation were shown to reduce the number of epidermal nerve fibers, to normalize imbalances in the expression levels of nerve elongation factors and nerve repulsion factors in lesional skin with AD or psoriasis, and to inhibit pruritus [4, 5, 32]. Recently, excimer lamp treatment was shown to be the most effective form of UV-based therapy for intraepidermal nerve fibers [33].

Adjunctive Therapies

Some patients with AD use adjunctive therapies, including primrose oil supplements, Chinese herbal medicines, and acupuncture, in the treatment of eczema. Evening primrose oil and borage oil supplements have been used orally be-

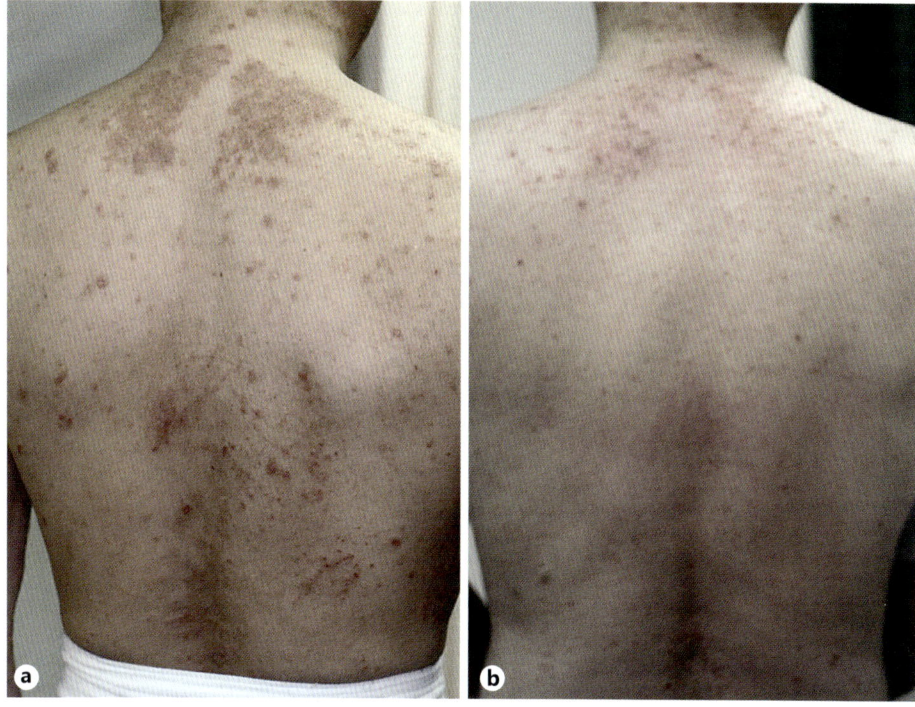

Fig. 2. Effect of CyA in an AD patient. **a** Male 35-year-old patient with AD (SCORAD 43, VAS 80). **b** After 1 month of therapy with oral CyA (3 mg/kg/day). CyA significantly reduced the VAS score and then improved SCORAD (SCORAD 18, VAS 15).

cause of their natural sources of γ-linolenic acid, and these oils are considered to have an anti-inflammatory effect [34, 35]. However, a Cochrane systematic review found no evidence that either evening primrose oil or borage oil were effective in treatment of eczema [34]. Chinese herbal medicines, such as shohusan and yokukansan, were also found to inhibit scratching behavior in AD model mice [36]. Acupuncture is a type of traditional Chinese medicine that involves stimulation of specific points on the skin using needlepoints, pressure, and/or heat. Acupuncture treatment of AD patients significantly reduced the mean visual analogue score (VAS) score compared with control AD patients [37]. However, the evidence is confined to small studies of limited quality.

New Antipruritic Approaches

Histamine H_4 receptor has been shown to play a role in inflammatory responses [16]. A recent report indicated that the H_4-antihistamine JNJ39758979 improved itch in patients with AD [38]. Administration of anti-NGF-neutralizing antibody or the TrkA inhibitors AG879 and K252a to AD model mice significantly attenuated both epidermal nerve fiber density and scratching behavior [40, 41]. Recombinant Sema3A replacement therapies in AD model mice were also found to inhibit scratching behavior and to improve dermatitis [3, 11, 41]. Thus, NGF, Sema3A, and their receptors may be antipruritic targets in patients with pruritic skin diseases such as AD. Dupilumab, a fully human monoclonal antibody

Table 1. Antipruritic therapy of AD

Therapeutic method	Mechanisms of antipruritic effect
Topical treatment	
Calcineurin inhibitor [12–14] Tacrolimus, pimecrolimus	Regulation of T-cell activation Inhibition of release of inflammatory cytokines
Corticosteroids [6, 12]	Inhibition of release of inflammatory cytokines Reduction of local inflammation (indirect effect)
Emollients [4, 9, 10, 11] Heparinoid	Reduction of epidermal nerve density
Systemic treatment	
Aprepitant [26]	Neurokinin 1 receptor antagonist → Inhibition of substance P
Calcineurin inhibitor [6, 22–25] CyA	Regulation of T-cell activation Inhibition of release of inflammatory cytokines
H_1-antihistamines [15–21]	Weak evidence
Neurotrophin [27–29]	Reduction of epidermal nerve density
Phototherapy	

Phototherapy [5, 30–33]
    UVA, PUVA
    NB-UVB
    Excimer lamp
	Immunosuppressive effects
	Reduction of epidermal nerve density
	    Indirect effect: normalization of expression levels
	    of axon guidance molecules
	    Direct effect (e.g. excimer lamp)

Adjunctive treatment	
Acupuncture [37] Chinese herbal medicine [35, 36] Primrose oil [34, 35]	Weak evidence
New therapeutic approaches	
Histamine H_4 receptor antagonist [38] JNJ 39758979	Inhibition of histamine H_4 receptor → Block of inflammatory responses
Recombinant Sema3A replacement therapy [3, 11, 41]	Reduction of epidermal nerve density

Anti-NGF therapy [39, 40]
    Anti-NGF neutralizing antibody
    TrkA inhibitor
	Inhibition of NGF signaling
	→ Reduction of epidermal nerve density

Dupilumab [42, 43]	Anti-IL-4 and IL-13 antibody → Block signaling of both IL-4 and IL-13
CIM331[44]	Anti-IL-31 receptor A antibody → Block signaling of IL-31
SVmab1[45]	Anti-voltage-gated sodium channel Nav1.7-specific antibody → Block signaling of Nav1.7
Naltrexone [47]	μ-Opioid receptor antagonist → Block signaling of μ-opioid
Minocycline [49]	Inhibitor of activated microglia → Inhibition of microglial activation
AG490 [50]	Inhibitor of STAT3 activator Janus kinase → Inhibition of STAT3-dependent reactive astrocyte
Neurotransplant [48]	Compensation of spinal inhibitory interneurons

that blocks signaling from both IL-4 and IL-13, also significantly reduced the severity and pruritus score in AD [42, 43]. Similar results were obtained using CIM331, a humanized anti-human IL-31 receptor A monoclonal antibody [44]. In addition, SVmab1, a voltage-gated sodium channel Nav1.7-specific antibody, was found to attenuate scratching behavior in mouse models [45]. Peripheral opioid systems may also play important roles in pruritus [46]. For example, μ-opioid receptor antagonists (e.g. naltrexone) significant relieved pruritus in patients with AD [47]. More recently, Basbaum and Bráz [48] reported that transplants of inhibitory interneuron are effective in a chronic neuropathic itch model in which there was a significant loss of dorsal horn inhibitory interneurons. Intrathecal administration of activated microglia inhibitor (e.g. minocycline) dose- and time-dependently suppressed scratching behavior and improved dermatitis in Dfb-treated NC/Nga mice [49]. Shiratori-Hayashi et al. [50] has described that signal transducer and activator of transcription (STAT) 3-dependent reactive astrocytes act as critical amplifiers of itching. Intrathecal administration of AG490 (inhibitor of the STAT3 activator Janus kinase) abolished the increase in gastrin-releasing peptide-evoked scratching in AD model mice [50]. These new strategies may also be effective in patients with AD.

Conclusion

This chapter describes recent knowledge regarding the control of pruritus in patients with AD (table 1). Currently, the most effective treatments for pruritus with AD primarily target inflammation (e.g. tacrolimus and CyA). Treatment with anti-NGF agents, Sema3A replacement, and other treatments such as UV-based therapy may normalize epidermal nerve fiber density. New therapeutic approaches are required to improve the quality of life of patients with AD and intractable itch.

References

1 Weidinger S, Novak N: Atopic dermatitis. Lancet 2016;387:1109–1122.
2 Ikoma A, Steinhoff M, Ständer S, Yosipovitch G, Schmelz M: The neurobiology of itch. Nat Rev Neurosci 2006;7:535–547.
3 Tominaga M, Takamori K: Itch and nerve fibers with special reference to atopic dermatitis: therapeutic implications. J Dermatol 2014;41:205–212.
4 Kamo A, Tominaga M, Negi O, Tengara S, Ogawa H, Takamori K: Topical application of emollients prevents dry skin-inducible intraepidermal nerve growth in acetone-treated mice. J Dermatol Sci 2011;62:64–66.
5 Tominaga M, Tengara S, Kamo A, Ogawa H, Takamori K: Psoralen-ultraviolet A therapy alters epidermal Sema3A and NGF levels and modulates epidermal innervation in atopic dermatitis. J Dermatol Sci 2009;55:40–46.
6 Mollanazar NK, Smith PK, Yosipovitch G: Mediators of chronic pruritus in atopic dermatitis: getting the itch out? Clin Rev Allergy Immunol 2015, DOI: 10.1007/s12016-015-8488-5.
7 Yarbrough KB, Neuhaus KJ, Simpson EL: The effects of treatment on itch in atopic dermatitis. Dermatol Ther 2013;26:110–119.
8 Sher LG, Chang J, Patel IB, Balkrishnan R, Fleischer AB Jr: Relieving the pruritus of atopic dermatitis: a meta-analysis. Acta Derm Venereol 2012;92:455–461.
9 Horimukai K, Morita K, Narita M, Kondo M, Kitazawa H, Nozaki M, Shigematsu Y, Yoshida K, Niizeki H, Motomura K, Sago H, Takimoto T, Inoue E, Kamemura N, Kido H, Hisatsune J, Sugai M, Murota H, Katayama I, Sasaki T, Amagai M, Morita H, Matsuda A, Matsumoto K, Saito H, Ohya Y: Application of moisturizer to neonates prevents development of atopic dermatitis. J Allergy Clin Immunol 2014;134:824–830.
10 Simpson EL, Chalmers JR, Hanifin JM, Thomas KS, Cork MJ, McLean WH, Brown SJ, Chen Z, Chen Y, Williams HC: Emollient enhancement of the skin barrier from birth offers effective atopic dermatitis prevention. J Allergy Clin Immunol 2014:134:818–823.
11 Negi O, Tominaga M, Tengara S, Kamo A, Taneda K, Suga Y, Ogawa H, Takamori K: Topically applied semaphorin 3A ointment inhibits scratching behavior and improves skin inflammation in NC/Nga mice with atopic dermatitis. J Dermatol Sci 2012;66:37–43.
12 Elmariah SB, Lerner EA: Topical therapies for pruritus. Semin Cutan Med Surg 2011;30:118–126.
13 Ständer S, Schürmeyer-Horst F, Luger TA, Weisshaar E: Treatment of pruritic diseases with topical calcineurin inhibitors. Ther Clin Risk Manag 2006;2:213–218.

14 Cury Martins J, Martins C, Aoki V, Gois AF, Ishii HA, da Silva EM: Topical tacrolimus for atopic dermatitis. Cochrane Database Syst Rev 2015;7:CD009864.

15 Kawashima M, Tango T, Noguchi T, Inagi M, Nakagawa H, Harada S: Addition of fexofenadine to a topical corticosteroid reduces the pruritus associated with atopic dermatitis in a 1-week randomized, multicentre, double-blind, placebo-controlled, parallel-group study. Br J Dermatol 2003;148:1212–1221.

16 Ohsawa Y, Hirasawa N: The role of histamine H_1 and H_4 receptors in atopic dermatitis: from basic research to clinical study. Allergol Int 2014;63:533–542.

17 Ring J, Alomar A, Bieber T, Deleuran M, Fink-Wagner A, Gelmetti C, Gieler U, Lipozencic J, Luger T, Oranje AP, Schäfer T, Schwennesen T, Seidenari S, Simon D, Ständer S, Stingl G, Szalai S, Szepietowski JC, Taïeb A, Werfel T, Wollenberg A, Darsow U; European Dermatology Forum (EDF); European Academy of Dermatology and Venereology (EADV); European Federation of Allergy (EFA); European Task Force on Atopic Dermatitis (ETFAD); European Society of Pediatric Dermatology (ESPD); Global Allergy and Asthma European Network (GA2LEN): Guidelines for treatment of atopic eczema (atopic dermatitis) part I. J Eur Acad Dermatol Venereol 2012;26:1045–1060.

18 Weisshaar E, Szepietowski JC, Darsow U, Misery L, Wallengren J, Mettang T, Gieler U, Lotti T, Lambert J, Maisel P, Streit M, Greaves MW, Carmichael AJ, Tschachler E, Ring J, Ständer S: European guideline on chronic pruritus. Acta Derm Venereol 2012;92:563–581.

19 Simons FE, Simons KJ: Histamine and H_1-antihistamines: celebrating a century of progress. J Allergy Clin Immunol 2011;128:1139–1150.

20 Thurmond RL, Kazerouni K, Chaplan SR, Greenspan AJ: Peripheral neuronal mechanism of itch: histamine and itch. Carstens E and Akiyama T (eds): Itch: Mechanisms and Treatment. Boca Raton, CRC Press/Taylor & Francis, 2014.

21 Apfelbacher CJ, van Zuuren EJ, Fedorowicz Z, Jupiter A, Matterne U, Weisshaar E: Oral H_1 antihistamines as monotherapy for eczema. Cochrane Database Syst Rev 2013;2:CD007770.

22 Roekevisch E, Spuls PI, Kuester D, Limpens J, Schmitt J: Efficacy and safety of systemic treatments for moderate-to-severe atopic dermatitis: a systematic review. J Allergy Clin Immunol 2014;133:429–438.

23 Azzi JR, Sayegh MH, Mallat SG: Calcineurin inhibitors: 40 years later, can't live without. J Immunol 2013;191:5785–5791.

24 Ko KC, Tominaga M, Kamata Y, Umehara Y, Matsuda H, Takahashi N, Kina K, Ogawa M, Ogawa H, Takamori K: Possible anti-pruritic mechanism of cyclosporine A in atopic dermatitis. Acta Derm Venereol 2016, in press.

25 Harper JI, Ahmed I, Barclay G, Lacour M, Hoeger P, Cork MJ, Finlay AY, Wilson NJ, Graham-Brown RA, Sowden JM, Beard AL, Sumner MJ, Berth-Jones J: Cyclosporin for severe childhood atopic dermatitis: short course versus continuous therapy. Br J Dermatol 2000;142:52–58.

26 Ständer S, Siepmann D, Herrgott I, Sunderkötter C, Luger TA: Targeting the neurokinin receptor 1 with aprepitant: a novel antipruritic strategy. PLoS One 2010;5:e10968.

27 Yoshii H, Suehiro S, Watanabe K, Yanagihara Y: Immunopharmacological actions of an extract isolated from inflamed skin of rabbits inoculated with vaccinia virus (neurotropin); enhancing effect on delayed type hypersensitivity response through the induction of Lyt-1+2– T cells. Int J Immunopharmacol 1987;9:443–451.

28 Kaku H, Fujita Y, Yago H, Naka F, Kawakubo H, Nakano K, Nishikawa K, Suehiro S: Study on pruritus in hemodialysis patients and the antipruritic effect of neurotropin: plasma levels of substance P, somatostatin, IgE, PTH and histamine. Nihon Jinzo Gakkai Shi 1990;32:319–326.

29 Kamo A, Tominaga M, Taneda K, Ogawa H, Takamori K: Neurotropin inhibits the increase in intraepidermal nerve density in the acetone-treated dry-skin mouse model. Clin Exp Dermatol 2013;38:665–668.

30 Rivard J, Lim HW: Ultraviolet phototherapy for pruritus. Dermatol Ther 2005;18:344–354.

31 Garritsen FM, Brouwer MW, Limpens J, Spuls PI. Photo(chemo)therapy in the management of atopic dermatitis: an updated systematic review with implications for practice and research. Br J Dermatol 2014;170:501–513.

32 Wallengren J, Sundler F: Phototherapy reduces the number of epidermal and CGRP-positive dermal nerve fibres. Acta Derm Venereol 2004;84:111–115.

33 Kamo A, Tominaga M, Kamata Y, Kaneda K, Ko KC, Matsuda H, Kimura U, Ogawa H, Takamori K: The excimer lamp induces cutaneous nerve degeneration and reduces scratching in a dry-skin mouse model. J Invest Dermatol 2014;134:2977–2984.

34 Bamford JT, Ray S, Musekiwa A, van Gool C, Humphreys R, Ernst E: Oral evening primrose oil and borage oil for eczema. Cochrane Database Syst Rev 2013;4:CD004416.

35 Sidbury R, Tom WL, Bergman JN, Cooper KD, Silverman RA, Berger TG, Chamlin SL, Cohen DE, Cordoro KM, Davis DM, Feldman SR, Hanifin JM, Krol A, Margolis DJ, Paller AS, Schwarzenberger K, Simpson EL, Williams HC, Elmets CA, Block J, Harrod CG, Smith Begolka W, Eichenfield LF: Guidelines of care for the management of atopic dermatitis: section 4. Prevention of disease flares and use of adjunctive therapies and approaches. J Am Acad Dermatol 2014;71:1218–1233.

36 Yamashita H, Tanaka H, Inagaki N: Treatment of the chronic itch of atopic dermatitis using standard drugs and kampo medicines. Biol Pharm Bull 2013;36:1253–1257.

37 Ma C, Sivamani RK: Acupuncture as a treatment modality in dermatology: a systematic review. J Altern Complement Med 2015;21:520–529.

38 Murata Y, Song M, Kikuchi H, Hisamichi K, Xu XL, Greenspan A, Kato M, Chiou CF, Kato T, Guzzo C, Thurmond RL, Ohtsuki M, Furue M: Phase 2a, randomized, double-blind, placebo-controlled, multicenter, parallel-group study of a H_4R-antagonist (JNJ-39758979) in Japanese adults with moderate atopic dermatitis. J Dermatol 2015;42:129–139.

39 Takano N, Sakurai T, Kurachi M: Effects of anti-nerve growth factor antibody on symptoms in the NC/Nga mouse, an atopic dermatitis model. J Pharmacol Sci 2005;99:277–286.

40 Takano N, Sakurai T, Ohashi Y, Kurachi M: Effects of high-affinity nerve growth factor receptor inhibitors on symptoms in the NC/Nga mouse atopic dermatitis model. Br J Dermatol 2007;156:241–246.

41 Yamaguchi J, Nakamura F, Aihara M, Yamashita N, Usui H, Hida T, Takei K, Nagashima Y, Ikezawa Z, Goshima Y: Semaphorin3A alleviates skin lesions and scratching behavior in NC/Nga mice, an atopic dermatitis model. J Invest Dermatol 2008;128:2842–2849.

42 Beck LA, Thaçi D, Hamilton JD, Graham NM, Bieber T, Rocklin R, Ming JE, Ren H, Kao R, Simpson E, Ardeleanu M, Weinstein SP, Pirozzi G, Guttman-Yassky E, Suárez-Fariñas M, Hager MD, Stahl N, Yancopoulos GD, Radin AR: Dupilumab treatment in adults with moderate-to-severe atopic dermatitis. N Engl J Med 2014;371: 130–139.

43 Thaçi D, Simpson EL, Beck LA, Bieber T, Blauvelt A, Papp K, Soong W, Worm M, Szepietowski JC, Sofen H, Kawashima M, Wu R, Weinstein SP, Graham NM, Pirozzi G, Teper A, Sutherland ER, Mastey V, Stahl N, Yancopoulos GD, Ardeleanu M: Efficacy and safety of dupilumab in adults with moderate-to-se-

vere atopic dermatitis inadequately controlled by topical treatments: a randomised, placebo-controlled, dose-ranging phase 2b trial. Lancet 2016;387: 40–52.

44 Nemoto O, Furue M, Nakagawa H, Shiramoto M, Hanada R, Matsuki S, Imayama S, Kato M, Hasebe I, Taira K, Yamamoto M, Mihara R, Kabashima K, Ruzicka T, Hanifin J, Kumagai Y: The first trial of CIM331, a humanized anti-human IL-31 receptor A antibody, for healthy volunteers and patients with atopic dermatitis to evaluate safety, tolerability and pharmacokinetics of a single dose in a randomised, double-blind, placebo-controlled study. Br J Dermatol 2016;174:296–304.

45 Lee JH, Park CK, Chen G, Han Q, Xie RG, Liu T, Ji RR, Lee SY: A monoclonal antibody that targets a NaV1.7 channel voltage sensor for pain and itch relief. Cell 2014;157:1393–1404.

46 Tominaga M, Ogawa H, Takamori K: Possible roles of epidermal opioid sys-

tems in pruritus of atopic dermatitis. J Invest Dermatol 2007;127:2228–2235.

47 Phan NQ, Bernhard JD, Luger TA, Ständer S: Antipruritic treatment with systemic μ-opioid receptor antagonists: a review. J Am Acad Dermatol 2010;63: 680–688.

48 Basbaum AI, Bráz JM: Cell transplants to treat the 'disease' of neuropathic pain and itch. Pain 2016;157(suppl 1):S42–S47.

49 Torigoe K, Tominaga M, Ko KC, Takahashi N, Matsuda H, Hayashi R, Ogawa H, Takamori K: Intrathecal minocycline suppresses itch-related behavior and improves dermatitis in a mouse model of atopic dermatitis. J Invest Dermatol 2016;136:879–881.

50 Shiratori-Hayashi M, Koga K, Tozaki-Saitoh H, Kohro Y, Toyonaga H, Yamaguchi C, Hasegawa A, Nakahara T, Hachisuka J, Akira S, Okano H, Furue M, Inoue K, Tsuda M: STAT3-dependent reactive astrogliosis in the spinal dorsal horn underlies chronic itch. Nat Med 2015;21:927–931.

Kenji Takamori, MD, PhD
Department of Dermatology, Juntendo University Urayasu Hospital
2-1-1 Tomioka Urayasu, Chiba 279-0021 (Japan)
E-Mail ktakamor@juntendo.ac.jp

Szepietowski JC, Weisshaar E (eds): Itch – Management in Clinical Practice.
Curr Probl Dermatol. Basel, Karger, 2016, vol 50, pp 94–101 (DOI: 10.1159/000446049)

Prurigo Nodularis Management

Athanasios Tsianakas · Claudia Zeidler · Sonja Ständer

Department of Dermatology and Center for Chronic Pruritus, University Hospital Münster, Münster, Germany

Abstract

Characterized by the clinical presentation of individual to multiple symmetrically distributed, hyperkeratotic, and intensely itchy papules and nodules, prurigo nodularis (PN) is a rare disease that emerges in patients with chronic pruritus due to continuous scratching over a long period of time. The itching and scratching of the lesions contribute to the vicious cycle that makes this disease difficult to treat, thus reducing the quality of life of affected patients. The pathogenesis of PN is ambiguous, although immunoneuronal crosstalk is implicated. Its etiology was found to be heterogenous. It can emerge as the symptom of various dermatological, neurological, psychiatric, and systemic diseases. There is currently no approved therapy for PN. However, contemporary therapies consist of calcineurin inhibitors, capsaicin, topical steroids, UV therapy, and a systemic application of antihistamines, anticonvulsants, μ-opioid receptor antagonists, and immunosuppressants. Multimodal therapy should be utilized in order to achieve optimal results, including topical and systemic symptomatic therapies.

Prurigo nodularis (PN) is a disease identified by the appearance of individual or multiple symmetrically distributed, hyperkeratotic, and erosive papules and nodules on the surface of the skin. There is currently no epidemiological data regarding the incidence and prevalence of PN. Affected patients seldom present in the daily clinical practice, thus making it difficult to document the many contributing factors. All age groups are impacted by PN, including the elderly (the most frequently affected group) and children [1, 2]. Long-term scratching in patients with chronic pruritus is the reason for the development of PN. The resulting lesions are intensely itchy, perpetuating the vicious itch-scratch cycle that makes PN difficult to treat and reducing patient quality of life. PN has various causes. 50% of patients with PN also suffer from atopic predisposition or atopic eczema [3]. Other diseases also contribute to the emergence of PN, including inflammatory dermatoses (e.g. bullous pemphigoid, lichen planus, nummular eczema), internal diseases (e.g. diabetes mellitus, chronic kidney disease), infections (e.g. HIV, hepatitis C), lymphoma (e.g. Hodgkin's lymphoma), carcinomas, and neurological/psychiatric diseases.

Therapy of Prurigo Nodularis

Establishing treatments for PN remains challenging and is made only more difficult by the small amount of randomized clinical trials (RCTs) available. In order to achieve optimal results, a multimodal therapy consisting of topical and systemic symptomatic therapies should be implemented [4]. Various factors must also be taken into consideration when creating an individual treatment plan. These include age, comorbidities, severity, impaired quality of life, and expected side effects. Washing exclusively with mild soaps and shower oils and maintaining a moisturizing basis therapy are recommended basic care procedures. A causal therapy strategy is very important and implements treatment of a potentially underlying disease which can lead to the improvement or sometimes even healing of PN (e.g. intensive therapy of diabetes in diabetogenic PN) [5]. Physicians should aim for two goals concerning symptomatic therapy: itch prevention and the complete healing of PN lesions. These normally require a combined therapy, considering the aspects mentioned above (for PN treatment options in clinical trials see table 1).

Topical Therapy of PN
Topical steroids, calcipotriol, and pimecrolimus have previously been analyzed in RCTs with regards to topical PN therapies. All remaining substances have been described in case series.

Topical Steroids
Topical steroids can produce an antipruritic effect and flatten nodules attributed to PN [6]. The occlusive application of betamethasone 0.1% cream on one side of the body and a moisturizing, antipruritic cream on the other was observed over 4 weeks in an RCT involving 12 patients with PN. A significant reduction in pruritus was noted in both treated areas, but its intensity was markedly reduced on the half of the body treated with betamethasone [visual analogue scale (VAS) before: 8.8, VAS after: 3.9; in comparison to the moisturizing, antipruritic cream, VAS 5.6 afterwards].

Clinical improvement was also observed following the direct injection of triamcinolone acetonide into the nodules [7]. This can be promising if the clinical picture of PN only shows few lesions.

Topical Calcineurin Inhibitors
Topical calcineurin inhibitors, in contrast to topical steroids, represent an intermittent, long-term therapeutic opportunity. The antipruritic effect of pimecrolimus on PN was recently determined in an RCT consisting of 30 participants, during which pimecrolimus was applied to one half of the patient's bodies, and hydrocortisone on the other. Both halves of the body yielded positive results after 10 days (VAS before 7.1, VAS after pimecrolimus 4.4, p < 0.001; VAS after hydrocortisone 4.5, p < 0.001) [8]. This treatment was used consistently for 8 weeks and resulted in a distinct improvement, according to findings. In daily practice, calcineurin inhibitors are used after failure of, or in case of contraindications for, topical steroids.

Topical Calcipotriol
Topical calcipotriol has also been proven to be effective in treating PN. A 50-µg/g calcipotriol ointment was applied to one half of the body and 0.1% betamethasone ointment to the other in an RCT consisting of 10 patients. Treatment with the calcipotriol ointment proved more successful. Two weeks of using this ointment resulted in less PN lesions than 4 weeks of treatment with betamethasone valerate [9].

Conclusion

PN is a disease representing a therapeutic challenge. Despite this, current RCTs conducted on novel targets, including neurokinin 1 inhibitors and opioid receptors, offer hope in providing targeted treatment for this intensely itchy disease.

Acknowledgements

We thank Emily Burnett for the help in preparation of the manuscript. This chapter was funded by the German Federal Ministry of Education and Research (BMBF; No. 01KG1305).

References

1 Iking A, Grundmann S, Chatzigeorgakidis E, et al: Prurigo as a symptom of atopic and non-atopic diseases: aetiological survey in a consecutive cohort of 108 patients. J Eur Acad Dermatol Venereol 2013;27:550–557.

2 Amer A, Fischer H: Prurigo nodularis in a 9-year-old girl. Clin Pediatr 2009;48:93–95.

3 Tanaka M, Aiba S, Matsumura N, et al: Prurigo nodularis consists of two distinct forms: early-onset atopic and late-onset non-atopic. Dermatology 1995;190:269–276.

4 Weisshaar E, Szepietowski JC, Darsow U, et al: European guideline on chronic pruritus. Acta Derm Venereol 2012;92:563–581.

5 Ko M, Chiu H, Jee S, et al: Postprandial blood glucose is associated with generalized pruritus in patients with type 2 diabetes. Eur J Dermatol 2013;23:688–693.

6 Saraceno R, Chiricozzi A, Nisticò SP, et al: An occlusive dressing containing betamethasone valerate 0.1% for the treatment of prurigo nodularis. J Dermatolog Treat 2010;21:363–366.

7 Richards RN: Update on intralesional steroid: focus on dermatoses. J Cutan Med Surg 2010;14:19–23.

8 Siepmann D, Lotts T, Blome C, et al: Evaluation of the antipruritic effects of topical pimecrolimus in non-atopic prurigo nodularis: results of a randomized, hydrocortisone-controlled, double-blind phase II trial. Dermatology 2013;227:353–360.

9 Wong SS, Goh CL: Double-blind, right/left comparison of calcipotriol ointment and betamethasone ointment in the treatment of prurigo nodularis. Arch Dermatol 2000;136:807–808.

10 Ständer S, Luger T, Metze D: Treatment of prurigo nodularis with topical capsaicin. J Am Acad Dermatol 2001;44:471–478.

11 Ständer S, Moormann C, Schumacher M, et al: Expression of vanilloid receptor subtype 1 in cutaneous sensory nerve fibers, mast cells, and epithelial cells of appendage structures. Exp Dermatol 2004;13:129–139.

12 Griffin JR, Davis, Mark DP: Amitriptyline/ketamine as therapy for neuropathic pruritus and pain secondary to herpes zoster. J Drugs Dermatol 2015;14:115–118.

13 Schulz S, Metz M, Siepmann D, et al: Antipruritische Wirksamkeit einer hoch dosierten Antihistaminikatherapie. Ergebnisse einer retrospektiv analysierten Fallserie. Hautarzt 2009;60:564–568.

14 Shintani T, Ohata C, Koga H, et al: Combination therapy of fexofenadine and montelukast is effective in prurigo nodularis and pemphigoid nodularis. Dermatol Ther 2014;27:135–139.

15 Hammes S, Hermann J, Roos S, et al: UVB 308-nm excimer light and bath PUVA: combination therapy is very effective in the treatment of prurigo nodularis. J Eur Acad Dermatol Venereol 2011;25:799–803.

16 Tamagawa-Mineoka R, Katoh N, Ueda E, et al: Narrow-band ultraviolet B phototherapy in patients with recalcitrant nodular prurigo. J Dermatol 2007;34:691–695.

17 Bruni E, Caccialanza M, Piccinno R: Phototherapy of generalized prurigo nodularis. Clin Exp Dermatol 2010;35:549–550.

18 Sorenson E, Levin E, Koo J, et al: Successful use of a modified Goeckerman regimen in the treatment of generalized prurigo nodularis. J Am Acad Dermatol 2015;72:e40–e42.

19 Paghdal KV, Schwartz RA: Topical tar: back to the future. J Am Acad Dermatol 2009;61:294–302.

20 Gunal AI, Ozalp G, Yoldas TK, et al: Gabapentin therapy for pruritus in haemodialysis patients: a randomized, placebo-controlled, double-blind trial. Nephrol Dial Transplant 2004;19:3137–3139.

21 Gencoglan G, Inanir I, Gunduz K: Therapeutic hotline: treatment of prurigo nodularis and lichen simplex chronicus with gabapentin. Dermatol Ther 2010;23:194–198.

22 Mazza M, Guerriero G, Marano G, et al: Treatment of prurigo nodularis with pregabalin. J Clin Pharm Ther 2013;38:16–18.

23 Scheinfeld N: The role of gabapentin in treating diseases with cutaneous manifestations and pain. Int J Dermatol 2003;42:491–495.

24 Phan NQ, Lotts T, Antal A, et al: Systemic kappa opioid receptor agonists in the treatment of chronic pruritus: a literature review. Acta Derm Venereol 2012;92:555–560.

25 Bergasa NV: The pruritus of cholestasis: facts. Hepatology 2015;61:2114.

26 Brune A, Metze D, Luger TA, et al: Antipruritische Therapie mit dem oralen Opiatrezeptorantagonisten Naltrexon. Offene, nicht placebokontrollierte Anwendung bei 133 Patienten. Hautarzt 2004;55:1130–1136.

27 Dawn AG, Yosipovitch G: Butorphanol for treatment of intractable pruritus. J Am Acad Dermatol 2006;54:527–531.

28 Hawi A, Alcorn H, Berg J, et al: Pharmacokinetics of nalbuphine hydrochloride extended release tablets in hemodialysis patients with exploratory effect on pruritus. BMC Nephrol 2015;16:47.

29 Ständer S, Böckenholt B, Schürmeyer-Horst F, et al: Treatment of chronic pruritus with the selective serotonin re-uptake inhibitors paroxetine and fluvoxamine: results of an open-labelled, two-arm proof-of-concept study. Acta Derm Venereol 2009;89:45–51.

30 Siepmann D, Luger TA, Ständer S: Antipruritic effect of cyclosporine microemulsion in prurigo nodularis: results of a case series. J Dtsch Dermatol Ges 2008; 6:941–946.

31 Spring P, Gschwind I, Gilliet M: Prurigo nodularis: retrospective study of 113 cases managed with methotrexate. Clin Exp Dermatol 2014;39:468–473.

32 Andersen TP, Fogh K: Thalidomide in 42 patients with prurigo nodularis Hyde. Dermatology 2011;223:107–112.

33 Taefehnorooz H, Truchetet F, Barbaud A, et al: Efficacy of thalidomide in the treatment of prurigo nodularis. Acta Derm Venereol 2011;91:344–345.

34 Sharma D, Kwatra SG: Thalidomide for the treatment of chronic refractory pruritus. J Am Acad Dermatol 2016;74: 363–369.

35 Kanavy H, Bahner J, Korman NJ: Treatment of refractory prurigo nodularis with lenalidomide. Arch Dermatol 2012; 148:794–796.

36 Liu H, Gaspari A, Schleichert R: Use of lenalidomide in treating refractory prurigo nodularis. J Drugs Dermatol 2013; 12:360–361.

37 Feldmeyer L, Werner S, Kamarashev J, et al: Atopic prurigo nodularis responds to intravenous immunoglobulins. Br J Dermatol 2012;166:461–462.

38 Ständer S, Siepmann D, Herrgott I, et al: Targeting the neurokinin receptor 1 with aprepitant: a novel antipruritic strategy. PloS One 2010;5:e10968.

39 Hawi A, Alcorn H Jr, Berg J, Hines C, Hait H, Sciascia T: Pharmacokinetics of nalbuphine hydrochloride extended release tablets in hemodialysis patients with exploratory effect on pruritus. BMC Nephrol 2015;16:47.

40 Sharma AD: Oral ketotifen and topical antibiotic therapy in the management of pruritus in prurigo nodularis: a randomized, controlled, single-blind, parallel study. Indian J Dermatol 2013;58:355–359.

41 Väätäinen N, Hannuksela M, Karvonen J: Local photochemotherapy in nodular prurigo. Acta Derm Venereol 1979;59: 436–437.

42 Nakashima C, Tanizaki H, Otsuka A, Miyachi Y, Kabashima K: Intractable prurigo nodularis successfully treated with combination therapy with a newly developed excimer laser and topical steroids. Dermatol Online J 2014;20:pii: 13030/qt9xp4640d.

43 Metze D, Reimann S, Beissert S, Luger T: Efficacy and safety of naltrexone, an oral opiate receptor antagonist, in the treatment of pruritus in internal and dermatological diseases. J Am Acad Dermatol 1999;41:533–539.

44 Metze D, Reimann S, Luger TA: Effective treatment of pruritus with naltrexone, an orally active opiate antagonist. Ann NY Acad Sci 1999;885:430–432.

45 Brune A, Metze D, Luger TA, Ständer S: Antipruritic therapy with the oral opiod receptor antagonist naltrexone. Open, non-placebo controlled administration in 133 patients (in German). Hautarzt 2004;55:1130–1136.

46 Halvorsen JA, Aasebø W: Oral tacrolimus treatment of pruritus in prurigo nodularis. Acta Derm Venereol 2015;95: 866–867.

47 Hann SK, Cho MY, Park YK: UV treatment of generalized prurigo nodularis. Int J Dermatol 1990;29:436–437.

Prof. Dr. Dr. Sonja Ständer
Department of Dermatology and Center for Chronic Pruritus, University Hospital Münster
Von-Esmarch-Strasse 58
DE–48149 Münster (Germany)
E-Mail sonja.staender@uni-muenster.de

Szepietowski JC, Weisshaar E (eds): Itch – Management in Clinical Practice.
Curr Probl Dermatol. Basel, Karger, 2016, vol 50, pp 102–110 (DOI: 10.1159/000446050)

Itch in Psoriasis Management

Jacek C. Szepietowski · Adam Reich

Department of Dermatology, Venereology and Allergology, Wrocław Medical University, Wrocław, Poland

Abstract

Psoriasis is a common chronic inflammatory skin disease observed in about 1–3% of the general population. About 60–90% of patients with psoriasis suffer from itching. Interestingly, in the past itch was not considered as an important symptom of psoriasis. Despite the high frequency of itch in psoriasis, the pathogenesis of this symptom is still not fully elucidated. Although most studies indicate neurogenic inflammation and the role of neuropeptides, other mediators may be important as well. The majority of psoriatic patients consider itch as the most bothersome symptom of the disease as it significantly alters daily functioning and psychosocial well-being. Patients with itch showed greater impairment of their health-related quality of life compared to those without itch, and the intensity of itch correlated with the degree of quality-of-life reduction. However, treatment options for itch in psoriasis are limited. Therapy of itch in patients with psoriasis should be directed toward the resolution of skin lesions, as disease remission usually is linked with itch relief. Recent studies have clearly pointed to an important role of apremilast and biologic agents in itch intensity reduction in subjects suffering from psoriasis. Other treatment modalities include antihistamines, especially with a sedative effect, narrowband ultraviolet B, and antidepressants (doxepin, mirtazapine, paroxetine). Support by family members and/or health professionals may also be of importance in helping psoriatic subjects cope with itch.

© 2016 S. Karger AG, Basel

Definition and Clinical Characteristics

Psoriatic itch is defined as an itch sensation occurring in patients suffering from psoriasis. According to the International Forum for the Study of Itch (IFSI), it is placed in the group of itch on diseased skin in the category of dermatologic itch [1].

Epidemiology
For many years itch was considered an uncommon symptom of psoriasis, and many older textbooks considered even lack of itching as a good parameter for differentiating psoriasis from other chronic inflammatory dermatoses. However, newer studies have clearly documented that itch is in fact a very frequent sensation in psoriasis which affects the vast majority of patients with this disease and is commonly quite severe [2, 3].

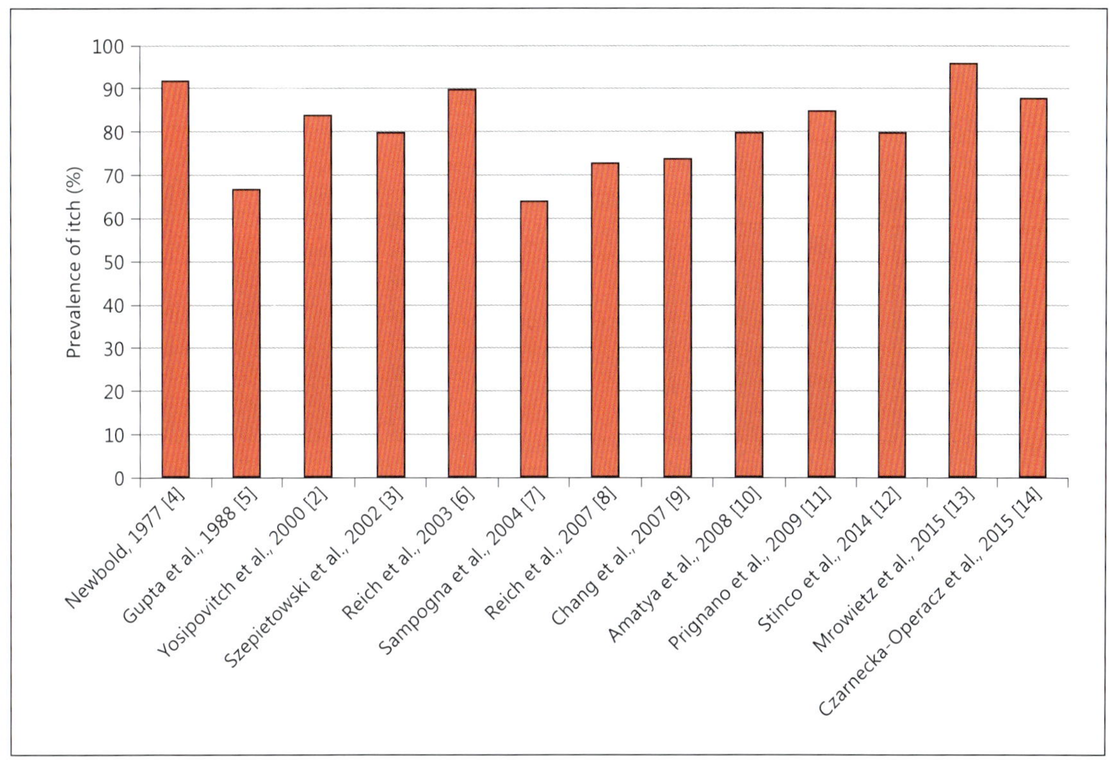

Fig. 1. Prevalence of itch in psoriatic patients.

In 1977, Newbold [4] described itch in 92% of 200 consecutively hospitalized patients with psoriasis. Subsequently, other authors assessing the prevalence of itch in patients with psoriasis confirmed a very high frequency of itch in this group of patients, ranging from 64 to 96% depending on the analyzed populations [2, 3, 5–14] (fig. 1). However, many of the abovementioned studies were not true prevalence studies with differing study populations, and itch was frequently reported among other study outcome measures. In addition, most of them did not consider the IFSI classification concerning the definition of chronic itch and may have also documented acute itch. Nevertheless, itch was the most commonly reported subjective sensation of psoriasis [7] and psoriatic individuals considered itch as the most bothersome disease symptom [15]. The high prevalence of itch in psoriasis in contemporary patients may be possibly related to changes in the lifestyle, higher daily stress, and greater exposure to pollutants [16].

There could be several reasons why itch was not considered as an important symptom of psoriasis in the past. First, it seems that physicians did not ask for this symptom because (according to the previous generally accepted scientific knowledge) it was not considered as part of the disease. Secondly, psoriasis patients are rather inert and hesitant (e.g. in contrast to patients with atopic dermatitis) and frequently do not report symptoms when not directly asked about them. Finally, the itch intensity is rather mild to moderate and other symptoms like scaling dominate much more.

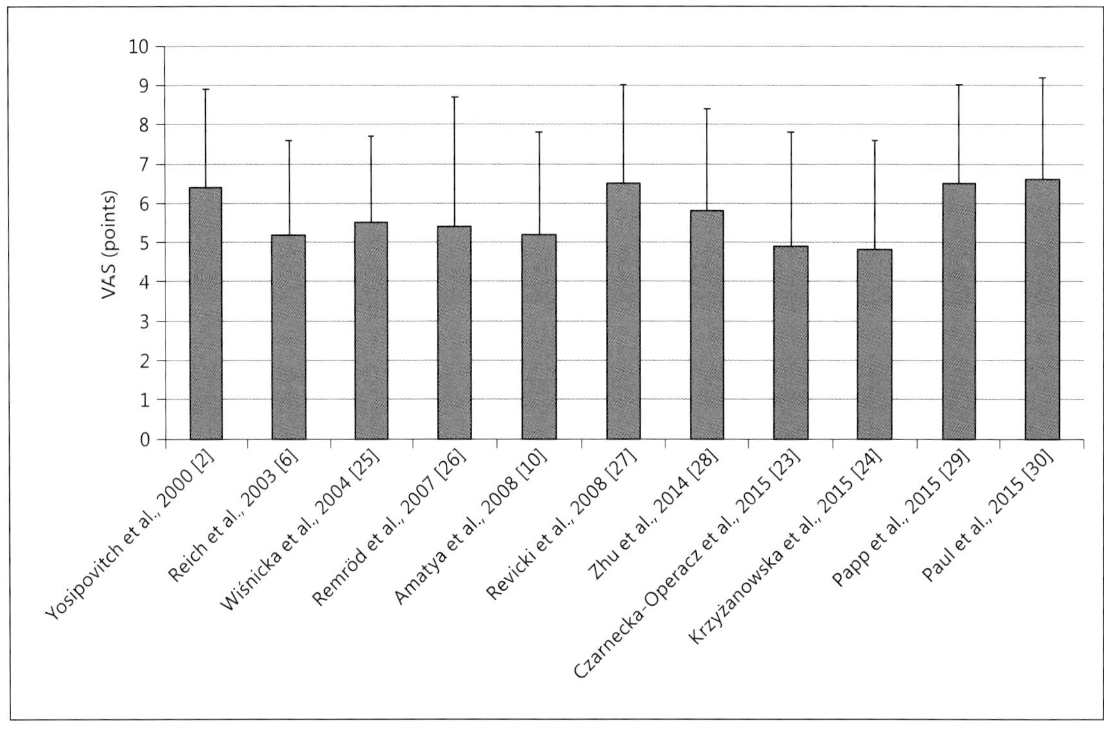

Fig. 2. Mean intensity of pruritus in psoriasis according to the VAS in various clinical studies.

Clinical Manifestation

Itch in psoriasis may involve any body area; however, the face and neck are frequently spared [2, 3, 17]. Itch is usually limited to lesional skin, but in a significant proportion of subjects it may also affect uninvolved skin and in some patients generalized itch is observed involving the entire body surface [6, 7, 10, 18]. Itch, sometimes together with burning sensations, may also be present in the genital area, especially in women [19, 20]. Remarkably, vulvar itch is not always accompanied by the presence of psoriatic plaques on the vulva [19]. Another frequent localization of itch in psoriasis is the scalp [21]. Itch in this area is commonly responsible for a poor treatment outcome due to severe scratching and subsequent Koebnerization [22].

According to the visual analogue scale (VAS) itching in psoriasis is usually of moderate severity (fig. 2) [2, 6, 10, 23–30]; however, sometimes it could be very severe, leading to extensive scratching and secondary scratch lesions (fig. 3). It should be underlined that these studies did not distinguish acute itch from chronic one. As mentioned above, scratching of the skin may result in formation of new skin lesions due to the Koebner phenomenon. Therefore, the presence of itch and subsequent scratching may lead to a vicious cycle during development of psoriatic lesions because of the Koebner phenomenon and occurrence of new skin plaques within the excoriations, which again can be quite itchy. The significant relation between psoriasis severity and pruritus intensity has been observed in many, albeit not in all, studies on itch in psoriasis [2, 3, 7, 9, 18, 31]. More-

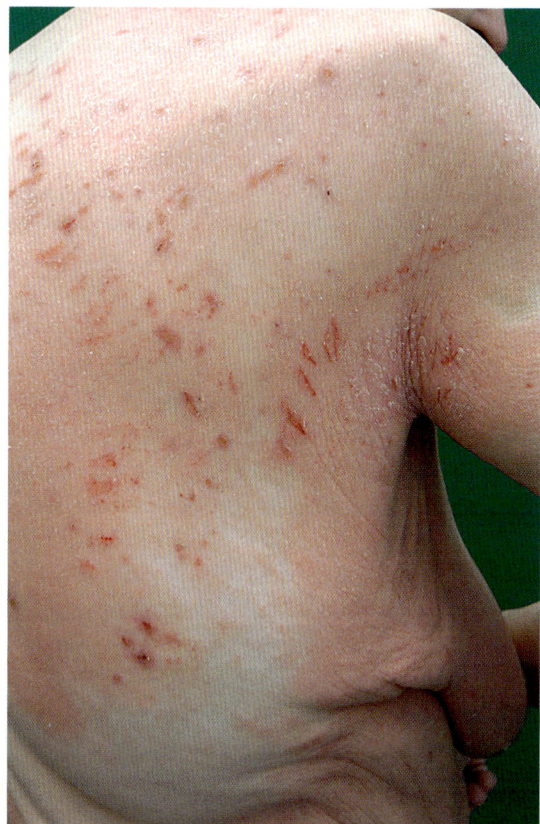

Fig. 3. Extensive scratch lesions due to severe pruritus in a patient with psoriasis.

over, the most intensive itching was usually observed during the appearance of new skin lesions or when psoriatic plaques extended further [3]. Itch relief was often associated with a complete resolution of psoriatic lesions [3].

In about three quarters of patients with psoriasis, itch appears on a daily basis and itch episodes usually last longer than 10 min [2, 10]. Itch severity is usually scored higher at night and during the winter [7, 10]. The most important factors exacerbating itch is heat, skin dryness, hot water, sweating, and emotional stress. In contrast, reduction or alleviation of itch is often caused by sleep and cold showers [2].

Influence on Patients' Well-Being

Patients with psoriasis demonstrate significantly reduced quality of life [32]. For many patients with psoriasis, itch is the most bothersome symptom of the disease [15, 33]. Importantly, patients with itch show greater impairment of their health-related quality of life compared to those without itch, and the intensity of itch correlates with the degree of quality of life reduction [34]. Many psoriatic individuals consider itch as annoying or unbearable [10] and for many of them this sensation is one of the most relevant factors contributing to perceived disease severity [33]. Amatya et al. [10] reported that the majority of patients with psoriasis handled itch as a symptom negatively influencing various aspects of their quality of life, like mood, concentration, sleep, sexual desire, and appetite. In another study, due to itch, 35% of psoriatic patients became more agitated, 24% depressed, 30% showed concentration difficulties, 23% changed their eating habits, and 35% reported their sexual function to be decreased or nonexistent [2]. Psoriatic subjects with itch also demonstrate more depressive symptoms than those without itching, and itch intensity significantly influences the severity of depressive symptoms and the degree of stigmatization [34]. Interestingly, psoriasis patients are more embarrassed due to itch than subjects with atopic dermatitis, a very itchy dermatosis which is usually believed to be accompanied by the most intensive itch [35]. Patients with psoriasis who suffer from itch also demonstrate significant problems with sleeping [2, 36] and itch intensity is associated with worse physical functioning [36].

Itch also alters the work productivity of psoriasis patients. Almost half of psoriatic individuals indicate itch as the most relevant disease symptom negatively interfering with the work activity, and the intensity of itch significantly correlates with the decreased work ability [37]. The impaired work productivity of itch psoriatic subjects may be mediated, at least partially, by sleeping problems; however, both factors appear to have independent negative effects on work [38].

Itch influences disease-coping strategies in patients with psoriasis. Severe itch is significantly associated with four personality traits: somatic trait anxiety, embitterment, mistrust, and physical trait aggression [39]. Less intense itch and fewer itch episodes are also linked to the stronger fighting spirit among patients with psoriasis [36]. In another study, psoriasis patients with the most frequent pruritus appraised their underlying disease significantly more frequently in terms of a threat, obstacle/loss, and harm, as compared with the patients with less frequent pruritus, and subjects with psoriasis who experienced pruritus all the time more often developed 'resignation' and 'self-blame' as coping strategies with the disease [40]. As a consequence, patients suffering from itch frequently withdraw from various daily activities [41]. Consequently, it seems that patients with psoriasis and more severe itch might have a more vulnerable psychological constitution. Thus, they may probably achieve greater benefit from psychological interventions compared to the rest of the patients [16].

Pathogenesis

The exact pathogenesis of itch in psoriasis is still not fully elucidated, but the majority of researchers support the idea that itching originates as a consequence of neurogenic inflammation [22]. It is also generally accepted that itch in psoriasis is influenced by the emotional stress [6, 23]. The exact mechanism how emotions interplay with the feeling of itch remains poorly understood, but it cannot be excluded that the retrograde activation of sensory nerves and release of proinflammatory and pruritogenic mediators from dermal nerve endings may be important.

Various neuropeptides released from dermal nerve endings, keratinocytes, and dermal cells seem to be good candidates for itch mediators in psoriasis [42]. Several neuropeptides have been shown to be abnormally expressed in lesional and nonlesional psoriatic skin as well as in the plasma of patients suffering from itch, including substance P (SP), calcitonin gene-related peptide, somatostatin, β-endorphin, neuropeptide Y, vasoactive intestinal peptide, and pituitary adenylate cyclase-activating polypeptide [43–45]. These substances show a number of immunomodulatory properties like activation of dendritic cells, lymphocytes, macrophages, and neutrophils; stimulation of keratinocyte hyperproliferation; degranulation of dermal mast cells; stimulation of angiogenesis, and modulation of the expression of adhesion molecules on the endothelial cells [44]. A significant correlation between itch intensity and the number of SP-positive nerve fibers and number of neurokinin 2 receptor (one of the SP receptors) immunoreactive cells were found in lesional psoriatic skin [45]. Patients with psoriasis suffering from itch have also shown higher expression of receptors for SP and calcitonin gene-related peptide [9]. Future studies should therefore be undertaken to prove whether SP-pathway blockade with available neurokinin inhibitors (e.g. aprepitant) would decrease itch in psoriasis. Indeed, such studies would also provide data of whether SP is a key mediator of psoriatic itch.

Another hypothesis regarding the pathogenesis of itch in psoriasis is related to abnormal skin innervation. A number of studies have documented increased expression of nerve growth factor (NGF) and its receptors in lesional itchy psoriatic skin, which correlated with itch intensity [9, 43]. In contrast, the dermal expression of semaphorin-3A, an axon-guidance molecule that inhibits neurite outgrowth of sensory C-fibers, was decreased in psoriasis with itch, and the level of semaphorin-3A expression negatively correlated with itch intensity assessed with the VAS [31, 46]. It could be suggested that downregulation of semaphorin-3A in combination with upregulation of NGF in psoriatic skin might be a trigger for hyperinnervation of C-fibers in the epidermis, a phenomenon involved in itch elucidation [46]. A significant role of nerve density and NGF in itch accompanying psoriasis is also supported by the recently published phase IIB clinical study in which the topical application of CT327, an inhibitor of the 140-kDa high-affinity NGF receptor, effectively reduced itch in psoriasis [18]. Increased epidermal nerve density was also shown to be involved in the development of itch in scalp psoriasis [21]. However, it is still unclear whether itch in psoriasis is evoked by direct activation of NGF receptors on dermal nerve endings or is rather related to decreased sensory threshold for itchy stimuli due to skin hyperinnervation induced by NGF overexpression [24]. Thus, further studies are still needed to verify these hypotheses.

Neurogenic inflammation and increased nerve density in psoriatic skin may not be the only underlying cause of itch. Some recent data have indicated that itch perception may be evoked or at least modulated by the endogenous opioid system. It was postulated that the presence of itch may be related to imbalance of μ- and κ-opioid receptors: the μ-opioid pathway is considered as itch promoting, while the κ-opioid pathway exerts the opposite effect. Supporting the role of the endogenous opioid system in itch perception, Taneda et al. [31] found significantly decreased expression of κ-opioid receptors in lesional epidermis of psoriatic patients with itch compared to those without itch. This phenomenon was accompanied by the reduced expression of its agonist, dynorphin A, while the expression of μ-opioid receptors remained unchanged, suggesting an increased μ-opioid tone in itchy subjects. Similar observations were made by our group showing reduced expression of κ-opioid receptors in psoriatic patients having itch which was inversely correlated with itch intensity [47].

In addition, some other itch mediators have also been postulated in psoriasis by other authors, including, but not limited to, γ-aminobutyric acid (GABA), interleukin (IL)-2, IL-31, E-selectin, and vascular adhesion protein 1; however, these observations have usually been made in single studies and need to be confirmed by other authors on larger groups of patients [42, 43, 48–50].

Management

Therapy of itch in psoriasis could be very challenging as very few studies have assessed the effect of currently available treatment options on itch and to date there is no single antipruritic therapy dedicated specifically to treating itch in psoriasis. As in other itchy conditions, patients with psoriasis might benefit from general antipruritic measures like proper skin moisturizing with emollients, wearing of light, airy clothes, avoiding hot and dry air, and applying calamine lotions or menthol preparation.

However, durable improvement or alleviation of itch is usually connected with the clearance of skin lesions [3]. Thus, the antipruritic treatment strategies in psoriatic itch should be directed toward the resolution of skin lesions. One study documented the efficacy of narrowband ultraviolet B (UVB) therapy in treating psoriatic itch [50]. However, it must be underlined that in some patients narrowband UVB may even aggravate itch by increasing skin dryness; therefore, patients on UVB therapy should be instructed to properly moisturize their skin as a preventive measure of skin dryness [51].

In addition, several recently published studies have documented that effective treatment with apremilast or biologics, like etanercept, secukinumab, adalimumab, ixekizumab, and brodalumab, may also be of value to reduce itch intensity [13, 27–30, 52].

Regarding other treatment modalities, some relief of itch, usually moderate, was observed during antihistamine therapy, particularly if it caused sedation [53]. In more severe cases unresponsive to antihistamines, oral antidepressants like mirtazapine (15 mg at night), doxepin (10–20 mg 3 times daily), or paroxetine (20–30 mg/day) may be tried. Mirtazapine was shown to relieve itch even in severe itch associated with erythrodermic psoriasis [51]. Mirtazapine exerts a sedative effect due to its H_1-antihistamine properties, but it also acts as an antagonist of noradrenergic α_2-receptors and 5-HT_2 and 5-HT_3 serotonin receptors [51]. Support given by the family and/or health professionals is also of great importance as it may increase the ability of patients to cope with itching [16].

As mentioned above, Roblin et al. [18] recently demonstrated in a randomized, double-blind, vehicle-controlled, phase IIb clinical trial on 160 subjects that CT327, that a 140-kDa high-affinity NGF receptor inhibitor might be of some benefit in the treatment of itch in psoriasis. Hopefully, this observation will be confirmed in subsequent studies and this compound will become freely available for pruritic psoriatics in the near future.

In conclusion, itch is a very prevalent and significant symptom of psoriasis. Despite the high frequency of itch in psoriasis, its pathogenesis is still not fully elucidated, and consequently available treatment options are quite limited. The majority of psoriatic patients consider itch as the most bothersome symptom of the disease and it significantly alters their quality of life. Therapy of psoriatic itch should be directed toward the resolution of skin lesions, as disease remission usually is linked with significant itch relief.

References

1 Ständer S, Weisshaar E, Mettang T, Szepietowski JC, Carstens E, Ikoma A, Bergasa NV, Gieler U, Misery L, Wallengren J, Darsow U, Streit M, Metze D, Luger TA, Greaves MW, Schmelz M, Yosipovitch G, Bernhard JD: Clinical classification of itch: a position paper of the International Forum for the Study of Itch. Acta Derm Venereol 2007;87:291–294.

2 Yosipovitch G, Goon A, Wee J, Chan YH, Goh CL: The prevalence and clinical characteristics of itch among patients with extensive psoriasis. Br J Dermatol 2000;143:969–973.

3 Szepietowski JC, Reich A, Wiśnicka B: Itching in patients suffering from psoriasis. Acta Dermatovenereol Croat 2002;10:221–226.

4 Newbold PCH: Itch in psoriasis; in Farber EM, Cox AJ (eds): Psoriasis. Proceedings of the Second International Symposium. New York, Yorke Medical Books, 1977, pp 334–336.

5 Gupta MA, Gupta AK, Kirkby S, Weiner HK, Mace TM, Schork NJ, Johnson EH, Ellis CN, Voorhees JJ: Pruritus in psoriasis. A prospective study of some psychiatric and dermatologic correlates. Arch Dermatol 1988;124:1052–1057.

6 Reich A, Szepietowski JC, Wiśnicka B, Pacan P: Does stress influence itching in psoriatic patients? Dermatol Psychosom 2003;4:151–155.

7 Sampogna F, Gisondi P, Melchi CF, Amerio P, Girolomoni G, Abeni D; IDI Multipurpose Psoriasis Research on Vital Experiences Investigators: Prevalence of symptoms by patients with different clinical types of psoriasis. Br J Dermatol 2004;151:594–599.

8 Reich A, Orda A, Wiśnicka B, Szepietowski JC: Plasma neuropeptides and perception of itch in psoriasis. Acta Derm Venereol 2007;87:299–304.

9 Chang SE, Han SS, Jung HJ, Choi JH: Neuropeptides and their receptors in psoriatic skin in relation to itch. Br J Dermatol 2007;156:1272–1277.

10 Amatya B, Wennersten G, Nordlind K: Patients' perspective of itch in chronic plaque psoriasis: a questionnaire-based study. J Eur Acad Dermatol Venereol 2008;22:822–826.

11 Prignano F, Ricceri F, Pescitelli L, Lotti T: Itch in psoriasis: epidemiology, clinical aspects and treatment options. Clin Cosmet Investig Dermatol 2009;2:9–13.

12 Stinco G, Trevisan G, Piccirillo F, Pezzetta S, Errichetti E, di Meo N, Valent F, Patrone P: Pruritus in chronic plaque psoriasis: a questionnaire-based study of 230 Italian patients. Acta Dermatovenerol Croat 2014;22:122–128.

13 Mrowietz U, Chouela EN, Mallbris L, Stefanidis D, Marino V, Pedersen R, Boggs RL: Itch and quality of life in moderate-to-severe plaque psoriasis: post hoc explorative analysis from the PRISTINE study. J Eur Acad Dermatol Venereol 2015;29:1114–1120.

14 Czarnecka-Operacz M, Polańska A, Klimańska M, Teresiak-Mikołajczak E, Molińska-Glura M, Adamski Z, Jenerowicz D: Itching sensation in psoriatic patients and its relation to body mass index and IL-17 and IL-31 concentrations. Postepy Dermatol Alergol 2015;32:426–430.

15 Reich A, Welz-Kubiak K, Rams L: Apprehension of the disease by patients suffering from psoriasis. Postepy Dermatol Alergol 2014;31:289–293.

16 Reich A, Mędrek K, Szepietowski JC: Interplay of itch and psyche in psoriasis: an update. Acta Derm Venereol 2016, DOI 10.2340/00015555-2374.

17 Reich A, Welz-Kubiak K, Szepietowski JC: Pruritus differences between psoriasis and lichen planus. Acta Derm Venereol 2011;91:605–606.

18 Roblin D, Yosipovitch G, Boyce B, Robinson J, Sandy J, Mainero V, Wickramasinghe R, Anand U, Anand P: Topical TrkA kinase inhibitor CT327 is an effective, novel therapy for the treatment of itch due to psoriasis: results from experimental studies, and efficacy and safety of CT327 in a phase 2b clinical trial in patients with psoriasis. Acta Derm Venereol 2015;95:542–548.

19 Zamirska A, Reich A, Berny-Moreno J, Salomon J, Szepietowski JC: Vulvar itch and burning sensation in women with psoriasis. Acta Derm Venereol 2008;88: 132–135.

20 Meeuwis KA, de Hullu JA, Massuger LF, van de Kerkhof PC, van Rossum MM: Genital psoriasis: a systematic literature review on this hidden skin disease. Acta Derm Venereol 2011;91:5–11.

21 Kim TW, Shim WH, Kim JM, Mun JH, Song M, Kim HS, Ko HC, Kim MB, Kim BS: Clinical characteristics of itch in patients with scalp psoriasis and their relation with intraepidermal nerve fiber density. Ann Dermatol 2014;26:727–732.

22 Szepietowski JC, Reich A: Pruritus in psoriasis: an update. Eur J Pain 2016;20: 41–46.

23 Czarnecka-Operacz M, Polańska A, Klimańska M, Teresiak-Mikołajczak E, Molińska-Glura M, Adamski Z, Jenerowicz D: Itching sensation in psoriatic patients and its relation to body mass index and IL-17 and IL-31 concentrations. Postepy Dermatol Alergol 2015; 32:426–430.

24 Krzyżanowska M, Muszer K, Chabowski K, Reich A: Assessment of the sensory threshold in patients with atopic dermatitis and psoriasis. Postepy Dermatol Alergol 2015;32:94–100.

25 Wiśnicka B, Szepietowski JC, Reich A, Orda A: Histamine, substance P and calcitonin gene-related peptide plasma concentration and pruritus in patients suffering from psoriasis. Dermatol Psychosom 2004;5:73–78.

26 Remröd C, Lonne-Rahm S, Nordlind K: Study of substance P and its receptor neurokinin-1 in psoriasis and their relation to chronic stress and itch. Arch Dermatol Res 2007;299:85–91.

27 Revicki D, Willian MK, Saurat JH, Papp KA, Ortonne JP, Sexton C, Camez A: Impact of adalimumab treatment on health-related quality of life and other patient-reported outcomes: results from a 16-week randomized controlled trial in patients with moderate to severe plaque psoriasis. Br J Dermatol 2008; 158:549–557.

28 Zhu B, Edson-Heredia E, Guo J, Maeda-Chubachi T, Shen W, Kimball AB: Itching is a significant problem and a mediator between disease severity and quality of life for patients with psoriasis: results from a randomized controlled trial. Br J Dermatol 2014;171:1215–1219.

29 Papp K, Reich K, Leonardi CL, Kircik L, Chimenti S, Langley RG, Hu C, Stevens RM, Day RM, Gordon KB, Korman NJ, Griffiths CE: Apremilast, an oral phosphodiesterase 4 (PDE4) inhibitor, in patients with moderate to severe plaque psoriasis: results of a phase III, randomized, controlled trial (Efficacy and Safety Trial Evaluating the Effects of Apremilast in Psoriasis [ESTEEM] 1). J Am Acad Dermatol 2015;73:37–49.

30 Paul C, Cather J, Gooderham M, Poulin Y, Mrowietz U, Ferrandiz C, Crowley J, Hu C, Stevens RM, Shah K, Day RM, Girolomoni G, Gottlieb AB: Efficacy and safety of apremilast, an oral phosphodiesterase 4 inhibitor, in patients with moderate-to-severe plaque psoriasis over 52 weeks: a phase III, randomized controlled trial (ESTEEM 2). Br J Dermatol 2015;173:1387–1399.

31 Taneda K, Tominaga M, Negi O, Tengara S, Kamo A, Ogawa H, Takamori K: Evaluation of epidermal nerve density and opioid receptor levels in psoriatic itch. Br J Dermatol 2011;165:277–284.

32 Krueger G, Koo J, Lebwohl M, Menter A, Stern RS, Rolstad T: The impact of psoriasis on quality of life: results of a 1998 National Psoriasis Foundation patient-membership survey. Arch Dermatol 2001;137:280–284.

33 Lebwohl MG, Bachelez H, Barker J, Girolomoni G, Kavanaugh A, Langley RG, Paul CF, Puig L, Reich K, van de Kerkhof PC: Patient perspectives in the management of psoriasis: results from the population-based Multinational Assessment of Psoriasis and Psoriatic Arthritis Survey. J Am Acad Dermatol 2014;70: 871–881.e1–e30.

34 Reich A, Hrehorów E, Szepietowski JC: Itch is an important factor negatively influencing the well-being of psoriatic patients. Acta Derm Venereol 2010;90: 257–263.

35 O'Neill JL, Chan YH, Rapp SR, Yosipovitch G: Differences in itch characteristics between psoriasis and atopic dermatitis patients: results of a web-based questionnaire. Acta Derm Venereol 2011;91:537–540.

36 Ograczyk A, Miniszewska J, Kępska A, Zalewska-Janowska A: Itch, disease coping strategies and quality of life in psoriasis patients. Postepy Dermatol Alergol 2014;31:299–304.

37 Zimoląg I, Reich A, Szepietowski JC: Influence of psoriasis on the ability to work. Acta Derm Venereol 2009;89: 575–576.

38 Kimball AB, Edson-Heredia E, Zhu B, Guo J, Maeda-Chubachi T, Shen W, Bianchi MT: Understanding the relationship between pruritus severity and work productivity in patients with moderate-to-severe psoriasis: sleep problems are a mediating factor. J Drugs Dermatol 2016;15:183–188.

39 Remröd C, Sjöström K, Svensson A: Pruritus in psoriasis: a study of personality traits, depression and anxiety. Acta Derm Venereol 2015;95:439–443.

40 Janowski K, Steuden S, Bogaczewicz J: Clinical and psychological characteristics of patients with psoriasis reporting various frequencies of pruritus. Int J Dermatol 2014;53:820–829.

41 Verhoeven L, Kraaimaat F, Duller P, van de Kerkhof P, Evers A: Cognitive, behavioral, and physiological reactivity to chronic itching: analogies to chronic pain. Int J Behav Med 2006;13:237–243.

42 Reich A, Szepietowski JC: Mediators of pruritus in psoriasis. Mediators Inflamm 2007;2007:64727.

43 Nakamura M, Toyoda M, Morohashi M: Pruritogenic mediators in psoriasis vulgaris: comparative evaluation of itch-associated cutaneous factors. Br J Dermatol 2003;149:718–730.

44 Saraceno R, Kleyn CE, Terenghi G, Griffiths CE: The role of neuropeptides in psoriasis. Br J Dermatol 2006;155: 876–882.

45 Amatya, B, El-Nour H, Holst M, Theodorsson E, Nordlind K: Expression of tachykinins and their receptors in plaque psoriasis with itch. Br J Dermatol 2011;164:1023–1029.

46 Kou K, Nakamura F, Aihara M, Chen H, Seto K, Komori-Yamaguchi J, Kambara T, Nagashima Y, Goshima, Y, Ikezawa Z: Decreased expression of semaphorin-3A, a neurite-collapsing factor, is associated with itch in psoriatic skin. Acta Derm Venereol 2012;92:521–528.

47 Kupczyk P, Reich A, Wysokińska E, Gajda M, Hołysz M, Hwang T, Kobuszewska A, Nowakowska B, Drukała J, Szepietowski JC: Opioid receptors expression and PGP 9.5-positive epidermal nerve fiber density in psoriasis – relationship with itch. Folia Neuropathol 2014;52:340–341.

48 Madej A, Reich A, Orda A, Szepietowski JC: Vascular adhesion protein-1 (VAP-1) is overexpressed in psoriatic patients. J Eur Acad Dermatol Venereol 2007;21: 72–78.

49 Nigam R, El-Nour H, Amatya B, Nordlind K: GABA and GABA(A) receptor expression on immune cells in psoriasis: a pathophysiological role. Arch Dermatol Res 2010;302:507–515.

50 Narbutt J, Olejniczak I, Sobolewska-Sztychny D, Sysa-Jedrzejowska A, Slowik-Kwiatkowska I, Hawro T, Lesiak A: Narrow band ultraviolet B irradiations cause alteration in interleukin-31 serum level in psoriatic patients. Arch Dermatol Res 2012;305:191–195.

51 Dawn A, Yosipovitch G: Treating itch in psoriasis. Dermatol Nurs 2006;18:227–233.

52 Sobell JM, Foley P, Toth D, Mrowietz U, Girolomoni G, Goncalves J, Day RM, Chen R, Yosipovitch G: Effects of apremilast on pruritus and skin discomfort/pain correlate with improvements in quality of life in patients with moderate to severe plaque psoriasis. Acta Derm Venereol 2016;96:514–520.

53 Domagała A, Reich A: Antihistamines in the treatment of psoriatic pruritus: a double-blind placebo-controlled pilot study. Acta Derm Venereol 2015;95:885.

Prof. Jacek C. Szepietowski, MD, PhD
Department of Dermatology, Venereology and Allergology, Wrocław Medical University
Ul. Chałubińskiego 1
PL–50-368 Wrocław (Poland)
E-Mail jacek.szepietowski@umed.wroc.pl

Szepietowski JC, Weisshaar E (eds): Itch – Management in Clinical Practice.
Curr Probl Dermatol. Basel, Karger, 2016, vol 50, pp 111–115 (DOI: 10.1159/000446051)

Itch in Special Skin Locations Management

Laurent Misery

Department of Dermatology, University Hospital of Brest, and Laboratory of Neurosciences of Brest, University of Western Brittany, Brest, France

Abstract

Itch management can be particularly complicated in some small areas like the scalp or the anogenital region for many reasons: the frequently poor diagnosis of the causes of itch in these areas, the dense innervation of these areas, and the symbolic value of these areas for the human psyche. The diagnosis of itchy scalp is easier than that of anogenital pruritus. Clinical examination and a careful inventory of all diseases of the patient and of the local environment are necessary. Localized treatments are frequently used at both sites, whereas specific pharmaceutical formulations are necessary for the pilose or the mucous environment. Nonetheless, systemic treatments or psychological interventions can be very useful.

© 2016 S. Karger AG, Basel

Itch management can be particularly complex in some small areas like the scalp or the anogenital region for many reasons: the frequently poor diagnosis of the causes of itch in these areas, the dense innervation of these areas, and the symbolic value of these areas for the human psyche.

Because these areas are small, localized treatments are frequently used at both sites, whereas specific pharmaceutical formulations are necessary for the pilose or the mucous environment. Nonetheless, systemic treatments or psychological interventions can be very useful. These therapeutic options are detailed in the chapters by Misery, Metz and Staubach, and Pongcharoen and Fleischer [this vol., pp. 35–39, 40–45, 46–53, respectively], and specific aspects will be discussed here.

Scalp

Definition and Clinical Manifestations

Itching on the scalp is very frequent and is reported by more than 20% of the French population [1]. The scalp has a complex neuroanatomy with an abundance of sensorineural end organs in the pilosebaceous unit [2]. However, there is a significant insensitivity of C-nerve fibers of the scalp to warmth, heat pain, itch (histamine-induced or cowhage-induced), and neurogenic inflammation by comparison with the forearm [3].

Seborrheic dermatitis (dandruff) as well as sensitive scalp (only subjective symptoms and sometimes erythema) are the most frequent causes of itchy scalp [1, 2, 4, 5], but there are many others: lice, psoriasis (erythematosquamous lesions), tinea capitis (alopecia, squames, fungi), scarring alopecias, neuropathic itch (itch in a specific nerve area), psychogenic itch (exacerbation by stress or rest), etc. All these diseases have specific treatments, and the diagnosis is usually obvious due to the clinical characteristics.

Management

In the presence of chronic pruritus on the scalp, a symptomatic treatment may be the use of polidocanol, a protease-activated receptor-2 antagonist, which is included in shampoos or lotions. Etiological treatments are obviously needed if possible: shampoos containing fungistatic and keratolytic substances for seborrheic dermatitis, corticosteroids and salicylic acid for psoriasis, fungistatics for tinea, corticosteroids for scarring alopecias, etc.

Stress is frequently accompanied by a consecutive scratching of the scalp, possibly because it is easily accessible or because this area is close to our brain and consequently to our mind. In any case, the scalp is a frequent localization of scratching excoriations, and psychological interventions are sometimes useful to stop a vicious cycle in skin conditions. Serotonin reuptake inhibitors may also be indicated.

Genital Area

Definition and Clinical Manifestations

Pruritus is also frequent in the external genital area in men and women, and is typically intensely perceived because of its dense innervation and symbolic value. Although there are numerous common features of the causes and perceptions of itch, sex-related differences are obviously related to the anatomy of the genital organs, as well as to differences in the functional organization of the peripheral and central nervous system [6, 7] and psychological specificities [8].

There are numerous causes of genital pruritus [9, 10]. They vary across the ages [11], with lichens and intraepithelial neoplasias being frequent in elderly patients, and the sexes, with candidosis being more frequent in women. The clinical examination usually leads to a diagnosis, but laboratory tests may be necessary. Clinical characteristics are summarized in table 1.

Candidosis is the most frequent infectious cause of genital pruritus, but others are possible: dermatophytoses, pediculosis pubis, scabies, pinworm infection, trichomoniasis, herpes, erythrasma, or rarer causes (molluscum contagiosum, infection with streptococcus or intestinal bacteria, schistosomiasis). Inflammatory dermatoses are frequently localized in the genital area, especially psoriasis. Specific genital localizations of lichen simplex, lichen sclerosus, or lichen planus are well known. Other inflammatory causes of genital pruritus can be contact dermatitis or Hailey-Hailey disease. Benign tumors like Fox-Fordyce disease or syringomas are also frequently itchy. Intraepithelial neoplasia or Paget disease may also induce pruritus.

In some cases, there is no skin finding. Genital pruritus can be considered as idiopathic, but the so-called 'sensitive skin' in the genital area needs to be eliminated. This condition is underestimated since a study showed that 57% of women and 37% of men perceived their genital skin as sensitive [12]. In contrast, the diagnosis of psychogenic pruritus is made too often and too easily, whereas restrictive criteria are necessary [13]. Neuropathic pruritus [14] may also occur in the genital area in cases of postherpetic neuralgia, pudendal neuralgia, or a Tarlov cyst, which is a sacral nerve root cyst.

Management

There are specific treatments for all these conditions (table 1). Cosmetic products can be used for symptomatic treatment. It is important to avoid

Table 1. Differential diagnosis and main treatments of anogenital pruritus

Diagnosis	Main symptoms	Main treatments
Candidosis	erythema, pustules	antifungals
Dermatophytoses	light erythema	antifungals
Pediculosis pubis	lice on hairs	pesticides
Scabies	furrows	pesticides
Pinworm infection	small worms	pesticides
Trichomoniasis	green flow	metronidazole
Herpes	cluster of vesicles	antiviral drugs
Erythrasma	erythema	azole and macrolide
Molluscum contagiosum	translucid papules	cryotherapy
Bacterial infection	erythema	antibiotics
Schistosomiasis	erythema	antischistosomal drugs
Psoriasis	erythema	topical steroids
Lichen simplex	whitish erythema	topical steroids
Lichen sclerosus	erythema and atrophy	topical steroids
Lichen planus	erythema	topical steroids
Contact dermatitis	erythema and vesicles	topical steroids
Hailey-Hailey disease	erythema and fissures	laser
Fox-Fordyce disease	papules	various
Syringomas	papules	laser
Intraepithelial neoplasia	erosive erythema	laser
Sensitive skin	no visible lesion	soothing topicals
Psychogenic pruritus	induction by stress	psychotherapy
Neuropathic pruritus	nerve territory	antiepileptic drugs

all irritant contacts and tight clothing. Syndets or alkaline soaps are indicated.

Although the strictly psychogenic pruritus is rare, aggravation of itch by stress is common, and psychological consequences of chronic genital pruritus are frequent. Psychological support and sometimes psychotherapies or psychotropic drugs can be very helpful in patients.

Anal and Perianal Area

Definition and Clinical Manifestations
Pruritus ani affects 1–5% of the population, is 4 times more common in men, and is most frequent between the fourth and sixth decades of life [15]. All causes that have been reported above for the genital area can occur in the anal and perianal area, especially contact eczema or psoriasis, but there are many specific proctological etiologies.

Any coexisting anal conditions can precipitate or exacerbate itch, with hemorrhoids being the commonest [15], but anal or colorectal cancer, functional bowel disorders, and posttraumatic lesions may also induce pruritus.

Fecal contamination causing pruritus ani is not simply a matter of prolonged contact with a moist substance or a hygiene issue, nor is it inevitable. Fecal contamination or soiling may be overt or occult. Occult soiling is often not perceptible for an individual to be aware of, but may be sufficient to initiate itch and scratching [15].

Foods have been implicated in idiopathic pruritus ani such as caffeinated drinks, alcohol, milk products, peanuts, spices, citrus fruits, grapes,

Table 2. Differential diagnosis and main treatments of specific causes of anal and perianal pruritus

Diagnosis	Main symptoms	Main treatments
Hemorrhoids	blue tumors	surgery
Cancer	mucosal tumors	surgery
Irritable bowel syndrome	pain, diarrhea, constipation	various
Posttraumatic lesions	scars	topical steroids
Fecal contamination	fecal contamination	hygiene
Irritation by food	anamnesis	elimination of irritants
Irritation by laxatives	anamnesis	exclusion
Irritation by drugs	anamnesis	exclusion

tomatoes (histamine), and chocolate; some researchers have shown a decrease in itch within 14 days if these are avoided [15].

Management

Diagnosed conditions should be treated appropriately (tables 1, 2). Management consists of 3 components which function in parallel – elimination of irritants and scratching, general control measures, and active treatment measures [15]. Patients have to eliminate irritants such as creams, soaps, bubble baths, toilet paper, scratching, and certain foods and drinks. Perineal cleansing should ideally be carried out in the squatting position so that the anal canal can be washed of retained feces [15]. Hygiene is fundamental, but excessive hygiene is counterproductive, just as in genital pruritus. Active treatment measures are related to the etiology (or etiologies).

Potent topical steroids are used sparingly as they can cause thinned skin, acute dermatitis and contact dermatitis from sensitization [15]. There is also the rebound itch after cessation that requires further steroid use, which has been described as an addiction [16]. Some orally ingested medications such as laxatives, Colpermin, colchicine, quinidine, peppermint oil, and some antibiotics also seem to lead to perianal itch [15].

Just like genital pruritus, pruritus ani can be exacerbated by stress and certain personality traits, anxiety, and depression. However, it is important to find somatic causes that induce or aggravate pruritus by the examination, anamnesis, and eventually some laboratory tests.

References

1 Misery L, Rahhali N, Duhamel A, Taieb C: Epidemiology of dandruff, scalp pruritus and associated symptoms. Acta Derm Venereol 2013;93:80–81.
2 Bin Saif GA, Ericson ME, Yosipovitch G: The itchy scalp – scratching for an explanation. Exp Dermatol 2011;20:959–968.
3 Bin Saif GA, Alajroush A, MacMichael A, Kwatra SG, Chan SG, MacGlone F, Yosipovitch G: Aberrant C nerve fibre function of the healthy scalp. Br J Dermatol 2012;167:485–489.
4 Misery L, Sibaud V, Ambronati M, Macy G, Boussetta S, Taieb C: Sensitive scalp: does this condition exist? An epidemiological study. Contact Dermatitis 2008; 58:234–238.
5 Elewski BE: Clinical diagnosis of common scalp disorders. J Invest Dermatol Symp Proc 2005;10:190–193.
6 Ständer S, Stumpf A, Osada N, Wilp S, Chatzigeorgakidis E, Pfleiderer B: Gender differences in chronic pruritus: women present different morbidity, more scratch lesions and higher burden. Br J Dermatol 2013;168:1273–1280.
7 Stumpf A, Burgmer M, Schneider G, Heuft G, Schmelz M, Phan NQ, et al: Sex differences in itch perception and modulation by distraction – an fMRI pilot study in healthy volunteers. PLoS One 2013;8:e79123.

8 Stumpf A, Stånder S, Warlich B, Fritz F, Bruland P, Pfleiderer B, Heuft G, Schneider G: Relations between the characteristics and psychological comorbidities of chronic pruritus differ between men and women: women are more anxious than men. Br J Dermatol 2015;172:1323–1328.

9 Welsh B, Howard A, Cook K: Vulval itch. Aust Fam Physician 2004;33:505–510.

10 Eichmann AR: Dermatoses of the male genital area. Dermatology 205;210:150–156.

11 Bohl TG: Overview of vulvar pruritus through the life cycle. Clin Obstet Gynecol 2005;48:786–807.

12 Farage MA: Perceptions of sensitive skin of the genital area. Curr Probl Dermatol 2011;40:142–154.

13 Misery L, Alexandre S, Dutray S, Chastaing M, Consoli SG, Audra H, Bauer D, Bertolus S, Callot V, Cardinaud F, Corrin E, Feton-Danou N, Malet R, Touboul S, Consoli SM: Functional itch disorder or psychogenic pruritus: suggested diagnosis criteria from the French Psychodermatology Group. Acta Derm Venereol 2007;87:341–344.

14 Misery L, Brenaut E, Le Garrec R, Abasq C, Genestet S, Marcorelles P, Zagnoli F: Neuropathic pruritus. Nat Rev Neurol 2014;10:408–416.

15 Siddqi S, Vijav V, Ward M, Mahendran R, Warren S: Pruritus ani. Ann R Coll Surg Engl 2008;90:457–463.

16 Kligman AM, Frosch PJ: Steroid addiction. Int J Dermatol 1979;18:23–31.

Prof. Laurent Misery
Service de dermatologie et de vénéréologie, CHU Brest
2, avenue Foch
FR–29200 Brest (France)
E-Mail laurent.misery@chu-brest.fr

Szepietowski JC, Weisshaar E (eds): Itch – Management in Clinical Practice.
Curr Probl Dermatol. Basel, Karger, 2016, vol 50, pp 116–123 (DOI: 10.1159/000446053)

Neurologic Itch Management

Ekin Şavk

Department of Dermatology, Faculty of Medicine, Adnan Menderes University, Aydın, Turkey

Abstract

Neurologic itch is defined as pruritus resulting from any dysfunction of the nervous system. Itch arising due to a neuroanatomic pathology is seen to be neuropathic. Causes of neuropathic itch range from localized entrapment of a peripheral nerve to generalized degeneration of small nerve fibers. Antipruritic medications commonly used for other types of itch such as antihistamines and corticosteroids lack efficacy in neuropathic itch. Currently there are no therapeutic options that offer relief in all types of neuropathic pruritus, and treatment strategies vary according to etiology. It is best to decide on the appropriate tests and procedures in collaboration with a neurologist during the initial work-up. Treatment of neuropathic itch includes general antipruritic measures, local or systemic pharmacotherapy, various physical modalities, and surgery. Surgical intervention is the obvious choice of therapy in cases of spinal or cerebral mass, abscess, or hemorrhagic stroke, and may provide decompression in entrapment neuropathies. Symptomatic treatment is needed in the vast majority of patients. General antipruritic measures should be encouraged. Local treatment agents with at least some antipruritic effect include capsaicin, local anesthetics, doxepin, tacrolimus, and botulinum toxin A. Current systemic therapy relies on anticonvulsants such as gabapentin and pregabalin. Phototherapy, transcutaneous electrical nerve stimulation, and physical therapy have also been of value in selected cases. Among the avenues to be explored are transcranial magnetic stimulation of the brain, new topical cannabinoid receptor agonists, various modes of acupuncture, a holistic approach with healing touch, and cell transplantation to the spinal cord.

The first and possibly most crucial step in management of neurologic itch is paved by the clinician's suspicion that the pruritic condition is of neurologic origin.

Definition and Clinical Characteristics

Neurologic itch is defined as pruritus resulting from any dysfunction of the nervous system. A further distinction between a solely functional and an anatomical pathology as the cause of this type of itch has been made by some authors and the terms 'neurogenic itch' and 'neuropathic itch' have been coined [1, 2]. Two other terms, 'neurochemical itch' and 'neuroanatomic itch', which have also been introduced in an attempt to classify itch pathophysiologically, may be considered synonyms of neurogenic and neuropathic itch, respectively [3]. Neurogenic itch has been described as itch arising as a consequence of altered neurochemical activity. The disinhibition of itch in cholestatic hepatic disease as a result of increased opioidergic tone is currently the prototype of this type of itch. Neuropathic itch has been defined as itch arising due to a neuroanatomic pathology. In other words, any damage to the neurons involved in the conduction and processing of the pruritic sensation is considered to be neuropathic. This category encompasses a much wider selection of examples than neurogenic itch. As cholestatic itch treatment will be discussed elsewhere in this book, this chapter will focus on management of various forms of neuropathic itch.

The causes of neuropathic itch range from localized entrapment of a peripheral nerve to generalized degeneration of small nerve fibers [4]. A recently recognized clinical phenomenon is generalized itch triggered by a localized disorder, namely brachioradial pruritus (BRP) [5]. Although the exact mechanism of this shift is not yet elucidated, central sensitization is thought to play an important role. Whether localized or generalized, all forms of neuropathic itch share two common denominators. Firstly, pruritus is accompanied by various paresthetic sensations including a feeling of electrical current, prickling, tingling, burning, and numbness – all of which are important clues in the diagnosis of neuro-

pathic itch [3, 6]. Neuropathic itch is also often associated with findings of central sensitization such as allodynia (pain resulting from a normally nonpainful stimulus), hyperalgesia (increased pain response to a painful stimulus), alloknesis (itch arising from a normally nonpruriceptive stimulus), and hyperknesis (increased itch response to a pruritic stimulus) [7]. The second characteristic common in all forms of neuropathic itch is the lack of efficacy of antipruritic medications commonly used for other types of itch. The list of these medications is led by antihistamines and topical corticosteroids [8]. Unfortunately, it is only this unresponsiveness to conventional antipruritic agents that is shared by different forms of neuropathic itch. Currently there are no therapeutic options that offer relief in all types of neuropathic pruritus, and treatment strategies vary according to etiology. Table 1 shows a list of clinical entities characterized by neuropathic itch and some treatment options suggested in the literature.

Diagnostics

The diagnostic approach to a patient with suspected neuropathic itch should start by excluding dermatological and other systemic diseases. Once these are eliminated, a neurological basis should be searched for beginning with history and neurological examination. It is best to consult a neurologist at this stage and decide on the appropriate tests and procedures in collaboration.

There is no single diagnostic test for neuropathic itch. Electromyography and nerve conduction studies are useful for showing a polyneuropathy which may be associated with itch, but normal findings do not rule out a neuropathic disorder as the abovementioned neurophysiological modalities cannot measure C-fiber activity which is responsible for itch. Measuring various sensory thresholds is far from being rewarding as such

Table 1. Conditions with neuropathic pruritus and some suggested therapies

Diagnosis	Treatment options
Neuropathic itch of specific localization	
BRP	Capsaicin patch, amitriptyline/ketamine cream, gabapentin, botulinum toxin A
Cheiralgia paresthetica	Decompression with surgery and other measures
Genitoanal pruritus	Intralesional corticosteroid + lidocaine if radiculopathy present, tacrolimus, local anesthetics
Glossodynia	Capsaicin oral rinse, gabapentin
Gonyalgia paresthetica	Reassurance
Meralgia paresthetica	Decompression with surgery and other measures
NP	Capsaicin patch, physical therapy, oxcarbazepine, botulinum toxin A, UVB phototherapy
Scalp dysesthesia	Pregabalin
Trigeminal trophic syndrome	Gabapentin, tacrolimus
Neuropathic itch of dermatological origin	
Postherpetic pruritus	Gabapentin, amitriptyline/ketamine gel
Scars/keloids	Pregabalin
Postburn pruritus	Doxepin cream, local anesthetics, gabapentin
Neuropathic itch with variable clinical presentation	
Abscess	Surgery + antimicrobials
Creutzfeldt-Jakob disease	Disease-modifying treatment
Multiple sclerosis	Disease-modifying treatment
Neuromyelitis optica	Disease-modifying treatment
Phantom itch of amputation	Scratching prosthetic limb
Stroke	Disease-modifying treatment
Syringomyelia	Surgery, gabapentin
Traumatic spinal injury	Pregabalin
Tumors (spinal, cerebral)	Surgery, gabapentin
Small fiber neuropathy	Gabapentin

tests do not always provide objective findings and no diagnostically meaningful patterns have been observed in patients with neuropathic pain [9]. Histopathological examination of the skin to demonstrate changes in cutaneous innervation is usually reserved for research purposes. This is largely due to the need for intricate tissue processing and difficulties in making a quantitative assessment of nerve density. Comparison of lesional samples with contralateral nonlesional skin is suggested [9, 10].

Currently the most frequently used diagnostic tool in the diagnosis of neuropathic itch is radioimaging. Radiologic modalities ranging from simple X-rays to computerized tomography and magnetic resonance imaging have been quite useful in detecting cerebral and spinal tumors, infarcts, various inflammatory lesions, and vertebral pathologies as causes of neuronal impingement [8, 9, 11–16]. Newer techniques offering accurate determination and localization of symptomatic nerve entrapment are magnetic resonance neurography and high-resolution ultrasound. These high-resolution nerve imaging methods enable images at the level of individual nerve fascicles and help discriminate between focal and nonfocal neuropathies. They have not yet been utilized in the evaluation of neuropathic itch, but hold great promise as the range of anatomic abnormalities they can detect include fibrous, muscular, and vascular entrapment; hypertrophic and ischemic neuropathy; neoplastic or granulomatous infiltration, and scar tissue [9, 17].

Treatment

Treatment of neuropathic itch includes general antipruritic measures, local or systemic pharmacotherapy, various physical modalities, and surgery. Discovery and elimination of the underlying pathology should be the initial aim. Unfortunately neuropathic itch is still an orphan entity and much of the published data on therapeutics are in the form of case reports, with very few randomized and controlled studies.

When the etiology is a spinal or cerebral mass, abscess, or hemorrhagic stroke, the obvious choice of therapy is surgical removal of the offending factor. Entrapment of specific peripheral nerves such as the superficial branch of the radial nerve in the hand which results in cheiralgia paresthetica, the lateral femoral cutaneous nerve of the lateral thigh which presents as meralgia paresthetica, cervical or thoracic spinal nerves causing BRP in the dorsolateral parts of the arms, or notalgia paresthetica (NP) in the back may also benefit from decompression of the affected nerves by surgical intervention, especially in severe cases [15, 18–20]. Physical therapy for muscle strengthening and postural adjustment coupled with elimination of the constricting factors such as bracelets, tight clothes, and excess weight are other recommendations [21, 22]. Collaboration with radiologists, neurologists, and neurosurgeons may not be easy when neuropathic itch is not accompanied by other clinical findings. Awareness about itch originating from neural disease is not yet common among these specialties. It may also be difficult to convince a surgeon to operate on a patient suffering from itch as this symptom is frequently not taken as seriously as pain.

In a great majority of patients with neuropathic itch, it is not possible to eradicate the cause and sometimes even after successful surgery there is only partial regression of itch; therefore, symptomatic treatment is needed [15, 23]. General antipruritic measures which should be enforced independently of the diagnosis are led by an effort to improve skin barrier function which is damaged by continuous scratching [23, 24]. Use of emollients and cleansers with low pH should be encouraged to break the itch-scratch cycle. Gentle massaging during application of an emollient has been suggested to improve anti-itch efficacy [25]. Other helpful adjustments are avoidance of warm ambient temperature, wearing loose fitting clothes, cutting nails short, and in certain cases using protective garments such as mittens or a helmet [1, 9, 23, 24, 26].

Good and long-lasting communication with the patient is crucial for treatment success of this notoriously frustrating symptom [6]. Cognitive behavioral therapy to help break the itch-scratch cycle or at least educating the patient about less destructive methods of scratching are rewarding to some extent [9, 26]. In milder cases, for example, many patients with NP are simply content with reassurance that their itch is not a reflection of a malignancy and that they are not imagining it. In contrast, BRP patients fervently ask for itch treatment. Cold application in the form of ice packs is of transient benefit and considered to be pathognomonic for this disorder [27].

Local Pharmacotherapy

Local symptomatic pharmacotherapy with a number of topical or intralesional agents has been used in various forms of localized neuropathic itch; however, only data from case reports exist so far. The list of medications with at least some effect includes capsaicin, local anesthetics, doxepin, tacrolimus, and botulinum toxin A [28]. Capsaicin, a compound found in chili peppers desensitizes sensory nerve fibers by binding to vanilloid receptor subtype 1 (TRPV1), which in return sends signals to the central nervous system resulting in a similar sensation to that of excessive heat. Following this initial 'burning' and with prolonged exposure to capsaicin, neuropeptides including substance P are depleted and TRPV1 inactivated at the sensory terminals of skin and mucosae [7]. Capsaicin cream in low concentrations (0.025–0.1%) was reported to improve pruritus in patients with NP and BRP [29, 30]. Capsaicin in the form of an oral rinse brought some relief to a group of patients with burning mouth syndrome [31]. Very recently, a newly introduced single-dose high-concentration patch containing 8% capsaicin was shown to have a long-lasting effect in a small group of patients with neuropathic pruritus refractory to other treatment [32]. Other local anesthetics such as pramoxine, lidocaine, a eutectic mixture of prilocaine and lidocaine, and amitriptyline/ketamine were reported to have short-term efficacy in NP, BRP, and postherpetic pruritus [14, 24, 26, 28, 33]. At present they are recommended as an additional short-term therapy [28].

Emerging anatomical, neurophysiological, and pharmacological evidence supports the involvement of neuropathic mechanisms in chronic pruritus of burns [34]. In contrast to the early inflammatory and proliferative phases of wound healing when histamine is among the main mediators of itch signaling, the late remodeling phase which takes place after wound closure is unresponsive to antihistamines and anti-inflammatory agents such as corticosteroids. Topical doxepin, which is a tricyclic antidepressant with potent antihistamine properties, has been used with moderate success for healed burn wounds with persistent itching [35]. However, the risk of developing contact dermatitis upon prolonged exposure and the lack of availability in several countries have limited further experience with this agent.

Tacrolimus is a calcineurin inhibitor which increases intracellular calcium ion concentrations of TRPV1 and enhances discharges of heat-sensitive cutaneous C-fibers similarly to capsaicin. Topical tacrolimus was reported to benefit one patient with NP and another patient with trigeminal trophic syndrome when used in combination with a systemic agent [36, 37]. Another agent with a proposed mode of action similar to that of capsaicin is botulinum toxin A. Treatment with 0.3- to 4-IU injections 1.5–2 cm apart has given variable results in a very limited number of patients with NP, BRP, meralgia paresthetica, and postherpetic pruritus [26, 38, 39].

Systemic Pharmacotherapy

Systemic pharmacotherapy of neuropathic itch is indicated in cases where local therapy is not effective or is difficult to apply. With no help from corticosteroids or antihistamines, except perhaps some soporific effect by the latter, the list of systemic medications which provide relief is largely made up of anticonvulsants. A major factor that hinders any kind of systemic pharmacotherapy is that with only short-term efficacy, any drug providing some relief of neuropathic pruritus needs to be taken either continuously or at least in repetitive cycles. This, coupled with the fact that in many countries few of these medications are approved or reimbursed for itch treatment, prevents the attainment of long-term results. Therefore, today systemic pharmacotherapy of neuropathic itch largely depends on off-label use of various medications [8]. The general recommendation is to start with a single agent at a low dose and increase the dose until antipruritic efficacy or intolerable side effects are observed. A combination of medications should only be attempted once the highest dose tolerable by a single drug has been exhausted.

Gabapentin and pregabalin are both structural analogues of γ-aminobutyric acid (GABA), which is an inhibitory neurotransmitter. Pregabalin was developed as a successor to gabapentin and binds more strongly to receptors than its predecessor. Both are recognized as pain modulators and have proven to be useful in neuropathic pain syndromes [23, 24, 26]. Gabapentin is considered to be a safe drug with generally mild side effects such as sedation, dizziness, weight gain, and peripheral edema. Case reports of a variety of patients with neuropathic itch ranging from BRP and NP to postherpetic itch and postburn pruritus responding to gabapentin at daily doses between 300 and 1,800 mg are encouraging [23, 24, 26, 40, 41]. Pregabalin at a daily dose of 150 mg was shown to be effective in chronic pruritus. However, experience with neuropathic itch is scarce and currently limited to two case reports: one of a patient with Brown-Séquard syndrome and the other a patient with scalp pruritus [26, 42]. The current European expert recommendation for systemic therapy of neuropathic itch includes only these two agents [28]. Another anticonvulsant which has shown efficacy in a small number of NP cases is oxcarbazepine, which is a keto-analogue of carbamazepine with a similar analgesic efficacy and a better side-effect profile [43]. Although antidepressants such as mirtazapine, paroxetine, lamotrigine, doxepin, and amitriptyline have been used in the treatment of neuropathic pain and their use in neuropathic itch is recommended by some experts, there is currently no published data regarding their efficacy [4, 24].

Other Therapeutic Modalities

Other therapeutic modalities with promising results on a limited number of cases are phototherapy, transcutaneous electrical nerve stimulation, physical therapy, and acupuncture [14, 22, 28, 44–46]. Both narrowband UVB cabin phototherapy [44] and local UVB phototherapy (unpubl. clinical experience) have provided some relief in small numbers of NP patients. Transcutaneous electrical nerve stimulation and physical therapy have also been of value in selected cases of local neuropathic itch [14, 22, 45]. All of these options are quite safe and offer the possibility to be combined with pharmaceutical treatment.

Among avenues to be explored in the future are noninvasive transcranial magnetic stimulation of the brain, new topical cannabinoid receptor agonists, κ-opioid receptor agonists and μ-opioid receptor antagonists, various modes of acupuncture, and a holistic approach with healing touch [23, 24, 26]. Finally in a very recent study, transplantation of GABAergic progenitor cells to the spinal cords of mice with genetically induced neuropathic itch resulting from loss of dorsal horn GABAergic interneurons, which normally inhibits transmission of the itch signal, has been shown to restore spinal cord inhibitory controls and ameliorate neuropathic itch. Such cell-mediated intervention that manages to help repair spinal damage holds promise not just as anti-itch therapy, but also as a modifier of the etiological spinal pathology [47].

In conclusion, our current armamentarium against neuropathic itch is evidence that in order for a complete cure, this enigmatic entity needs to be further explored by neuroscience enthusiasts, including dermatologists. With advanced medical technology in hand, compassion for the itching at heart, and a growing interest in itch in the cerebrum, this will surely be a rewarding expedition for the entire investigative dermatology community to embark upon.

References

1 Twycross R, Greaves MW, Handwerker H, Jones EA, Libretto SE, Szepietowski JC, Zylicz Z: Itch: scratching more than the surface. QJM 2003;96:7–26.

2 Ständer S, Weisshaar E, Mettang T, Szepietowski JC, Carstens E, Ikoma A, Bergasa NV, Gieler U, Misery L, Wallengren J, Darsow U, Streit M, Metze D, Luger TA, Greaves MW, Schmelz M, Yosipovitch G, Bernhard JD: Clinical classification of itch: a position paper of the International Forum for the Study of Itch. Acta Derm Venereol 2007;87:291–294.

3 Bernhard JD: Itch and pruritus: what are they, and how should itches be classified? Dermatol Ther 2005;18:288–291.

4 Stumpf A, Ständer S: Neuropathic itch: diagnosis and management. Dermatol Ther 2013;26:104–109.

5 Kwatra SG, Ständer S, Bernhard JD, Weisshaar E, Yosipovitch G: Brachioradial pruritus: a trigger for generalization of itch. J Am Acad Dermatol 2013;68:870–873.

6 Bernhard JD: Not all itches arise in the skin. Br J Dermatol 2015;172:309–311.

7 Ikoma A: Updated neurophysiology of itch. Biol Pharm Bull 2013;36:1235–1240.

8 Ständer S, Zeidler C, Magnolo N, Raap U, Mettang T, Kremer AE, Weisshaar E, Augustin M: Clinical management of pruritus. J Dtsch Dermatol Ges 2015;13:101–115.

9 Oaklander AL: Neuropathic Itch; in Carstens E, Akiyama T (eds): Itch: Mechanisms and Treatment. Boca Raton, CRC Press/Taylor and Francis, 2014.

10 Savk E, Dikicioğlu E, Culhaci N, Karaman G, Sendur N: Immunohistochemical findings in notalgia paresthetica. Dermatology 2002;204:88–93.

11 Savk E, Savk O, Bolukbasi O, Culhaci N, Dikicioğlu E, Karaman G, Sendur N: Notalgia paresthetica: a study on pathogenesis. Int J Dermatol 2000;39:754–759.

12 Savk O, Savk E: Investigation of spinal pathology in notalgia paresthetica. J Am Acad Dermatol 2005;52:1085–1087.

13 Marziniak M, Phan NQ, Raap U, Siepmann D, Schürmeyer-Horst F, Pogatzki-Zahn E, Niederstadt T, Ständer S: Brachioradial pruritus as a result of cervical spine pathology: the results of a magnetic resonance tomography study. J Am Acad Dermatol 2011;65:756–762.

14 Mirzoyev SA, Davis MD: Brachioradial pruritus: Mayo Clinic experience over the past decade. Br J Dermatol 2013;169:1007–1015.

15 Soltani-Arabshahi R, Vanderhooft S, Hansen CD: Intractable localized pruritus as the sole manifestation of intramedullary tumor in a child: case report and review of the literature. JAMA Dermatol 2013;149:446–449.

16 Thornsberry LA, English JC 3rd: Scalp dysesthesia related to cervical spine disease. JAMA Dermatol 2013;149:200–203.

17 Pham M, Bäumer T, Bendszus M: Peripheral nerves and plexus: imaging by MR-neurography and high-resolution ultrasound. Curr Opin Neurol 2014;27:370–379.

18 Tosun N, Tuncay I, Akpinar F: Entrapment of the sensory branch of the radial nerve (Wartenberg's syndrome): an unusual cause. Tohoku J Exp Med 2001;193:251–254.

19 Binder A, Fölster-Holst R, Sahan G, Koroschetz J, Stengel M, Mehdorn HM, Schwarz T, Baron R: A case of neuropathic brachioradial pruritus caused by cervical disc herniation. Nat Clin Pract Neurol 2008;4:338–342.

20 Gohar A: Neuropathic hand pruritus. Indian J Dermatol Venereol Leprol 2009;75:531–532.

21 Massey EW: Sensory mononeuropathies. Semin Neurol 1998;18:177–183.

22 Fleischer AB, Meade TJ, Fleischer AB: Notalgia paresthetica: successful treatment with exercises. Acta Derm Venereol 2011;91:356–357.

23 Grundmann S, Ständer S: Chronic pruritus: clinics and treatment. Ann Dermatol 2011;23:1–11.

24 Yosipovitch G, Bernhard JD: Clinical practice. Chronic pruritus. N Engl J Med 2013;368:1625–1634.

25 Zachariah JR, Rao AL, Prabha R, Gupta AK, Paul MK, Lamba S: Post burn pruritus – a review of current treatment options. Burns 2012;38:621–629.

26 Dhand A, Aminoff MJ: The neurology of itch. Brain 2014;137:313–322.

27 Bernhard JD, Bordeaux JS: Medical pearl: the ice-pack sign in brachioradial pruritus. J Am Acad Dermatol 2005;52:1073.

28 Weisshaar E, Szepietowski JC, Darsow U, Misery L, Wallengren J, Mettang T, Gieler U, Lotti T, Lambert J, Maisel P, Streit M, Greaves MW, Carmichael AJ, Tschachler E, Ring J, Ständer S: European guideline on chronic pruritus. Acta Derm Venereol 2012;92:563–581.

29 Wallengren J, Klinker M: Successful treatment of notalgia paresthetica with topical capsaicin. vehicle controlled, double-blind, crossover study. J Am Acad Dermatol 1995;32:287–289.

30 Wallengren J: Brachioradial pruritus: a recurrent solar dermopathy. J Am Acad Dermatol 1998;39:803–806.

31 de Moraes M, do Amaral Bezerra BA, da Rocha Neto PC, de Oliveira Soares AC, Pinto LP, de Lisboa Lopes Costa A: Randomized trials for the treatment of burning mouth syndrome: an evidence-based review of the literature. J Oral Pathol Med 2012;41:281–287.

32 Misery L, Erfan N, Castela E, Brenaut E, Lantéri-Minet M, Lacour JP, Passeron T: Successful treatment of refractory neuropathic pruritus with capsaicin 8% patch: a bicentric retrospective study with long-term follow-up. Acta Derm Venereol 2015;95:864–865.

33 Griffin JR, Davis MD: Amitriptyline/ketamine as therapy for neuropathic pruritus and pain secondary to herpes zoster. J Drugs Dermatol 2015;14:115–118.

34 Goutos I: Neuropathic mechanisms in the pathophysiology of burns pruritus: redefining directions for therapy and research. J Burn Care Res 2013;34:82–93.

35 Goutos I, Dziewulski P, Richardson PM: Pruritus in burns: review article. J Burn Care Res 2009;30:221–228.

36 Nakamizo S, Miyachi Y, Kabashima K: Treatment of neuropathic itch possibly due to trigeminal trophic syndrome with 0.1% topical tacrolimus and gabapentin. Acta Derm Venereol 2010;90:654–655.

37 Ochi H, Tan LX, Tey HL: Notalgia paresthetica: treatment with topical tacrolimus. J Eur Acad Dermatol Venereol 2016;30:452–454.

38 Wallengren J, Bartosik J: Botulinum toxin type A for neuropathic itch. Br J Dermatol 2010;163:424–426.

39 Pérez-Pérez L, García-Gavín J, Allegue F, Caeiro JL, Fabeiro JM, Zulaica A: Notalgia paresthetica: treatment using intradermal botulinum toxin A. Actas Dermosifiliogr 2014;105:74–77.

40 Loosemore MP, Bordeaux JS, Bernhard JD: Gabapentin treatment for notalgia paresthetica, a common isolated peripheral sensory neuropathy. J Eur Acad Dermatol Venereol 2007;21:1440–1441.

41 Bueller HA, Bernhard JD, Dubroff LM: Gabapentin treatment for brachioradial pruritus. J Eur Acad Dermatol Venereol 1999;13:227–228.

42 Sarifakioglu E, Onur O: Women with scalp dysesthesia treated with pregabalin. Int J Dermatol 2013;52:1417–1418.

43 Savk E, Bolukbasi O, Akyol A, Karaman G: Open pilot study on oxcarbazepine for the treatment of notalgia paresthetica. J Am Acad Dermatol 2001;45:630–632.

44 Pérez-Pérez L, Allegue F, Fabeiro JM, Caeiro JL, Zulaica A: Notalgia paresthesica successfully treated with narrowband UVB: report of five cases. J Eur Acad Dermatol Venereol 2010;24:730–732.

45 Savk E, Savk O, Sendur F: Transcutaneous electrical nerve stimulation offers partial relief in notalgia paresthetica patients with a relevant spinal pathology. J Dermatol 2007;34:315–319.

46 Carlsson CP, Wallengren J: Therapeutic and experimental therapeutic studies on acupuncture and itch: review of the literature. J Eur Acad Dermatol Venereol 2010;24:1013–1016.

47 Braz JM, Juarez-Salinas D, Ross SE, Basbaum AI: Transplant restoration of spinal cord inhibitory controls ameliorates neuropathic itch. J Clin Invest 2014;124:3612–3616.

Ekin Şavk
Department of Dermatology, Faculty of Medicine, Adnan Menderes University
Aytepe
TR–09100, Aydın (Turkey)
E-Mail esavk@adu.edu.tr

Szepietowski JC, Weisshaar E (eds): Itch – Management in Clinical Practice.
Curr Probl Dermatol. Basel, Karger, 2016, vol 50, pp 124–132 (DOI: 10.1159/000446055)

Psychogenic Itch Management

Jacek C. Szepietowski · Radomir Reszke

Department of Dermatology, Venereology and Allergology, Wrocław Medical University, Wrocław, Poland

Abstract

Pruritus is a bothersome and prevalent symptom reported by patients suffering from both cutaneous and extracutaneous diseases. Psychogenic pruritus, also referred to as functional itch disorder, is a distinct clinical entity. According to the definition proposed by the French Psychodermatology Group (FPDG) in 2007, the disorder is characterized by pruritus which is the chief complaint and psychologic factors that contribute to eliciting, worsening, and sustaining the symptoms. Specific diagnostic criteria were proposed, including 3 compulsory and 7 optional, of which 3 have to be met in order to establish the diagnosis. Psychogenic pruritus may require cooperation between dermatologists, psychiatrists, and psychologists. Psychotherapy and psychopharmacotherapy are mainstays of managing the disease. However, publications regarding psychogenic itch management are uncommon. Initially, general measures have to be taken, including avoiding irritating factors, preventing skin dryness, and frequent application of emollients. As in pruritus of other causes, several drugs are used, with more emphasis on substances that influence central nervous system: H_1-antihistamines (hydroxyzine, chlorpheniramine, cyproheptadine, diphenhydramine, promethazine), tricyclic antidepressants (doxepin), tetracyclic antidepressants (mirtazapine), selective serotonin reuptake inhibitors (citalopram, escitalopram, fluoxetine, fluvoxamine, paroxetine, sertraline), antipsychotic drugs (pimozide), anticonvulsants (topiramate), and benzodiazepines (alprazolam), preferably depending on the coexisting symptoms. © 2016 S. Karger AG, Basel

Definition and Clinical Characteristics

Itch is regarded as the most common symptom in dermatology that significantly reduces the quality of life in affected patients. This bothersome symptom is frequently encountered in medical practice in other specialties as well. Possible underlying systemic causes involve endocrine, hematologic, hepatic, infectious, renal, or neurological diseases [1]. Occasionally, the origins of chronic pruritus reside in the psyche area principally, emphasized by the following statement: 'It is the brain that itches, not the skin' [2]. Pruritus is common among psychiatric patients (17.5–32%), whereas

Table 1. Psychogenic itch-related terms used in the literature

Functional itch disorder
Somatoform pruritus
Psychosomatic pruritus
Nonorganic pruritus
Itch disorder associated with psychological disorders

over 70% of dermatology inpatients suffering from chronic pruritus presented with psychiatric symptomatology [3–5]. Among 195 dermatologic outpatients, 10.3% presented with somatoform pruritus [6]. Psychogenic pruritus is considered as an independent clinical entity in which pruritus is the main symptom while psychogenic factors are crucial in eliciting, intensifying, and sustaining the disease [7]. The definition was proposed by the French Psychodermatology Group (FPDG) in 2007. The authors discussed several related terms (table 1) and suggested that functional itch disorder is the most appropriate one as it places the disorder in the 'functional' spectrum and does not include a 'psychogenic' element which may seem too interpretative. Nevertheless, the nomenclature remains controversial.

According to the FPDG, psychogenic pruritus is diagnosed based on several criteria, as described in the chapter by Reich and Szepietowski [this vol., pp. 24–28]. There are three compulsory criteria which encompass localized or generalized pruritus without primary skin lesions, at least 6 weeks' duration of symptoms, and the absence of somatic causes of itch. Additionally, 3 out of 7 optional criteria also need to be met. The latter are presented in figure 1 along with prevalence rates in patients suffering from psychogenic pruritus, as reported by Misery et al. [8]. Prior to establishing the diagnosis of psychogenic itch, it is necessary to exclude various possible cutaneous and extracutaneous causes, which may be time-consuming and costly. Importantly, psychogenic itch diagnosis is neither a synonym of idiopathic

pruritus (pruritus of unknown origin) nor of senile pruritus, although in every one of them conscientious exclusion of various contributing factors has to be performed. Moreover, psychogenic factors in general may influence pruritus notwithstanding the underlying cause. Although the FPDG diagnostic criteria are useful in clinical practice, 6 weeks' duration of symptoms appears controversial. Psychogenic etiology of acute pruritus was also reported [9].

Management

Despite characteristic features implying specific therapeutic modalities in psychogenic pruritus, the initial approach is similar in all pruritus subtypes. General clinical recommendations include avoiding dryness of the skin and contact with irritant factors [1]. Therefore, too frequent washing, hot baths, low air humidity, hot and spicy food and beverages, alcohol, compresses with Rivanol© or chamomile, woolen clothes, and contact with aeroallergens are contraindicated. Frequent application of emollients at least twice daily improves the skin barrier and reduces itching notwithstanding the underlying cause. Topical preparations with urea, tannin, menthol, polidocanol, lignocaine, and wet or fat-moist wrappings provide temporary relief from bothersome symptoms and break the vicious 'itch-scratch-itch cycle'.

A specific treatment approach targeted at psychogenic pruritus is an example of interdisciplinary cooperation between dermatologists, psychiatrists, psychosomatic medicine specialists, and psychologists. Fried [10] proposed a 'three-level approach' to psychogenic pruritus, concentrating on lesional, emotional, and cognitive levels. Establishing a trust-based relationship between the physician and patient is essential. In general, psychogenic pruritus is treated utilizing psychotherapy and psychopharmacotherapy. Psychotherapy of itch is a complex and clinically relevant issue

gender dependent, varying between 20 and 40 h [36]. Mirtazapine is extensively metabolized (mainly by CYP2D6 and CYP3A4 isoenzymes); over 75% of the dose is eliminated via urine. Typically, the drug is administered in doses extending from 7.5 to even 45 mg per day (for pruritic subjects most commonly 7.5–15 mg administered in the evening). Fawcett and Barkin [37] evaluated 359 patients treated with mirtazapine due to depression. The most common side effects encompassed dryness of the mouth, appetite alteration, drowsiness, excessive sedation, fatigue, constipation, and body weight increase. In comparison with TCA, sexual dysfunction and the risk of overdosing are rare. Besides treatment of depression disorders, mirtazapine is utilized as an itch-relieving treatment in advanced cancer, cholestasis, hepatic failure, renal failure, atopic eczema, lichen simplex chronicus, cutaneous T-cell lymphoma, and carcinoma en cuirasse [13, 38–41]. 5-HT_2-receptor antagonism of mirtazapine results in anxiolytic effects that alleviate itching notwithstanding the cause.

Selective Serotonin Reuptake Inhibitors
SSRIs are antidepressant drugs that preferentially bind to the presynaptic serotonin reuptake carrier in the central nervous system, thus increasing serotonin levels in the synaptic cleft [42]. Serotonin reuptake specificity varies among the group; noradrenaline reuptake and dopamine reuptake, along with dopamine, muscarinic, and adrenergic receptor affinity also contribute to clinical outcomes. Gastrointestinal absorption is high albeit slow. Fluvoxamine, fluoxetine, and paroxetine are characterized by nonlinear kinetics. As a result, increasing the dose results in a disproportionate increase in drug concentrations [43].

It is important that the clinical onset of action usually starts no sooner than 2–3 weeks after initiating the therapy with SSRIs. The maximum effect is observed approximately after 4–6 weeks of therapy. Besides treating depression, SSRIs are recommended in managing obsessive-compul-

sive disorder, generalized anxiety disorder, posttraumatic stress disorder, and eating disorders [44, 45]. As psychoemotional factors may influence itch threshold [2] and chronic pruritus patients present depressive symptoms in up to 10.1% of the cases [5], the use of antidepressants is justifiable. In a study by Ständer et al. [46], 72 patients suffering from chronic itch were treated with paroxetine or fluvoxamine: 49 patients (68%) experienced reduction of symptoms, with 40 patients in total (55.6%) reporting good or very good antipruritic effect. Biondi et al. [15] advocated the use of paroxetine in a patient with psychogenic pruritus.

Although several adverse effects may occur, the safety profile of SSRIs is significantly more favorable in comparison with TCA. Interestingly, SSRIs were reported as an eliciting factor of pruritus as well [47].

Notably, SSRIs are potent inhibitors of CYP enzymes (especially CYP2D6, CYP2C9, and CYP2C19) and are metabolized by CYP themselves. This information is clinically relevant as pharmacological interactions may occur, especially in polypharmacy patients. Pharmacological characteristics of SSRIs are given in table 3.

Pimozide
Among various treatment modalities utilized in patients suffering from psychodermatoses, antipsychotic drugs have also been evaluated. Pimozide is a potent dopamine receptor antagonist, preferentially blocking D_2 receptors in central nervous system. After oral administration, 50% bioavailability is reached, with a half-life of approximately 29 h [50]. Pimozide undergoes hepatic metabolism, and excretion occurs chiefly via urine. Apart from antidopaminergic activity, α-adrenergic blockade, voltage-dependent calcium channels inhibition, opiate antagonism, and 5-HT_2 antagonism were also reported [50, 51]. The typical dosage is 1–2 mg/day, increased daily or weekly by 1–2 mg, although Lorenzo and Koo [52] proposed a starting dose of 0.5–1.0 mg, in-

Active ingredient	Typical dose, mg/day	Bioavailability; half-life	Meta-bolism	Excretion	Adverse effects
Citalopram	20–60	100%; 36 h	yes	50% renal	asthenia, sweating, constipation, decreased appetite, dryness of mouth, nausea, anxiety, dizziness, nervousness, paresthesia, somnolence, tremor, ejaculation abnormalities, serotonin syndrome
Escitalopram (S-enantiomer of racemic citalopram)	10–20	80%; 32.5±14.2 h	yes	renal	
Fluoxetine	20–60	<90%; 24–96 h	yes	renal; 10% unchanged	
Fluvoxamine	50–200	>53%; 8–28 h	yes	renal	
Paroxetine	20–30	50%; 9.8–21 h	yes	36% metabolites via feces	
Sertraline	25–150	22.4–46.7 h	yes	renal; 50% metabolites via feces	

creased weekly by 1 mg. Several groups have reported the effectiveness of pimozide in managing delusions of parasitosis [53–55]. Hamann and Avnstorp [54] emphasized that pruritus diminished significantly in these patients. It is important to underline that pimozide is not registered in many countries and that patients with delusional parasitosis are also successfully managed with newer antipsychotics, like risperidone (1–3 mg/day) or olanzapine (2.5–10 mg/day) [56].

Potential adverse effects of pimozide include extrapyramidal reactions (akathisia, tremor, rigidity, salivation, masked facies), insomnia, anorexia, nausea, abdominal pain, diarrhea, constipation, hypotension, sedation, drowsiness, insomnia, anxiety, agitation, excitement, hallucinations, and dryness of mouth [57].

Alprazolam

BDZ are positive allosteric modulators of the γ-aminobutyric acid A (GABA$_A$) receptor, which is a ligand-gated chloride ion channel [58]. In general, GABA acts as an inhibitory molecule in the central nervous system, decreasing the excitability of neurons. Due to these properties, BDZ serve as potent anxiolytics, sedatives, hypnotics, anticonvulsants, and myorelaxants. Additionally, BDZ-induced amnesia is utilized in premedication by anesthesiologists. Alprazolam is a commonly used member of triazolobenzodiazepines.

Following oral administration, alprazolam is rapidly absorbed; the bioavailability reaches 84–92% [59]. The mean half-life ranges between 10 and 18 h. The drug is metabolized by hepatic microsomal enzymes and metabolites are excreted via urine. Although BDZ have a high therapeutic index and thus overdose symptoms are usually mild or moderate, potential adverse effects are rich in number and have to be taken into account by the physician. These include somnolence, diplopia, dysarthria, ataxia, and intellectual impairment [60]. Occasionally, life-threatening cardiopulmonary adverse effects may occur. Prolonged use is associated with the risk of dependence and withdrawal symptoms [61]. Interactions with other drugs exerting depressive effects on the central nervous system or alcohol are also possible.

As for psychodermatology, alprazolam administered in doses 0.25–0.5 mg three times daily is a supportive method in managing psychogenic pruritus or psychogenic excoriations in patients with prominent anxiety [10].

Topiramate

Topiramate is a sulfate-substituted monosaccharide that exerts its antiepileptic properties by several mechanisms, such as blocking voltage-sensitive sodium channels, increasing GABA$_A$-receptor-mediated chloride current, decreasing glutamate-mediated neurotransmission, increasing potassium conductance, inhibiting carbonic anhydrase isoenzyme, and interacting with protein kinase phosphorylation sites [62]. Besides neurological indications, psychiatric patients have also benefited from topiramate, especially those suffering from bipolar disorders, unipolar depression, schizophrenia, eating disorders, posttraumatic stress disorder, alcohol dependence, and Tourette's syndrome [63]. Typically, the daily dose varies between 50 and 400 mg. Following oral administration the bioavailability reaches 80%, with a half-life of approximately 19–23 h. Topiramate is excreted mostly unchanged in urine. Adverse effects include dizziness, headaches, paresthesia, ataxia, speech disturbances, somnolence, psychomotor slowing, nervousness, memory problems, and body weight loss [64].

Additionally, several papers have reported incitement of pruritus after topiramate intake [65–67]. On the other hand, an interesting case report by Calabrò et al. [68] raised the subject of an intractable psychogenic pruritus successfully treated with 150 mg of topiramate daily. As previously mentioned, publications focusing specifically on psychogenic pruritus management are very few in number.

In conclusion, psychogenic itch is a challenging clinical problem. Psychotherapeutic approach for those patients seems to be crucial; however, at least some of them may require psychopharmacotherapy as discussed above. It is important to underline that some agents, such as SSRIs, are also considered as second- or third-line therapy for other types of chronic itch.

References

1 Weisshaar E, Szepietowski JC, Darsow U, Misery L, Wallengren J, Mettang T, Gieler U, Lotti T, Lambert J, Maisel P, Streit M, Greaves MW, Carmichael AJ, Tschachler E, Ring J, Ständer S: European guideline on chronic pruritus. Acta Derm Venereol 2012;92:563–581.
2 Paus R, Schmelz M, Bíró T, Steinhoff M: Frontiers in pruritus research: scratching the brain for more effective itch therapy. J Clin Invest 2006;116:1174–1186.
3 Halvorsen JA, Dalgard F, Thoresen M, Thoresen M, Bjertness E, Lien L: Itch and mental distress: a cross-sectional study among late adolescents. Acta Derm Venereol 2009;89:39–44.
4 Mazeh D, Melamed Y, Cholostoy A, Aharonovitzch V, Weizman A, Yosipovitch G: Itching in the psychiatric ward. Acta Derm Venereol 2008;88:128–131.
5 Schneider G, Driesch G, Heuft G, Evers S, Luger TA, Ständer S: Psychosomatic cofactors and psychiatric comorbidity in patients with chronic itch. Clin Exp Dermatol 2006;31:762–767.
6 Stangier U, Köhnlein B, Gieler U: Somatoforme Störungen bei ambulanten dermatologischen Patienten. Psychotherapeut 2003;48:321–328.
7 Misery L, Alexandre S, Dutray S, Chastaing M, Consoli SG, Audra H, Bauer D, Bertolus S, Callot V, Cardinaud F, Corrin E, Feton-Danou N, Malet R, Touboul S, Consoli SM: Functional itch disorder or psychogenic pruritus: suggested diagnosis criteria from the French Psychodermatology Group. Acta Derm Venereol 2007;87:341–344.
8 Misery L, Wallengren J, Weisshaar E, Zalewska A; French Psychodermatology Group. Validation of diagnosis criteria of functional itch disorder or psychogenic pruritus. Acta Derm Venereol 2008;88:503–504.
9 Halvorson H, Crooks J, Lahart DA, Farrell KP: An outbreak of itching in an elementary school – a case of mass psychogenic response. J Sch Health 2008;78:294–297.
10 Fried RG: Evaluation and treatment of 'psychogenic' pruritus and self-excoriation. J Am Acad Dermatol 1994;30:993–999.
11 Harth W, Gieler U, Kusnir D, Tausk FA (eds): Clinical Management in Psychodermatology, ed 1. Berlin, Springer, 2009.
12 Harris BA, Sherertz EF, Flowers FP: Improvement of chronic neurotic excoriations with oral doxepin therapy. Int J Dermatol 1987;26:541–543.
13 Davis MP, Frandsen JL, Walsh D, Andresen S, Taylor S: Mirtazapine for pruritus. J Pain Symptom Manage 2003;25:288–291.
14 Shaw RJ, Dayal S, Good J, Bruckner AL, Joshi SV: Psychiatric medications for the treatment of pruritus. Psychosom Med 2007;69:970–978.
15 Biondi M, Arcangeli T, Petrucci RM: Paroxetine in a case of psychogenic pruritus and neurotic excoriations. Psychother Psychosom 2000;69:165–166.
16 Pukadan D, Antony J, Mohandas E, Cyriac M, Smith G, Elias A: Use of escitalopram in psychogenic excoriation. Aust NZ J Psychiatry 2008;42:435–436.
17 Koo JY, Ng TC: Psychotropic and neurotropic agents in dermatology: unapproved uses, dosages, or indications. Clin Dermatol 2002;20:582–594.
18 Church DS, Church MK: Pharmacology of antihistamines. World Allergy Organ J 2011;4(3 suppl):S22–S27.
19 Simons FE: Advances in H_1-antihistamines. N Engl J Med 2004;351:2203–2217.

20 Paton DM, Webster DR: Clinical pharmacokinetics of H_1-receptor antagonists (the antihistamines). Clin Pharmacokinet 1985;10:477–497.

21 Singh H, Becker PM: Novel therapeutic usage of low-dose doxepin hydrochloride. Expert Opin Investig Drugs 2007; 16:1295–1305.

22 Virtanen R, Scheinin M, Iisalo E: Single dose pharmacokinetics of doxepin in healthy volunteers. Acta Pharmacol Toxicol (Copenh) 1980;47:371–376.

23 Pentel PR, Benowitz NL: Tricyclic antidepressant poisoning. Management of arrhythmias. Med Toxicol 1986;1:101–121.

24 Smith PF, Corelli RL: Doxepin in the management of pruritus associated with allergic cutaneous reactions. Ann Pharmacother 1997;31:633–635.

25 Hoss D, Segal S. Scalp dysesthesia. Arch Dermatol 1998;134:327–330.

26 Pour-Reza-Gholi F, Nasrollahi A, Firouzan A, Nasli Esfahani E, Farrokhi F: Low-dose doxepin for treatment of pruritus in patients on hemodialysis. Iran J Kidney Dis 2007;1:34–37.

27 Smith KJ, Skelton HG, Yeager J, Lee RB, Wagner KF: Pruritus in HIV-1 disease: therapy with drugs which may modulate the pattern of immune dysregulation. Dermatology 1997;195:353–358.

28 Shohrati M, Tajik A, Harandi AA, Davoodi SM, Akmasi M: Comparison of hydroxyzine and doxepin in treatment of pruritus due to sulfur mustard. Skinmed 2007;6:70–72.

29 Berberian BJ, Breneman DL, Drake LA, Gratton D, Raimir SS, Phillips S, Sulica VI, Bernstein JE: The addition of topical doxepin to corticosteroid therapy: an improved treatment regimen for atopic dermatitis. Int J Dermatol 1999;38:145–148.

30 Drake LA, Fallon JD, Sober A: Relief of pruritus in patients with atopic dermatitis after treatment with topical doxepin cream. The Doxepin Study Group. J Am Acad Dermatol 1994;31:613–616.

31 Drake LA, Millikan LE: The antipruritic effect of 5% doxepin cream in patients with eczematous dermatitis. Doxepin Study Group. Arch Dermatol 1995;131: 1403–1408.

32 Breneman DL, Dunlap FE, Monroe EW, Schupbach CW, Shmunes E, Phillips SB: Doxepin cream relieves eczema-associated pruritus within 15 min and is not accompanied by a risk of rebound upon discontinuation. J Dermatol Treat 1997; 8:161–168.

33 Shelley WB, Shelley ED, Talanin NY: Self-potentiating allergic contact dermatitis caused by doxepin hydrochloride cream. J Am Acad Dermatol 1996;34: 143–144.

34 Bonnel RA, La Grenade L, Karwoski CB, Beitz JG: Allergic contact dermatitis from topical doxepin: Food and Drug Administration's postmarketing surveillance experience. J Am Acad Dermatol 2003;48:294–296.

35 Anttila SA, Leinonen EV: A review of the pharmacological and clinical profile of mirtazapine. CNS Drug Rev 2001;7: 249–264.

36 Timmer CJ, Sitsen JM, Delbressine LP: Clinical pharmacokinetics of mirtazapine. Clin Pharmacokinet 2000;38:461–474.

37 Fawcett J, Barkin RL: Review of the results from clinical studies on the efficacy, safety and tolerability of mirtazapine for the treatment of patients with major depression. J Affect Disord 1998;51: 267–285.

38 Hundley JL, Yosipovitch G: Mirtazapine for reducing nocturnal itch in patients with chronic pruritus: a pilot study. J Am Acad Dermatol 2004;50:889–891.

39 Bigatà X, Sais G, Soler F: Severe chronic urticaria: response to mirtazapine. J Am Acad Dermatol 2005;53:916–917.

40 Demierre MF, Taverna J: Mirtazapine and gabapentin for reducing pruritus in cutaneous T-cell lymphoma. J Am Acad Dermatol 2006;55:543–544.

41 Lee JJ, Girouard SD, Carlberg VM, Mostaghimi A: Effective use of mirtazapine for refractory pruritus associated with carcinoma en cuirasse. BMJ Support Palliat Care 2016;6:119–121.

42 van Harten J: Clinical pharmacokinetics of selective serotonin reuptake inhibitors. Clin Pharmacokinet 1993;24:203–220.

43 Hiemke C, Härtter S: Pharmacokinetics of selective serotonin reuptake inhibitors. Pharmacol Ther 2000;85:11–28.

44 Aigner M, Treasure J, Kaye W, Kasper S; WFSBP Task Force On Eating Disorders: World Federation of Societies of Biological Psychiatry (WFSBP) guidelines for the pharmacological treatment of eating disorders. World J Biol Psychiatry 2011; 12:400–443.

45 Bandelow B, Sher L, Bunevicius R, Hollander E, Kasper S, Zohar J, Möller HJ; WFSBP Task Force on Mental Disorders in Primary Care; WFSBP Task Force on Anxiety Disorders, OCD and PTSD: Guidelines for the pharmacological treatment of anxiety disorders, obsessive-compulsive disorder and posttraumatic stress disorder in primary care. Int J Psychiatry Clin Pract 2012;16:77–84.

46 Ständer S, Böckenholt B, Schürmeyer-Horst F, Weishaupt C, Heuft G, Luger TA, Schneider G: Treatment of chronic pruritus with the selective serotonin re-uptake inhibitors paroxetine and fluvoxamine: results of an open-labelled, two-arm proof-of-concept study. Acta Derm Venereol 2009;89:45–51.

47 Cederberg J, Knight S, Svenson S, Melhus H: Itch and skin rash from chocolate during fluoxetine and sertraline treatment: case report. BMC Psychiatry 2004; 4:36.

48 Rao N: The clinical pharmacokinetics of escitalopram. Clin Pharmacokinet 2007; 46:281–290.

49 Kaufman JM: Selective serotonin reuptake inhibitor (SSRI) drugs: more risks than benefits? J Am Physicians Surg 2009;14:7–12.

50 Tennyson H, Levine N: Neurotropic and psychotropic drugs in dermatology. Dermatol Clin 2001;19:179–197.

51 Cohen ML, Carpenter R, Schenck K, Wittenauer L, Mason N: Effect of nitrendipine, diltiazem, trifluoperazine and pimozide on serotonin2 (5-HT_2) receptor activation in the rat uterus and jugular vein. J Pharmacol Exp Ther 1986; 238:860–867.

52 Lorenzo CR, Koo J: Pimozide in dermatologic practice: a comprehensive review. Am J Clin Dermatol 2004;5:339–349.

53 Reilly TM, Jopling WH, Beard AW: Successful treatment with pimozide of delusional parasitosis. Br J Dermatol 1978; 98:457–459.

54 Hamann K, Avnstorp C: Delusions of infestation treated by pimozide: a double-blind crossover clinical study. Acta Derm Venereol 1982;62:55–58.

55 Zomer SF, De Wit RF, Van Bronswijk JE, Nabarro G, Van Vloten WA: Delusions of parasitosis. A psychiatric disorder to be treated by dermatologists? An analysis of 33 patients. Br J Dermatol 1998;138:1030–1032.

56 Lepping P, Freudenmann RW: Delusional parasitosis: a new pathway for diagnosis and treatment. Clin Exp Dermatol 2008;33:113–117.

57 Pinder RM, Brogden RN, Swayer R, Speight TM, Spencer R, Avery GS: Pimozide: a review of its pharmacological properties and therapeutic uses in psychiatry. Drugs 1976;12:1–40.

58 Griffin CE 3rd, Kaye AM, Bueno FR, Kaye AD: Benzodiazepine pharmacology and central nervous system-mediated effects. Ochsner J 2013;13:214–223.

59 Greenblatt DJ, Wright CE: Clinical pharmacokinetics of alprazolam. Therapeutic implications. Clin Pharmacokinet 1993;24:453–471.

60 Gaudreault P, Guay J, Thivierge RL, Verdy I: Benzodiazepine poisoning. Clinical and pharmacological considerations and treatment. Drug Saf 1991;6: 247–265.

61 Baldwin DS, Aitchison K, Bateson A, Curran HV, Davies S, Leonard B, Nutt DJ, Stephens DN, Wilson S: Benzodiazepines: risks and benefits. A reconsideration. J Psychopharmacol 2013;27: 967–971.

62 Guerrini R, Parmeggiani L: Topiramate and its clinical applications in epilepsy. Expert Opin Pharmacother 2006;7:811–823.

63 Arnone D: Review of the use of topiramate for treatment of psychiatric disorders. Ann Gen Psychiatry 2005;4:5.

64 Wong IC, Lhatoo SD: Adverse reactions to new anticonvulsant drugs. Drug Saf 2000;23:35–56.

65 Ochoa JG: Pruritus, a rare but troublesome adverse reaction of topiramate. Seizure 2003;12:516–518.

66 Aggarwal A, Kumar R, Sharma RC, Sharma DD: Topiramate induced pruritus in a patient with alcohol dependence. Indian J Dermatol 2011;56:421–422.

67 Signorelli MS, Cinconze M, Nasca MR, Marino M, Martinotti G, Di Giannantonio M, Aguglia E: Can topiramate induce pruritus? A case report and review of literature. CNS Neurol Disord Drug Targets 2015;14:309–312.

68 Calabrò RS, Bramanti P, Digangi G, Mondello S, Italiano D: Psychogenic itch responding to topiramate. Psychosomatics 2013;54:297–300.

Prof. Jacek C. Szepietowski, MD, PhD
Department of Dermatology, Venereology and Allergology, Wrocław Medical University
Ul. Chałubińskiego 1
PL–50-368 Wrocław (Poland)
E-Mail jacek.szepietowski@umed.wroc.pl

Szepietowski · Reszke

Szepietowski JC, Weisshaar E (eds): Itch – Management in Clinical Practice.
Curr Probl Dermatol. Basel, Karger, 2016, vol 50, pp 133–141 (DOI: 10.1159/000446056)

Uremic Itch Management

Thomas Mettang

DKD Helios Klinik, Wiesbaden, Germany

Abstract

Uremic itch is a frequent and sometimes very tormenting symptom in patients with advanced or end-stage renal failure, with a strong negative impact on the quality of life. According to a representative study, the point prevalence of chronic itch is 25% in hemodialysis patients but may reach more than 50% in single cohorts depending on the country and dialysis efficacy. Not much is known regarding the pathogenesis of uremic itch. Besides parathyroid hormone, histamine, tryptase, and alteration of the calcium-phosphate metabolism have been suspected. More recently, derangements in the opioid system and an inflammatory condition have been investigated as suspected players in the pathogenesis of uremic itch, but remain unproven so far. Treatment of chronic itch in dialysis patients remains difficult. Besides topical application of rehydrating or immunomodulating compounds, such as γ-linolenic acid or tacrolimus treatment with nalfurafine may be helpful. Apart from that, gabapentin and pregabalin are promising drugs to alleviate uremic itch. In many cases, UVB phototherapy is effective in reducing the intensity of itch. When treating patients, one should take into account that most of the drugs available are not licensed for the treatment of itch. Therefore, a deliberate use of therapeutic options aiming for a good risk-benefit relation should be adopted. In very severe and refractory cases, patients suitable for renal transplantation might be switched to 'high urgency' status, as successful renal transplantation cures uremic pruritus in most of the cases.   © 2016 S. Karger AG, Basel

Definition and Clinical Characteristics

Uremic itch, also called uremic pruritus or chronic kidney disease (CKD)-associated itch remains a frequent and sometimes tormenting problem in many patients with advanced or end-stage renal disease [1]. Management of chronic itch (CI) in these patients, especially in the most severely affected, has been shown to be extremely difficult.

The problem in the establishment of effective treatment modalities is the incomplete knowledge of the underlying pathophysiological mechanism and the great clinical heterogeneity of CKD-associated pruritus [2]. Systematically performed studies are hard to obtain and therefore sparse.

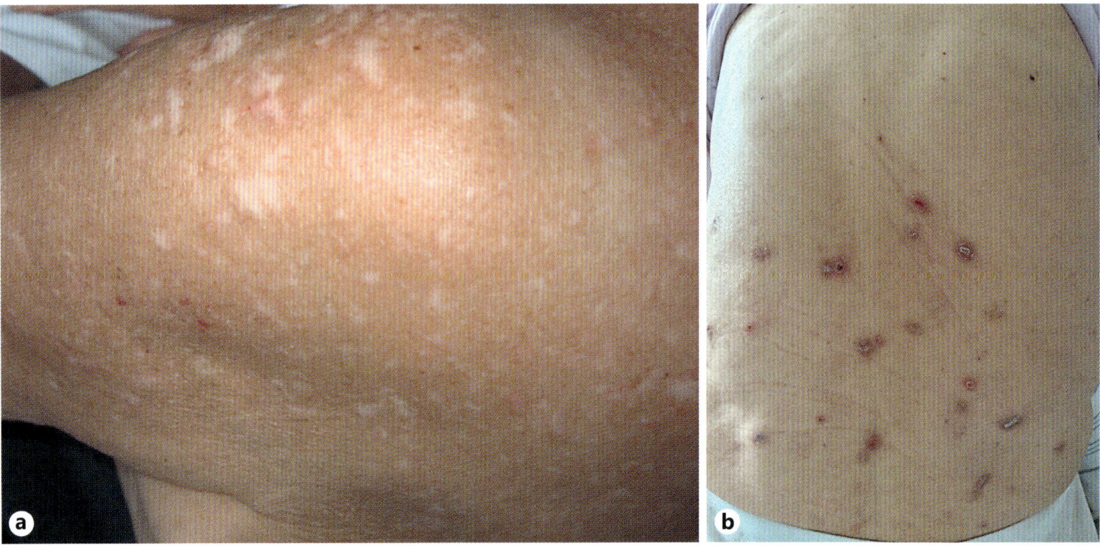

Fig. 1. Skin affections observed in patients with uremic itch. **a** Deep scars on the shoulder of a patient on hemodialysis. **b** Prurigo nodularis on the back of a patient on peritoneal dialysis.

The intensity of CKD-associated itch ranges widely from mild discomfort to complete restlessness during the day and at night. When uremic itch occurs, in most patients skin appearance is normal, except for common changes in skin color and a frequently observed xerosis. Scratch lesions like excoriation with or without impetigo ensue and in some cases prurigo nodularis is observed (fig. 1). The spatial distribution of CKD-associated itch varies: 25–50% complain about generalized itch [3, 4]. In a recent cross-sectional study in Germany (GEHIS), CI in hemodialysis patients was reported to be most frequent on the back, legs, and scalp, being worst during and directly after hemodialysis [1]. Another study reported itch to be most severe in direct association with the hemodialysis procedure in only 25% of patients [5].

The diagnosis of uremic itch might be difficult. Many patients with CKD in later stages (IV–V) suffer from other diseases, such as cardiovascular diseases, diabetes mellitus, chronic liver, or hematological diseases, which by themselves or by the medication given for treatment may provoke itch. Additionally, itchy skin diseases might be present. Hayani et al. [2] reported 18% of patients with CI in hemodialysis being affected by skin diseases.

Prevalence of Uremic Pruritus

It seems that the incidence of CI in hemodialysis has declined over the past 20 years. While in the early 1970s almost 85% of patients were affected [6] by CKD-associated itch, the incidence decreased to 50–60% in the late 1980s [7]. Many studies did report on the prevalence of CI in hemodialysis, and these had different criteria for diagnosis and patient selection, and mostly covered only one or a few hemodialysis centers. Data from the Dialysis Outcomes and Practice Patterns Study (DOPPS) in a very large cohort of patients on hemodialysis in different countries revealed that ~45% of patients suffer from CKD-associated itch [8]. The first nationwide representative cross-sectional study in Germany recently demonstrated a substantially lower prevalence of CI (25%) [1].

Interestingly, severe itch seems to be rarer in pediatric patients on dialysis (both peritoneal dialysis and hemodialysis). In a systematic review of all German pediatric dialysis centers involving 199 children, only 9.1% of the children on dialysis complained about itch. Moreover, the intensity reported was not very severe in the patients affected [9]. Another more recent study, however, reported the prevalence of CI in pediatric patients on peritoneal dialysis and hemodialysis to be 23% [10]

There are only scarce data on the prevalence of CI in patients undergoing peritoneal dialysis. The few reports available, however, may strengthen the notion that prevalence of CI in peritoneal dialysis is similar to that in hemodialysis [9, 11].

Pathophysiology

Many different hypotheses on the pathophysiology of CKD-associated itch have been generated. Parathormone was focused on because CI in hemodialysis patients seemed to be most severe in patients with pronounced hyperparathyroidism and resolved after parathyroidectomy [12, 13]. Other studies, however, could not confirm parathormone as an itch-inducing compound [14]. Neither skin deposition of calcium or phosphate salts nor serum levels of calcium-binding proteins are associated with CI in dialysis [15, 16]. Furthermore, although increased in uremia [17–19], there is no proof that histamie or tryptase induce itch in CKD [7, 18, 20]. Xerosis, which is a frequent symptom in patients with CKD, is likely to add to the intensity of itch in dialysis patient suffering from CI [21].

With regard to several observations and data from other studies, there is increasing evidence that uremic itch is a systemic instead of an isolated skin disease and that derangements of the immune system with a proinflammatory pattern may be involved in the pathogenesis of CKD-associated itch. In a study by Virga et al. [22], it could be demonstrated that hemodialysis patients with CKD-associated itch had significantly higher C-reactive protein levels than those without CKD-associated itch.

In a multicenter study we could demonstrate that T cell differentiation is more pronounced to Th1 in hemodialysis patients with CI than in patients without CKD-associated itch [23]. Additionally, C-reactive protein and interleukin (IL) levels in the blood of patients with CKD-associated itch were significantly increased. These results may support the hypothesis that an inflammatory state may convey or at least accompanies CKD-associated itch.

Management

Therapeutic options are sparse in CKD-associated itch. The most important treatment approaches are:
- Topical treatment with different ointments
- Systemic treatment with μ-opioid receptor antagonists and κ-agonists
- Drugs with anti-inflammatory properties
- Gabapentin and pregabalin
- Phototherapy
- Acupuncture

Table 1 summarizes the most important controlled trials in CI in dialysis.

Topical Treatment with Tacrolimus and γ-Linolenic Ointment

Daily topical treatment using rehydrating emollients should be regarded as baseline therapy. The addition of cooling substances such as menthol to emollients may further improve its antipruritic effect, but properly controlled studies are lacking.

Atopic dermatitis responds well to tacrolimus ointment and leads to complete or partial resolu-

Table 1. Important controlled trials in CI in dialysis

First author [Ref.], year	Intervention/medication	Design	Patients treated, n	Duration of treatment	Results
Gunal [38], 2004	gabapentin 300 mg p.o. 3 times a week	RCT	25	4 weeks	highly significant effect
Rhazeghi [39], 2009	gabapentin 100 mg p.o. 3 times a week	RCT crossover	34	4 weeks	highly significant effect
Wikstrom [31], 2005	nalfurafine 5 µg i.v. 3 times a week	meta-analysis of 2 RCTs	144	2–4 weeks	significant effect
Kumagai [32], 2010	nalfurafine 2.5 vs. 5 µg p.o. daily	RCT	337	2 weeks	significant effect
Peer [29], 1996	naltrexone 50 mg p.o. daily	RCT crossover	15	7 days	highly significant effect
Pauli-Magnus [30], 2000	naltrexone 50 mg p.o. daily	RCT crossover	23	28 days	no effect (no difference between placebo and treatment)
Silva [36], 1994	thalidomide 100 mg p.o. daily	RCT	29	7 days	moderate but significant effect (p < 0.05)
Duo [46], 1987	electroacupuncture 3× weekly	controlled (sham acupuncture)	6	2 weeks	significant effect
Che-Yi [47], 2005	acupuncture 3× weekly	controlled (sham acupuncture)	40	1 month	significant effect
Ko [44], 2011	phototherapy (narrowband UVB)	single-blinded	21	6 weeks	no significant effect
Duque [27], 2005	tacrolimus 0.01% ointment, 2× daily	vehicle-controlled	22	4 weeks	no significant difference between vehicle and treatment
Chen [28], 2006	2.2% γ-linolenic-acid-containing ointment 3× daily	RCT crossover	17	2 weeks	significant effect (p < 0.0001)

i.v. = Intravenous; p.o. = per os; RCT = randomized clinical trial.

tion of illness-related symptoms [24]. We reported on 3 patients on peritoneal dialysis with severe CKD-associated itch. The patients applied a 0.03% tacrolimus ointment twice daily to the most affected areas for a period of 7 days, which led to a substantial improvement of itch intensity [25]. In an uncontrolled prospective study, 25 patients treated with topical tacrolimus ointment for 6 weeks showed marked improvement in CI [26]. A double-blind, vehicle-controlled study in 22 hemodialysis patients with CI, however, revealed an impressive reduction of itch intensity in both the treatment and vehicle group of about 80% [27]. A difference between tacrolimus and vehicle could not be demonstrated. The authors, however, were not able to explain the improvement of CI by vehicle.

In a study by Chen et al. [28], a cream containing high concentrations of γ-linolenic acid and essential fatty acids was able to reduce itch in 17 patients suffering from severe CI. The authors speculated that the effect of this treatment was conveyed by the anti-inflammatory properties of γ-linolenic acid as a precursor of the prostaglandin system.

Systemic Treatment with μ-Opioid Receptor Antagonists and κ-Agonists

μ-Opioid Receptor Antagonists
The therapeutic use of opiate antagonists in patients with uremic itch was based on the assumption that endogenous opiate peptides may also be involved in the pathogenesis of uremic itch. A placebo-controlled clinical trial by Peer et al. [29] showed that administration of the oral μ-receptor antagonist naltrexone was associated with a significant decrease in itch perception in all of the treated patients with severe uremic itch.

We did a similar study (placebo-controlled, double-blind, crossover) with 50 mg of naltrexone per day in 23 patients on hemodialysis or peritoneal dialysis with persistent treatment-resistant itch over a 4-week period. Itch intensity was scored daily by a visual analogue scale (VAS) and weekly by a detailed score [30]. The difference between the naltrexone- and placebo-treatment periods was not statistically significant. The different results of the two studies are hard to explain. The studies had a similar design and merely differed as to the intensity of itch in the evaluated groups.

κ-Opioid Receptor Agonists
It was speculated that the activation of κ-opioid receptors expressed by dermal cells and lymphocytes may lead to the suppression of itch sensation. Therefore, when these receptors are not adequately stimulated or μ-receptors are overexpressed, patients may experience more severe itching. In line with this hypothesis it was tested whether κ-receptor agonists (nalfurafine) are able to reduce CKD-associated itch. These substances are likely to act on the spinal cord level by inhibiting the itch impulse transmitted by the first neuron.

Nalfurafine is a highly selective κ-opioid receptor agonist. In a meta-analysis of two randomized double-blind and placebo-controlled studies, 5 μg nalfurafine was administered as a short infusion following hemodialysis 3 times weekly for a total period of 2 or 4 weeks on 144 hemodialysis patients with CI. A moderate but significant effect of nalfurafine could be demonstrated [31]. In another randomized, prospective, placebo-controlled phase III study, a total of 337 hemodialysis patients with CI were treated orally with nalfurafine hydrochloride at doses of 2.5 or 5 μg daily for 2 weeks [32]. During treatment with nalfurafine, itch intensity (measured by VAS; 0–100 mm), significantly decreased by 22 mm (5 μg) and 23 mm (2.5 μg), respectively, after 7 days of application. During placebo, CI dropped by 13 mm. Adverse drug reactions (insomnia in particular) were substantially more frequent in both treatment groups (35.1% on 5 μg and 25% on 2.5 μg) compared to the placebo group (16.2%). Moreover, the effect of medication wore off fast once treatment was stopped. Similar results in terms of results and adverse drugs effects were obtained by an open-label long-term study with 5 mg nalfurafine given orally in 211 hemodialysis patients over a period of 52 weeks [33].

Whether butorphanol, a drug with both κ-agonistic and μ-antagonistic properties is effective in CKD-associated itch remains to be elucidated. Dawn and Yosipovitch [34] have used this drug in patients with 'intractable itch' with promising results.

Drugs with Anti-Inflammatory Properties

Thalidomide
Thalidomide, which is used as an immunomodulator to treat graft-versus-host reactions, suppresses tumor necrosis factor (TNF)-α production and leads to a predominant differentiation of Th2 lymphocytes with suppression of IL-2-pro-

Choice	Drug	Dose	Caveats	Evidence
1.	gabapentin	50–100 mg/day p.o.	dose reduction due to impaired renal elimination; no interaction	I A
2.	pregabalin	2 × 75 mg/week p.o.	dose reduction due to impaired renal elimination; no interaction	I B
3.	naltrexone	50 mg/day	withdrawal-like symptoms: increase dose cautiously; pain, disorientation	IIb B
4.	nalfurafine	2.5–5.0 mg/day p.o.	presently not licensed in Europe; sleep disturbance, nausea	I B
5.	phototherapy and topical treatment (see text)		in addition to other systemic treatment	IIb A–IIb C

Apart from specific medical therapy, all patients should receive daily topical treatment using rehydrating emollients as baseline therapy. p.o. = Per os.

ducing Th1 cells [35]. In a placebo-controlled, crossover, randomized double-blind study, thalidomide was used to treat refractory uremic itch. It turned out that CI improved in approximately 50% of patients treated with thalidomide [36]. Aside from the suppression of TNF-α, a centrally abating effect might be responsible for beneficial antipruritic effects.

Pentoxifylline
In an open study, 600 mg of pentoxifylline, a weak TNF-α inhibitor, was administered intravenously 3 times a week (at the end of each dialysis session) for 4 weeks to 7 hemodialysis patients with CI who did not respond to treatment with gabapentin or UVB phototherapy. The patients who tolerated the drug experienced an almost complete resolution of itch that continued for at least 4 weeks after cessation of therapy [37]. Considering the rather modest tolerance of the agent at least with the dose applied, this approach may only be recommended in severe refractory cases.

Gabapentin and Pregabalin

Gabapentin, which was originally designed as an anticonvulsant, has centrally acting calcium channel blocker properties with a pain-modulating effect in patients with neuropathic pain. Gunal et al. [38] treated 25 patients on hemodialysis with CKD-associated itch, applying 300 mg of gabapentin orally 3 times weekly for 4 weeks. It could be shown that the therapy was safe and highly effective in reducing itch. Itch intensity as determined by VAS dropped from 8.4 prior to treatment to 1.2 four weeks after the start of treatment. Similar results were obtained in another double-blind, controlled, crossover study treating 34 patients with 100 mg of gabapentin orally 3 times a week [39]. This drug, although not licensed for the treatment of itch, was largely well tolerated and can be considered as an effective treatment for CI in dialysis.

Pregabalin is a similar drug and has also been reported to reduce CI in dialysis. Therapy with 75 mg of pregabalin given orally twice weekly was compared either to ondansetron or placebo. While a significant effect of pregabalin could be documented, the use of ondansetron and placebo did not yield significant results [40]. In another paper, it was suggested that patients on dialysis not responding to or not tolerating gabapentin should be switched to pregabalin because of good effectiveness and tolerability [41].

Phototherapy

A series of studies have dealt with the effectiveness of phototherapy in CKD-associated itch, especially radiation with broadband UVB. Gilchrest et al. [42] showed that treating patients with UVB light led to relief of CKD-associated itch in a considerable number of patients. According to a meta-analysis by Tan et al. [43], UVB radiation remains the most promising therapy, whereas UVA does not seem to be effective.

Studies on the effectiveness of narrowband UVB radiation could not verify a significant antipruritic effect [44]. Furthermore, the risk for skin malignancies following UVB irradiation and long-term systemic immunosuppression should be kept in mind, especially concerning patients on dialysis who are scheduled for renal transplantation.

Acupuncture

Acupuncture was effectively used to control for pain in different situations [45]. The first report on acupuncture in dialysis patients with CI dates back to 1987 when electroacupuncture or sham-electrostimulation was applied to 6 patients on hemodialysis with severe CI in a blinded manner by Duo [46]. Patients on acupuncture showed a significantly higher reduction in itch determined by a score than the sham-treated patients. In another study, 40 patients with CKD-associated pruritus were treated with acupuncture either at the Quchi (LI11) acupoint or at a nonacupoint 2 cm lateral 3 times weekly for 1 month. Patients treated using the correct acupoint revealed a substantial reduction in itch using a score regarding severity, distribution, and sleep disturbance, whereas itch in patients with sham-acupuncture did not change substantially [47]. Given these results, acupuncture at least in experienced hands might be a useful tool in the treatment of CKD-associated pruritus.

When treating dialysis patients with CI, a stepwise approach is strongly recommended (table 2). Treatment should be initiated with maneuvers exhibiting the most favorable safety and efficacy profiles. Besides topical treatment, gabapentin, immunomodulatory drugs, and κ-receptor agonists may be helpful in severe cases. In desperate cases, patients principally eligible for a kidney transplant may be declared 'high urgency', which will decrease their waiting time. In most cases, successful kidney transplantation will relieve patients from CKD-associated pruritus [48].

References

1 Weiss M, Mettang T, Tschulena U, Passlick-Deetjen J, Weisshaar E: Prevalence of chronic itch and associated factors in haemodialysis patients: a representative cross-sectional study. Acta Derm Venereol 2015;95:816–821.

2 Hayani K, Weiss M, Weisshaar E: Clinical findings and provision of care in haemodialysis patients with chronic itch: new results from the German Epidemiological Haemodialysis Itch Study. Acta Derm Venereol 2016;96:361–366.

3 Morvay M, Marghescu S: Skin changes in hemodialysis patients (in German). Med Klin (Munich) 1988;83:507–510.

4 Ponticelli C, Bencini PL: Uremic pruritus: a review. Nephron 1992;60:1–5.

5 Gilchrest BA, Stern RS, Steinman TI, Brown RS, Arndt KA, Anderson WW: Clinical features of pruritus among patients undergoing maintenance hemodialysis. Arch Dermatol 1982;118:154–156.

6   Young AW Jr, Sweeney EW, David DS, Cheigh J, Hochgelerenl EL, Sakai S, et al: Dermatologic evaluation of pruritus in patients on hemodialysis. NY State J Med 1973;73:2670–2674.

7   Mettang T, Fritz P, Weber J, Machleidt C, Hübel E, Kuhlmann U: Uremic pruritus in patients on hemodialysis or continuous ambulatory peritoneal dialysis (CAPD). The role of plasma histamine and skin mast cells. Clin Nephrol 1990; 34:136–141.

8   Pisoni RL, Wikstrom B, Elder SJ, Akizawa T, Asano Y, Keen ML, et al: Pruritus in haemodialysis patients: International results from the Dialysis Outcomes and Practice Patterns Study (DOPPS). Nephrol Dial Transplant 2006;21:3495–3505.

9   Schwab M, Mikus G, Mettang T, Pauli-Magnus C, Kuhlmann U: Urämischer Pruritus im Kindes- und Jugendalter. Monatszeitschrift Kinderheilkunde 1999;147:232.

10 Wojtowicz-Prus E, Kilis-Pstrusinska K, Reich A, Zachwieja K, Miklaszewska M, Szczepanska M, et al: Disturbed skin barrier in children with chronic kidney disease. Pediatr Nephrol 2015;30:333–338.

11 Narita I, Alchi B, Omori K, Sato F, Ajiro J, Saga D, et al: Etiology and prognostic significance of severe uremic pruritus in chronic hemodialysis patients. Kidney Int 2006;69:1626–1632.

12 Massry SG, Popovtzer MM, Coburn JW, Makoff DL, Maxwell MH, Kleeman CR: Intractable pruritus as a manifestation of secondary hyperparathyroidism in uremia. Disappearance of itching after subtotal parathyroidectomy. N Engl J Med 1968;279:697–700.

13 Hampers CL, Katz AI, Wilson RE, Merrill JP: Disappearance of 'uremic' itching after subtotal parathyroidectomy. N Engl J Med 1968;279:695–697.

14 Stahle-Backdahl M, Hagermark O, Lins LE, Torring O, Hilliges M, Johansson O: Experimental and immunohistochemical studies on the possible role of parathyroid hormone in uraemic pruritus. J Intern Med 1989;225:411–415.

15 Blachley JD, Blankenship DM, Menter A, Parker TF 3rd, Knochel JP: Uremic pruritus: skin divalent ion content and response to ultraviolet phototherapy. Am J Kidney Dis 1985;5:237–241.

16 Mettang T, Matterne U, Roth HJ, Weisshaar E: Lacking evidence for calcium-binding protein fetuin-A to be linked with chronic kidney disease-related pruritus (CKD-rP). NDT Plus 2010;3:104–105.

17 Stockenhuber F, Kurz RW, Sertl K, Grimm G, Balcke P: Increased plasma histamine levels in uraemic pruritus. Clin Sci (Lond) 1990,79:477–482.

18 Dimkovic N, Djukanovic L, Radmilovic A, Bojic P, Juloski T: Uremic pruritus and skin mast cells. Nephron 1992;61:5–9.

19 Dugas-Breit S, Schopf P, Dugas M, Schiffl H, Rueff F, Przybilla B: Baseline serum levels of mast cell tryptase are raised in hemodialysis patients and associated with severity of pruritus. J Dtsch Dermatol Ges 2005;3:343–347.

20 Hiroshige K, Kabashima N, Takasugi M, Kuroiwa A: Optimal dialysis improves uremic pruritus. Am J Kidney Dis 1995; 25:413–419.

21 Szepietowski JC, Reich A, Schwartz RA: Uraemic xerosis. Nephrol Dial Transplant 2004;19:2709–2712.

22 Virga G, Visentin I, La, Milia, V, Bonadonna A: Inflammation and pruritus in haemodialysis patients. Nephrol Dial Transplant 2002;17:2164–2169.

23 Kimmel M, Alscher DM, Dunst R, Braun N, Machleidt C, Kiefer T, et al: The role of micro-inflammation in the pathogenesis of uraemic pruritus in haemodialysis patients. Nephrol Dial Transplant 2006;21:749–755.

24 Gianni LM, Sulli MM: Topical tacrolimus in the treatment of atopic dermatitis. Ann Pharmacother 2001;35:943–946.

25 Pauli-Magnus C, Klumpp S, Alscher DM, Kuhlmann U, Mettang T: Short-term efficacy of tacrolimus ointment in severe uremic pruritus. Perit Dial Int 2000;20:802–803.

26 Kuypers DR, Claes K, Evenepoel P, Maes B, Vanrenterghem Y: A prospective proof of concept study of the efficacy of tacrolimus ointment on uraemic pruritus (UP) in patients on chronic dialysis therapy. Nephrol Dial Transplant 2004; 19:1895–1901.

27 Duque MI, Yosipovitch G, Fleischer AB Jr, Willard J, Freedman BI: Lack of efficacy of tacrolimus ointment 0.1% for treatment of hemodialysis-related pruritus: a randomized, double-blind, vehicle-controlled study. J Am Acad Dermatol 2005;52:519–521.

28 Chen YC, Chiu WT, Wu MS: Therapeutic effect of topical gamma-linolenic acid on refractory uremic pruritus. Am J Kidney Dis 2006;48:69–76.

29 Peer G, Kivity S, Agami O, Fireman E, Silverberg D, Blum M, et al: Randomised crossover trial of naltrexone in uraemic pruritus. Lancet 1996;348:1552–1554.

30 Pauli-Magnus C, Mikus G, Alscher DM, Kirschner T, Nagel W, Gugeler N, et al: Naltrexone does not relieve uremic pruritus: results of a randomized, double-blind, placebo-controlled crossover study. J Am Soc Nephrol 2000;11:514–519.

31 Wikstrom B, Gellert R, Ladefoged SD, Danda Y, Akai M, Ide K, et al: Kappa-opioid system in uremic pruritus: multicenter, randomized, double-blind, placebo-controlled clinical studies. J Am Soc Nephrol 2005;16:3742–3747.

32 Kumagai H, Ebata T, Takamori K, Muramatsu T, Nakamoto H, Suzuki H: Effect of a novel kappa-receptor agonist, nalfurafine hydrochloride, on severe itch in 337 haemodialysis patients: a phase III, randomized, double-blind, placebo-controlled study. Nephrol Dial Transplant 2010;25:1251–1257.

33 Kumagai H, Ebata T, Takamori K, Miyasato K, Muramatsu T, Nakamoto H, et al: Efficacy and safety of a novel k-agonist for managing intractable pruritus in dialysis patients. Am J Nephrol 2012;36:175–183.

34 Dawn AG, Yosipovitch G: Butorphanol for treatment of intractable pruritus. J Am Acad Dermatol 2006;54:527–531.

35 McHugh SM, Rifkin IR, Deighton J, Wilson AB, Lachmann PJ, Lockwood CM, et al: The immunosuppressive drug thalidomide induces T helper cell type 2 (Th2) and concomitantly inhibits Th1 cytokine production in mitogen- and antigen-stimulated human peripheral blood mononuclear cell cultures. Clin Exp Immunol 1995;99:160–167.

36 Silva SR, Viana PC, Lugon NV, Hoette M, Ruzany F, Lugon JR: Thalidomide for the treatment of uremic pruritus: a crossover randomized double-blind trial. Nephron 1994;67:270–273.

37 Mettang T, Krumme B, Bohler J, Roeckel A: Pentoxifylline as treatment for uraemic pruritus – an addition to the weak armamentarium for a common clinical symptom? Nephrol Dial Transplant 2007;22:2727–2728.

38 Gunal AI, Ozalp G, Yoldas TK, Gunal SY, Kirciman E, Celiker H: Gabapentin therapy for pruritus in haemodialysis patients: a randomized, placebo-controlled, double-blind trial. Nephrol Dial Transplant 2004;19:3137–3139.

39 Razeghi E, Eskandari D, Ganji MR, Meysamie AP, Togha M, Khashayar P: Gabapentin and uremic pruritus in hemodialysis patients. Ren Fail 2009;31: 85–90.

40 Yue J, Jiao S, Xiao Y, Ren W, Zhao T, Meng J: Comparison of pregabalin with ondansetron in treatment of uraemic pruritus in dialysis patients: a prospective, randomized, double-blind study. Int Urol Nephrol 2015;47:161–167.

41 Rayner H, Baharani J, Smith S, Suresh V, Dasgupta I: Uraemic pruritus: relief of itching by gabapentin and pregabalin. Nephron Clin Pract 2013;122:75–79.

42 Gilchrest BA, Rowe JW, Brown RS, Steinman TI, Arndt KA: Ultraviolet phototherapy of uremic pruritus. Long-term results and possible mechanism of action. Ann Intern Med 1979;91:17–21.

43 Tan JK, Haberman HF, Coldman AJ: Identifying effective treatments for uremic pruritus. J Am Acad Dermatol 1991; 25:811–818.

44 Ko M, Yang J, Wu H, Hu F, Chen S, Tsai P, et al: Narrowband ultraviolet B phototherapy for patients with refractory uraemic pruritus: a randomized controlled trial. Br J Dermatol 2011;165: 633–639.

45 Zhang R, Lao L, Ren K, Berman BM: Mechanisms of acupuncture-electroacupuncture on persistent pain. Anesthesiology 2014;120:482–503.

46 Duo LJ: Electrical needle therapy of uremic pruritus. Nephron 1987;47:179–83.

47 Che-Yi C, Wen CY, Min-Tsung K, Chiu-Ching H: Acupuncture in haemodialysis patients at the Quchi (LI11) acupoint for refractory uraemic pruritus. Nephrol Dial Transplant 2005;20:1912–1915.

48 Altmeyer P, Kachel HG, Schäfer G, Fassbinder W: Normalization of uremic skin changes following kidney transplantation (in German). Hautarzt 1986;37: 217–221.

Thomas Mettang, MD, FASN
DKD Helios Klinik
Aukammallee 33
DE–65191 Wiesbaden (Germany)
E-Mail T_Mettang@t-online.de

Table 1. Medical therapy (therapeutic recommendations)

Approach	Drug therapy	Dosage	Evidence
ICP only	UDCA	10–15 mg/kg/day (p.o.)	I
1st line	cholestyramine	4–16 g/day (p.o.)	II-2
2nd line	rifampicin	300–600 mg/day (p.o.)	I
3rd line	naltrexone	50 mg/day (p.o.)	I
4th line	sertraline	100 mg/day (p.o.)	II-2

Categories of evidence (based on the GRADE system): I = randomized controlled trials; II-1 = controlled trials without randomization; II-2 = cohort or case-control analytic studies; II-3 = multiple time series, dramatic uncontrolled experiments; III = opinions of respected authorities, descriptive epidemiology.

forms of itch has added to our knowledge of cholestatic itch and might give us a new therapeutic target [16].

Management

Management of a patient with cholestatic itch can be considered under the following headings:

1 Establishing the diagnosis: to confirm that itch is being caused due to cholestasis, which requires demonstration of liver pathology and exclusion of other causes (dermatological/systemic) of itch
2 Treatment of primary liver pathology
3 Effective symptomatic treatment of itch

If the cause of cholestasis is reversible (e.g. some types of extrahepatic biliary obstruction), immediate intervention (i.e. relief of the obstruction) may be all that is needed. This may be achieved by procedures like stenting, nasobiliary or transcutaneous drainage, and biliodigestive anastomoses. Sometimes a potentially reversible cause (e.g. drug-induced cholestasis without ductopenia) requires that the cause be identified and removed in the hope that cholestasis will resolve spontaneously.

The therapeutic approach for symptomatic control of itch can either be medical or interventional (tables 1, 2). It is to be noted that the current treatment recommendations for itch in cholestasis are based on only a few well-designed randomized placebo-controlled trials and several cohort studies [17].

The rationale for any medical and interventional therapeutic approach can be any one of the following:

1 To remove the pruritogen(s) from the enterohepatic cycle by nonabsorbable anion exchange resins such as cholestyramine in mild itch or invasive interventions such as nasobiliary and transcutaneous drainage or external biliary diversion in desperate cases
2 To alter the metabolism of the presumed pruritogen(s) in the liver and/or the intestine by inducers of the hepatic biotransformation machinery such as rifampicin

Table 2. Invasive/surgical therapy

1 Plasmapheresis
2 Extracorporeal albumin dialysis: molecular adsorbent recirculating system
3 Plasma separation and anion adsorption
4 Partial external diversion of bile
5 Ileal diversion
6 Nasobiliary drainage
7 Liver transplantation – the ultimate option for refractory cases

3 To modulate central itch signaling by influencing the endogenous opioidergic and serotoninergic system via μ-opioid antagonists and selective serotonin reuptake inhibitors, respectively

4 To remove the potential pruritogen(s) from the systemic circulation by invasive methods such as anion absorption, plasmapheresis, or extracorporeal albumin dialysis if itch is intractable

Specific Therapeutic Agents for Treatment of Cholestatic Itch

Bile Acid Therapy

The drug in this class is UDCA. It exerts beneficial anticholestatic effects [18] and represents a baseline therapy for several cholestatic disorders such as primary biliary cirrhosis, pediatric cholestatic syndromes, and ICP. In ICP, UDCA improved itch and liver enzymes in several randomized placebo-controlled trials and is considered first-line treatment [19]. It forms up to 3% of the human bile pool. When given as a drug, it makes the bile pool more hydrophilic. Its benefits are attributed to its effects on transporters, detoxification of bile, antiapoptotic effect on hepatocytes and cholangiocytes, and stimulation of cholangiocyte secretion. The recommended dose is 10–15 mg/kg/day. This well-tolerated drug has been studied in several other chronic cholestatic disorders, but never with regard to itch as a primary end point [20].

Anion Exchange Resins

Except for IPC, in all other forms of itch associated with cholestasis where bile flow cannot be restored by invasive procedures, anion exchange resins are recommended as the first-line treatment. These agents are basically used to treat hypercholesterolemia and include cholestyramine, colestipol, and colesevelam [21]. These drugs act by enhancing the intestinal excretion of the pruritogens in bile. However, other mechanisms may also be involved, especially when cholestyramine is considered. This includes release of cholecystokinin, which also acts as an endogenous antiopiate [22], thereby suppressing opioid-mediated itch. Beneficial effects for cholestyramine have been reported in several uncontrolled case series [23, 24]. The recommended dose of cholestyramine is 4–16 g daily, initiated with 4 g administered orally before and after breakfast. Common adverse effects include bloating, constipation, malabsorption of nutrients, and complications including coagulopathy. The potential to interfere with absorption of other concurrent medications must be noted.

Hepatic Enzyme Inducers

Rifampicin is the drug in this class. It is regarded as a second-line treatment. Few prospective randomized placebo-controlled trials have proven the antipruritic efficacy of rifampicin [25, 26]. The mechanism of action of rifampicin is uncertain. It induces drug-metabolizing enzymes and transporters through activation of the pregnane X receptor. The enhanced metabolism and excretion of pruritogens is therefore suggested. Furthermore, it may also have antiopiate activity, thereby decreasing itch. The recommended dose for rifampicin is 150 mg twice daily if serum bilirubin is >3 mg/dl and 150 mg three times daily if serum bilirubin is <3 mg/dl. It is a safe short-term therapy for cholestatic itch; however, hepatotoxicity may occur in up to 13% of patients on longer use. For this reason, follow-up with liver function tests is necessary. The barbiturate phenobarbital is a ligand of the nuclear receptor CAR and induces isoenzymes of the cytochrome P450 family like rifampicin. Phenobarbital has been reported to relieve itch in cholestasis, but was clearly inferior to rifampicin in randomized crossover studies [27].

Opiate Antagonists

These are recommended as a third-line treatment. The drugs in this category include nal-

31 Turner IB, Rawlins MD, Wood P, James OF: Flumecinol for the treatment of pruritus associated with primary biliary cirrhosis. Aliment Pharmacol Ther 1994;8:337–342.

32 Watson JP, Jones DE, James OF, Cann PA, Bramble MG: Case report: oral antioxidant therapy for the treatment of primary biliary cirrhosis: a pilot study. J Gastroenterol Hepatol 1999;14:1034–1040.

33 Walt R, Daneshmed T, Fellows I: Effect of stanozolol on itching in primary biliary cirrhosis. Br Med J 1988;296:607.

34 Hanid MA, Levi AJ: Phototherapy for pruritus in primary biliary cirrhosis. Lancet 1980;2:530.

35 Bergasa NV, Link MJ, Keogh M, et al: Pilot study of bright light therapy reflected towards the eyes for the pruritus of chronic liver disease. Am J Gastroenterol 2001;96:1563–1570.

36 Cholen LB, Ambinder EP, Wolke AM, et al: Role of plasmapheresis in primary biliary cirrhosis. Gut 1985;26:29–294.

37 Macia M, Aviles J, Navarro J, et al: Efficacy of molecular absorbent recirculating system for the treatment of intractable pruritus in cholestasis. Am J Med 2003;114:62–64.

38 Pares A, Cisneros L, Salmeron JM, et al: Extracorporeal albumin dialysis: a procedure for prolonged relief of intractable pruritus in patients with primary biliary cirrhosis. Am J Gastroenterol 2004;99:1105–1110.

39 Kremer AE, Bolier R, van Dijk R, et al: Advances in pathogenesis and management of pruritus in cholestasis. Dig Dis 2014;32:637–645.

40 Clinical trial. Gov IBAT inhibitor A2450 for cholestatic pruritus. https://clinicaltrials.gov/ct2/show/NCT02360852?term=a4250&rank=1.

Dr. Asit Mittal, Professor and Consultant Dermatologist
Department of Dermatology, RNT Medical College and Associate Hospitals
House No. 62, Road No. 2, Ashok Nagar
Udaipur 313001 (India)
E-Mail asitmittal62@gmail.com

Szepietowski JC, Weisshaar E (eds): Itch – Management in Clinical Practice.
Curr Probl Dermatol. Basel, Karger, 2016, vol 50, pp 149–154 (DOI: 10.1159/000446060)

Paraneoplastic Itch Management

Brandon Rowe · Gil Yosipovitch

Department of Dermatology and Itch Center, Temple University School of Medicine, Philadelphia, Pa., USA

Abstract

Paraneoplastic itch occurs as the result of a systemic reaction to an underlying malignancy. Paraneoplastic itch is most commonly associated with lymphoproliferative malignancies and solid tumors that result in cholestasis. Paraneoplastic itch may occur in the absence of a primary rash or in association with dermatologic conditions such as erythroderma, acanthosis nigricans, dermatomyositis, Grover's disease, and eruptive seborrheic keratosis. Treatment of paraneoplastic itch is centered on targeting the underlying malignancy responsible for the systemic reaction. In cases of malignancy that are refractive to treatment, other therapies have been found to be effective for paraneoplastic itch, including selective serotonin reuptake inhibitors, mirtazapine, gabapentin, thalidomide, opioids, aprepitant, and histone deacetylase inhibitors. © 2016 S. Karger AG, Basel

Definition and Clinical Characteristics

Paraneoplastic itch is defined as pruritus that occurs either within the natural progression of malignancy or preceding the diagnosis of malignancy [1]. Direct mass invasion or compression by a tumor mass resulting in pruritus does not qualify as paraneoplastic itch. In 2015 the Special Interest Group of the International Forum on the Study of Itch defined paraneoplastic itch as 'the sensation of itch as a systemic (not local) reaction to the presence of a tumor or a hematological malignancy neither induced by the local presence of cancer cells nor by tumor therapy' [2].

There are limited epidemiologic data on the prevalence of paraneoplastic itch. One retrospective study evaluating 700 patients with solid tumor and hematologic malignancy reported a 13% prevalence of generalized pruritus in those with concurrent dermatologic conditions [3]. The largest prospective studies have evaluated patients suffering from chronic itch in the absence of observable skin manifestations. One study investigated 8,743 chronic itch patients in the absence of rash, and found that chronic itch without skin changes doubles the risk of developing a hematologic malignancy and triples the risk of developing a bile duct malignancy when compared to the general population [4]. A similar study following 12,813 patients diagnosed with chronic itch found a 13% increase in the overall incidence of developing cancer, and a 68% increase in hematologic malignancies compared to the general population over a 5-year period [5]. Paraneoplastic itch is most commonly reported in lymphoproliferative malignancies including multiple myeloma, non-Hodgkin's lymphoma (15% prevalence), and Hodgkin's lymphoma (25% prevalence) [6–8].

Paraneoplastic itch-associated hematologic malignancy and solid tumors resulting in cholestasis frequently occur without concurrent skin changes [1, 7]; however, several observable pruritic skin conditions can occur secondary to malignancy (fig. 1), including erythroderma [9], acanthosis nigricans, dermatomyositis (DM), Grover's disease, and eruptive seborrheic keratoses.

Acanthosis nigricans is a common skin condition characterized by velvety, hyperpigmented plaques that commonly occur in the neck and axilla. A retrospective analysis of 90 patients with acanthosis nigricans revealed that 17 (19%) suffered from an associated malignancy and 7 suffered from generalized pruritus, while generalized pruritus preceded the appearance of acanthosis nigricans in 3 patients [10].

DM is an autoimmune skin condition characterized by proximal muscle weakness, heliotrope rash, photosensitivity, and Gottron's papules. It has been associated with several malignancies including colon, ovarian, and breast cancer. A large-scale population-based study from Sweden evaluated 392 patients with DM and found that 59 patients (15%) had an associated cancer diagnosed at the time of or after the diagnosis of DM [11]. When compared to the general population, the relative risk of cancer was found to be 2.4 (95% CI: 1.6–3.6) for men and 3.4 (95% CI: 2.4–4.7) for women. A prospective study comparing the clinical characteristics of DM in the US and Singapore found 3 Singapore DM patients developed a malignancy over the course of 5 years, 2 of which were nasopharyngeal carcinoma [12].

One cross-sectional study investigating the prevalence of itch in patients with DM revealed that 85% of subjects suffered from some degree of pruritus and 58% suffered from moderate-to-severe pruritus [13]. Additional studies have confirmed that pruritus is a common complaint in DM [12, 14].

Transient acantholytic dermatosis (Grover's disease) is another category of pruritic skin lesions associated with malignancy. It is characterized by a pruritic papulovesicular rash involving the upper trunk [15]. Spontaneous remission typically occurs over the course of weeks to months. Grover's disease has been reported to appear concurrently or after the diagnosis of chronic and acute myelogenous leukemia, transitional cell carcinoma of the bladder and kidney, and multiple myeloma [16].

The Leser-Trélat sign is described as a sudden increase in size and number of seborrheic keratoses in the setting of an underlying internal malignancy [17]. Generalized pruritus has been reported to occur in patients who display the Leser-Trélat sign [18]. There is controversy as to whether the Leser-Trélat sign is a legitimate paraneoplastic sign, in part due to the fact that it is commonly associated with acanthosis nigricans [19]. As previously discussed, acanthosis nigricans is a paraneoplastic sign, which is a confounding factor when trying to determine the true prevalence of malignancy in patients that display the Leser-Trélat sign. It has also been noted that the Leser-Trélat sign is found predominately in the elderly population, the most common age group to develop malignancy. Further statistical analysis is needed to determine the true epidemiology of malignancy associated with the Leser-Trélat sign.

Management

The most effective treatment for paraneoplastic itch is to treat the underlying malignancy. For disease that is refractive to treatment or for malignancies that require time to resolve, a number of therapies have proven to be effective in reducing pruritus. We will discuss the therapeutic ladder of

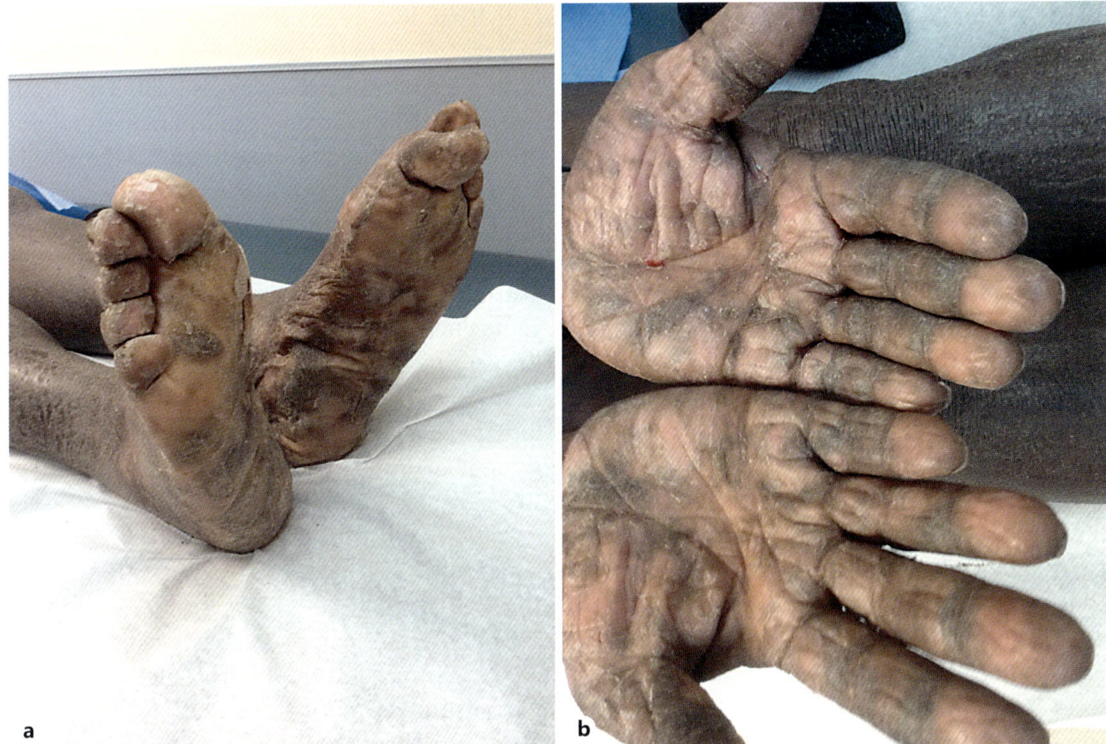

Fig. 1. a,b A 71-year old-male developed acquired palmoplantar keratoderma prior to the appearance of hyperpigmented patches over his legs diagnosed as mycosis fungoides. The patient reported intense generalized pruritus representing paraneoplastic itch secondary to mycosis fungoides, which improved with total skin electron beam radiation therapy.

treatments based on efficacy, side effect profile, and historical use. We will review the proposed mechanism of action, efficacy, and side effects of each treatment option.

Selective Serotonin Reuptake Inhibitors

Selective serotonin reuptake inhibitors selectively inhibit the reuptake of serotonin, thus enhancing the effects of serotonin release in the central nervous system. The mechanism for inhibiting pruritus is not well understood; however, one theory is that selective serotonin reuptake inhibitors' modulation of central opioid receptors results in

itch reduction [20]. A randomized clinical trial demonstrated a 50% reduction in paraneoplastic itch severity when patients were administered 20 mg of paroxetine daily for 7 days [20]. Selective serotonin reuptake inhibitors are well tolerated, with the main side effects being nausea and drowsiness reported for this dose.

Mirtazapine

Mirtazapine is an antagonist to a number of receptors, including central α_2-adrenergic presynaptic autoreceptors, 5-HT$_2$, 5-HT$_3$, and the antihistamine H$_1$ receptors. It is unclear which receptor is responsible for the antipruritic effects of mirtazapine. It has been found to be highly effective for paraneoplastic itch reduction or elimination at doses of 7.5–30 mg nightly [21]. Mirtazapine has been found to be particularly effective for nocturnal itch in the setting of chronic pruritus, which can be an important consideration for the medical management of paraneoplastic itch [22]. The major side effects of mirtazapine include sedation and weight gain [23, 24].

Gabapentin

Gabapentin is a structural analogue to γ-aminobutyric acid (GABA). It has long been used in the treatment of neuropathic pain by inhibiting neuronal calcium channels, resulting in reduction of intracellular glutamate levels and decreased neuronal excitability [25]. Inhibition of itch may work by a similar mechanism but has yet to be specifically investigated. Gabapentin has been reported to effectively treat itch induced by cutaneous T-cell lymphoma (CTCL), with a suggested starting dose of 300 mg nightly and a maximum dose of 2,400 mg daily [26]. Gabapentin is generally well tolerated, with the most commonly reported adverse effects including sleepiness (20%), ataxia (17%), nystagmus (15%), and weakness [27, 28].

Thalidomide

Thalidomide is notorious for its history of limb malformations from its historical use as a therapeutic agent for morning sickness in pregnancy. Since then it has gained favor as a chemotherapeutic agent and has shown efficacy for abolishing itch. Its mechanism of action is unknown, but it has been shown to inhibit tumor necrosis factor-α, interleukin (IL)-6, IL-10, and IL-12, and has a central depressant effect that may be responsible for its observed antipruritic properties [29]. Thalidomide has shown efficacy in treating itch secondary to Hodgkin's lymphoma [30], and is an excellent option for patient suffering from itch secondary to multiple myeloma, as thalidomide has been used to successfully treat multiple myeloma refractory to standard chemotherapy agents [31]. Special consideration must be taken when prescribing thalidomide to women of childbearing age due to its well-documented teratogenic effects on fetal limb formation. Screening for peripheral neuropathy should be carried out in any patient taking thalidomide for more than 3 months due to a 25–56% 2-year incidence of peripheral neuropathy [32].

Opioids

κ-Opioid agonists have demonstrated efficacy as antipruritic agents [33, 34]. The analgesic butorphanol, a mixed μ-opioid antagonist/κ-opioid agonist, has been reported to rapidly reduce itch secondary to non-Hodgkin's lymphoma [35]. A second opioid with similar properties is nalbuphine, a mixed μ-/κ-opioid agonist that has been shown to have efficacy as both an analgesic and antipruritic agent. A recent meta-analysis of randomized controlled clinical trials did not reveal a significant difference in pain relief between nalbuphine and morphine; however, patients taking morphine were 5 times more likely to suffer from itch than patients receiving nalbuphine [36]. Recent clinical studies have revealed efficacy of nalbuphine in controlling morphine-induced pruritus and uremic pruritus [37, 38]. As with other opioids, common side effects include nausea, sedation, and confusion.

Aprepitant

Aprepitant is a neurokinin 1 receptor inhibitor that was first used as an antiemetic agent for chemotherapy patients. Mouse models have demonstrated that neurokinin 1 receptor antagonists block itch produced by substance P, a sensory neuropeptide that has been found to correlate to eczema disease severity [39, 40]. An 80-mg daily dose of aprepitant has shown efficacy in reducing pruritus in patients with Sézary syndrome and hospitalized with severe pruritus-induced insomnia and depression [41]. Patients experienced a rapid response with an average itch severity reduction from 8 to 2.3 on a 10-point itch visual analogue scale after only 1 day of therapy. The most common side effects associated with aprepitant are nausea, diarrhea, and constipation.

produced by CD4 helper T cells, and has been found to correlate to pruritus in CTCL patients [42]. Reduction of serum IL-31 levels in patients with CTCL has been shown to correlate significantly with reduced itch [43]. Histone deacetylase inhibitors can be considered for CTCL patients suffering from severe pruritus to treat both the itch and the underlying malignancy. The most common adverse effects are nausea (81%) and fatigue (69%), while reports of elevated liver function enzymes, neutropenia, and viral reactivation require routine clinical and laboratory monitoring in patients treated with histone deacetylase inhibitors [44].

Histone Deacetylase Inhibitors

Histone deacetylase inhibitors such as vorinostat and romidepsin have recently been investigated for the treatment of CTCL. Histone formation is required for chromatin production, a critical process in rapidly dividing malignant T cells. Reduction in malignant T cells in turn reduces their output of chemokines, which have been implicated in the pathophysiology of paraneoplastic itch in CTCL patients. Specifically, IL-31 is a chemokine

Conclusion

Numerous therapies have shown efficacy for the treatment of paraneoplastic itch. We laid out a therapeutic ladder for the treatment of paraneoplastic itch arranged by efficacy, side effect profile, and novelty of the agent. More investigation into the pathophysiology of paraneoplastic itch will lead to more targeted therapies for patients.

References

1 Yosipovitch G: Chronic pruritus: a paraneoplastic sign. Dermatol Ther 2010;23: 590–596.
2 Weisshaar E, Weiss M, Mettang T, Yosipovitch G, Zylicz Z: Paraneoplastic itch: an expert position statement from the Special Interest Group (SIG) of the International Forum on the Study of Itch (IFSI). Acta Derm Venereol 2015;95: 261–265.
3 Kilic A, Gul U, Soylu S: Skin findings in internal malignant diseases. Int J Dermatol 2007;46:1055–1060.
4 Fett N, Haynes K, Propert KJ, Margolis DJ: Five-year malignancy incidence in patients with chronic pruritus: a population-based cohort study aimed at limiting unnecessary screening practices. J Am Acad Dermatol 2014;70:651–658.
5 Johannesdottir SA, Farkas DK, Vinding GR, et al: Cancer incidence among patients with a hospital diagnosis of pruritus: a nationwide Danish cohort study. Br J Dermatol 2014;171:839–846.
6 Erskine JG, Rowan RM, Alexander JO, Sekoni GA: Pruritus as a presentation of myelomatosis. Br Med J 1977;1:687–688.
7 Gobbi PG, Attardo-Parrinello G, Lattanzio G, Rizzo SC, Ascari E: Severe pruritus should be a B-symptom in Hodgkin's disease. Cancer 1983;51: 1934–1936.
8 Mandal S, Varma K, Jain S: Cutaneous manifestations in non-Hodgkin's lymphoma. Acta Cytologica 2007;51:853–859.
9 Robak E, Robak T: Skin lesions in chronic lymphocytic leukemia. Leuk Lymphoma 2007;48:855–865.
10 Brown J, Winkelmann RK: Acanthosis nigricans: a study of 90 cases. Medicine (Baltimore) 1968;47:33–51.
11 Sigurgeirsson B, Lindelof B, Edhag O, Allander E: Risk of cancer in patients with dermatomyositis or polymyositis. A population-based study. N Engl J Med 1992;326:363–367.
12 Yosipovitch G, Tan A, LoSicco K, et al: A comparative study of clinical characteristics, work-up, treatment, and association to malignancy in dermatomyositis between two tertiary skin centers in the USA and Singapore. Int J Dermatol 2013;52:813–819.

13 Shirani Z, Kucenic MJ, Carroll CL, et al: Pruritus in adult dermatomyositis. Clin Exp Dermatol 2004;29:273–276.

14 Hundley JL, Carroll CL, Lang W, et al: Cutaneous symptoms of dermatomyositis significantly impact patients' quality of life. J Am Acad Dermatol 2006;54: 217–220.

15 Grover RW: Transient acantholytic dermatosis. Arch Dermatol 1970;101:426–434.

16 Guana AL, Cohen PR: Transient acantholytic dermatosis in oncology patients. J Clin Oncol 1994;12:1703–1709.

17 Kurzrock R, Cohen PR: Cutaneous paraneoplastic syndromes in solid tumors. Am J Med 1995;99:662–671.

18 Holdiness MR: Pruritus and the Leser-Trélat sign. J Am Acad Dermatol 1988; 18:149.

19 Rampen HJ, Schwengle LE: The sign of Leser-Trélat: does it exist? J Am Acad Dermatol 1989;21:50–55.

20 Zylicz Z, Krajnik M, Sorge AA, Costantini M: Paroxetine in the treatment of severe non-dermatological pruritus: a randomized, controlled trial. J Pain Symptom Manage 2003;26:1105–1112.

21 Davis MP, Frandsen JL, Walsh D, Andresen S, Taylor S: Mirtazapine for pruritus. J Pain Symptom Manage 2003;25: 288–291.

22 Hundley JL, Yosipovitch G: Mirtazapine for reducing nocturnal itch in patients with chronic pruritus: a pilot study. J Am Acad Dermatol 2004;50:889–891.

23 Puzantian T: Mirtazapine, an antidepressant. Am J Health Syst Pharm 1998; 55:44–49.

24 Davis MP, Dickerson ED, Pappagallo M, Benedetti C, Grauer PA, Lycan J: Mirtazepine: heir apparent to amitriptyline? Am J Hosp Palliat Care 2001;18:42–46.

25 Rose MA, Kam PC: Gabapentin: pharmacology and its use in pain management. Anaesthesia 2002;57:451–462.

26 Demierre MF, Taverna J: Mirtazapine and gabapentin for reducing pruritus in cutaneous T-cell lymphoma. J Am Acad Dermatol 2006;55:543–544.

27 Magalhaes E, Mascarenhas AM, Kraychete DC, Sakata RK: Gabapentin to treat sacral perineural cyst-induced pain. Case report. Rev Bras Anestesiol 2004;54:73–77.

28 Dahl JB, Mathiesen O, Moiniche S: 'Protective premedication': an option with gabapentin and related drugs? A review of gabapentin and pregabalin in in the treatment of post-operative pain. Acta Anaesthesiol Scand 2004;48:1130–1136.

29 Singhal S, Mehta J: Thalidomide in cancer. Biomed Pharmacother 2002;56: 4–12.

30 Goncalves F: Thalidomide for the control of severe paraneoplastic pruritus associated with Hodgkin's disease. Am J Hosp Palliat Care 2010;27:486–487.

31 Singhal S, Mehta J, Desikan R, et al: Antitumor activity of thalidomide in refractory multiple myeloma. N Engl J Med 1999;341:1565–1571.

32 Bastuji-Garin S, Ochonisky S, Bouche P, et al: Incidence and risk factors for thalidomide neuropathy: a prospective study of 135 dermatologic patients. J Invest Dermatol 2002;119:1020–1026.

33 Cowan A, Kehner G, Inan S: Targeting itch with ligands selective for κ opioid receptors. Handb Exp Pharmacol 2015; 226:291–314.

34 Ko MC: Neuraxial opioid-induced itch and its pharmacological antagonism. Handb Exp Pharmacol 2015;226:315–335.

35 Dawn AG, Yosipovitch G: Butorphanol for treatment of intractable pruritus. J Am Acad Dermatol 2006;54:527–531.

36 Zeng Z, Lu J, Shu C, et al: A comparision of nalbuphine with morphine for analgesic effects and safety: meta-analysis of randomized controlled trials. Sci Rep 2015;5:10927.

37 Cohen SE, Ratner EF, Kreitzman TR, Archer JH, Mignano LR: Nalbuphine is better than naloxone for treatment of side effects after epidural morphine. Anesth Analg 1992;75:747–752.

38 Hawi A, Alcorn H Jr, Berg J, Hines C, Hait H, Sciascia T: Pharmacokinetics of nalbuphine hydrochloride extended release tablets in hemodialysis patients with exploratory effect on pruritus. BMC Nephrol 2015;16:47.

39 Andoh T, Nagasawa T, Satoh M, Kuraishi Y: Substance P induction of itch-associated response mediated by cutaneous NK1 tachykinin receptors in mice. J Pharmacol Exp Ther 1998;286:1140–1145.

40 Hon KL, Lam MC, Wong KY, Leung TF, Ng PC: Pathophysiology of nocturnal scratching in childhood atopic dermatitis: the role of brain-derived neurotrophic factor and substance P. Br J Dermatol 2007;157:922–925.

41 Duval A, Dubertret L: Aprepitant as an antipruritic agent? N Engl J Med 2009; 361:1415–1416.

42 Singer EM, Shin DB, Nattkemper LA, et al: IL-31 is produced by the malignant T-cell population in cutaneous T-cell lymphoma and correlates with CTCL pruritus. J Invest Dermatol 2013;133: 2783–2785.

43 Cedeno-Laurent F, Singer EM, Wysocka M, et al: Improved pruritus correlates with lower levels of IL-31 in CTCL patients under different therapeutic modalities. Clin Immunol 2015;158:1–7.

44 Bates SE, Eisch R, Ling A, et al: Romidepsin in peripheral and cutaneous T-cell lymphoma: mechanistic implications from clinical and correlative data. Br J Haematol 2015;170:96–109.

Gil Yosipovitch, MD
Department of Dermatology and Itch Center, Temple University School of Medicine
3322 North Broad Street, Medical Office Building, Suite 212
Philadelphia, PA 19140 (USA)
E-Mail gil.yosipovitch@tuhs.temple.edu

Szepietowski JC, Weisshaar E (eds): Itch – Management in Clinical Practice.
Curr Probl Dermatol. Basel, Karger, 2016, vol 50, pp 155–163 (DOI: 10.1159/000446084)

Drug-Induced Itch Management

Toshiya Ebata

Department of Dermatology, The Jikei University School of Medicine, Chitofuna Dermatology Clinic, Tokyo, Japan

Abstract

Drugs may cause itching as a concomitant symptom of drug-induced skin reactions or in the form of pruritus without skin lesions. Drug-induced itch is defined as generalized itching without skin lesions, caused by a drug. Itching associated with drug-induced cholestasis is among the common dermatologic adverse events (dAEs) that induce itching. Some drugs such as opioids, antimalarials, and hydroxyethyl starch are known to induce itching without skin lesions. The clinical features and underlying proposed mechanisms of itching caused by these drugs have been specifically investigated. The recent application of targeted anticancer drugs has increased the survival rate of cancer patients. These new agents cause significant dAEs such as acneiform rashes, dry skin, hand-foot syndrome, paronychia, and itching. Itching is a common side effect of epidermal growth factor receptor inhibitors. Though not life-threatening, these dAEs have a negative impact on a patient's quality of life, leading to dose reduction and possibly less effective cancer therapy. It is important to provide an effective supportive antipruritic treatment without interruption of the administration of these drugs. This chapter concludes by describing basic measures to be taken for diagnosis and treatment of drug-induced itch. The principle of treatment is discontinuation of suspected causative drugs in general except for anticancer medications. In case itching lasts long after drug withdrawal or the causative drug cannot be stopped, vigorous symptomatic antipruritic treatment and specific therapies for different types of drug-induced itch should be undertaken. © 2016 S. Karger AG, Basel

Drug-induced itch is defined as generalized itching without skin lesions, caused by a drug [1]. Localized itch induced by drugs can be included in this category [2]. Secondary changes such as excoriations, crusts, lichenifications, papules, and nodules induced by rubbing and scratching are often observed. Drugs may cause itching as a concomitant symptom of drug-induced skin reactions (drug eruptions) as well, and it is sometimes difficult to distinguish drug-induced itch from itching accompanying drug eruptions. Though the prevalence of drug-induced itch has not been fully investigated, a number of drugs induce itching as the result of drug-induced cholestasis and liver damage. Also some agents such as opioids, antimalarials, hydroxyethyl starch (HES), and targeted anticancer drugs are known to induce itching without skin lesions. The clinical features and underlying proposed mechanisms of itching caused by these drugs have been specifically investigated. This chapter presents general information on drug-induced itch, focusing on its management with the description of some specific drugs that cause itching.

Prevalence of Drug-Induced Itch

Any drug may induce itching through possible allergic reactions, and itching as a side effect is mentioned in the enclosed labels of many drugs. For example, if you search 'itching' listed as a side effect in package inserts of the prescribed drugs in Japan on the website of Pharmaceutical and Medical Devices Agency (PMDA; www.pmda.go.jp), you will receive 7,892 matches. As these include a number of generics and different formulations of the same brand drugs, the real number must be smaller, but still considerable. As details are not known for most of the reports here, it is almost impossible to name all the drugs that induce itching and to show the precise prevalence of drug-induced itch. Itching was mentioned as a common complaint in 31.3% of 3,671 cases of cutaneous adverse drug reactions (ADRs) [3]. Drug-induced itch without skin lesions is less common than drug eruptions with itch [4]. Two studies reported that 1.4 and 12.5% of cutaneous drug reactions were itching without skin lesions, respectively [5, 6]. Individually, a few drugs have been reported to induce itching fairly commonly. For example, the incidence of opioid-induced itch is between 30 and 100% after intrathecal and epidural administration [7]. Chloroquine, a widely prescribed antimalarial, evokes generalized itching in 60–70% in black Africans [8]. Table 1 lists the drugs that may cause itching without skin lesions.

Categories and Pathogenesis of Drug-Induced Itch

Drug-induced itch is categorized into acute and chronic itch [9]. In acute itch there is a clear temporal relationship between the drug intake and appearance of itching. Itching usually appears anywhere from a few days to a few weeks after the initiation of drug administration and may resolve shortly after drug discontinuation. Opioids, antimalarials, and serotonin reuptake inhibitors are drugs known to induce acute itch. On the other hand, itching may last longer than 6 weeks after drug withdrawal, which fulfils the definition of chronic itch [10]. For example, in HES-induced itch, neuronal storage of the substance evokes itch. After the withdrawal of HES administration, the remission of itching depends on the rate of degradation of the substance, which on average lasts longer than 6 weeks [11]. Itching concomitant with drug-induced cholestasis may appear several weeks after the start of the drugs and in a few cases persists for several months after discontinuation of the drugs [12].

The pathogenesis of drug-induced itch is not fully understood for all the causative agents. Postulated underlying mechanisms include immunological type I and type IV allergy; cholestasis; hepatotoxicity; photoallergy and phototoxicity; increased release of pruritogens such as histamine, serotonin, and neuropeptides; augmented pharmacologic actions; enzyme induction; xerosis of the skin; neuronal deposition of the substances in the skin; neurological alterations, and contact with water in case of aquagenic itch. Most of these mechanisms may also be involved with itching concomitant with drug-induced skin lesions.

Table 1. Drugs that may induce itching without skin lesions

Group of drugs	Examples
ACE inhibitors	captopril, enalapril, lisinopril
Alkaloid	atropine, papaverine
Antiarrhythmic drugs	amiodarone, disopyramide, flecainide
Antianxiety drugs	diazepam, nitrazepam, oxazepam
Antibiotics	amoxicillin, ampicillin, cefotaxime, erythromycin, josamycin, minocycline, ofloxacin, penicillin, tetracycline
Anticoagulant	ticlopidine
Antiepileptics	carbamazepine, clonazepam, gabapentin, lamotrigine
Antigout drugs	allopurinol, colchicine, probenecid
Antimalarials	amodiaquine, chloroquine, halofantrine, hydroxychloroquine
Antirheumatics	gold salts
Antitubercular drugs	isoniazid, rifampicin
Beta-adrenergic blockers	acebutolol, atenolol
Calcium antagonists	amlodipine, diltiazem, nifedipine, verapamil
Catecholamines	dobutamine
Cytokines	interleukin-2
Cytostatic drugs	bleomycin, peplomycin
Hormones	estrogens, insulin, oral contraceptives, tamoxifen
Neuroleptics	chlorpromazine, haloperidol, risperidone
Opioids	codeine, fentanyl, morphine
Plasma volume expanders	HES
Targeted anticancer drugs	cetuximab, erlotinib, panitumumab, vemurafenib

ACE = Angiotensin-converting enzyme.

Itching Associated with Drug-Induced Cholestasis and Hepatotoxicity

Drug-induced liver injury is one of the most common ADRs. They are classified into hepatocellular injury type, cholestatic type, mixed type, acute hepatic failure, and others. Drug-induced cholestasis frequently causes itching without skin lesions with or without jaundice. Though the incidence of itching for an individual drug may be low, the wide variety of drugs with the potential ability to cause cholestasis and itching makes this category the most common cause of drug-induced itch. Estrogens, phenothiazines, allopurinol, erythromycin, and oxypenicillins have been known to cause itch for many years. However, an increasingly large number of drugs such as ticlopidine, terbinafine, fluoroquinolones, statins, and amoxicillin-clavulanate have recently been reported to induce itching. The underlying mechanism of itching associated with cholestasis remains to be elucidated. Increased serum levels of bile salts, opioids, autotaxin enzyme, and its end product lysophosphatidic acid may be involved [12, 13]. Itching may resolve shortly after the discontinuation of the offending drug. Sometimes, however, antipruritic therapies such as ursodeoxycholic acid, rifampicin, cholestyramine, and ultraviolet B radiation may be necessary because of the persistence of itching. A few cases of prolonged cholestasis with chronic itch several months after drug withdrawal have also been reported [14].

Opioid-Induced Itch

Opioids are widely used for the treatment of acute and chronic pain. Itching has been known as a common side effect of neuraxial administration of opioids since the 1980s [15]. This delivers the drug intrathecally into the cerebrospinal fluid in close proximity to the spinal cord or epidurally into the epidural space to gain profound analgesia. The incidence of itching by neuraxial administration of opioids is much higher when compared with other routes of administration [7]. The mechanism of opioid-induced itch is postulated to be a centrally mediated process via μ-opioid receptors (MORs). Itching is more often seen with the use of opioids with high affinity to MORs, such as morphine and fentanyl, and in obstetric and postoperative patients. Opioid-induced itch is sometimes severe and lessens the value of neuraxial opioids for pain relief [16].

MOR antagonists such as naloxone and naltrexone, dopamine (D$_2$) receptor antagonists such as droperidol, serotonin (5-HT$_3$) receptor antagonists such as ondansetron, and sedating antihistamines are used for opioid-induced itch treatment with limited efficacy. The use of MOR antagonists is theoretically rational and they are reported to be effective in the prevention and treatment of neuraxial opioid-induced itch. However, these antagonists equally reverse analgesia attained by neuraxial opioids. Agonists acting at κ-opioid receptors are also analgesics, but they have potential antipruritic actions. Although there are controversies surrounding the usefulness of nalbuphine (partial κ-opioid receptor agonist and MOR antagonist) because of its sedative side effect and inconsistent efficacy, a recent systematic review suggests that nalbuphine is the best choice to treat opioid-induced itch [17].

Chloroquine-Induced Itch

Chloroquine has been used to prevent and treat malaria since the 1940s. It also has indications in amoebic liver abscess, rheumatoid arthritis, and lupus erythematosus. Serious side effects include eye reactions known as chloroquine retinopathy, seizures, and deafness. Chloroquine-induced itch is very common among black Africans, with incidence rates reaching 60–70% [8]. It is less common in other races. The incidence was reported to be 22% by a recent study in Brazil [18]. It seems to be a rare side effect in Asians (1.9% of over 1,000 malaria patients on chloroquine therapy in Thailand [19]) and in Caucasians [20]. Other antimalarial drugs such as amodiaquine, Fansidar, halofantrine, and hydroxychloroquine have been reported to induce itching as well.

Among the 'itchy reactors' to antimalarials, 40% claimed the itch to be unbearable and 21% to be severe. In 60% itching involved all parts of the body, and it was confined to the palms and soles in 36%. A stinging sensation was associated with the itching in some patients. The peak intensity of itching occurred 6–24 h after chloroquine dosing. The high concordance rate for itch in twins and siblings, and the varied distribution in the incidence of itch among the races suggest a genetic contribution to the susceptibility to itching. Histamine release by chloroquine, endogenous μ-opioid peptides [21], and slower metabolism of chloroquine leading to the higher concentration have all been postulated mechanisms of action. Antihistamines are commonly used with limited success. Prednisolone was reported to be more efficacious than antihistamines with no negative influence on malaria parasite clearance [22]. Naltrexone was shown to be effective in reducing chloroquine-induced itch to a similar extent as promethazine [21]. Recently Mrgprs (Mas-related G protein-coupled receptors), a family of G protein-coupled receptors expressed in peripheral sensory neurons, were reported to mediate itching caused by chloroquine [23]. This finding is expected to provide a novel therapeutic target for histamine-independent itch.

HES-Induced Itch

HES is a commonly infused artificial colloid for clinical fluid management in surgical and intensive care units. Among the documented side effects of HES such as coagulopathy, clinical bleeding, renal dysfunction and anaphylactoid reactions, severe persistent itching has been recognized since the 1980s. There have been numerous case reports and clinical studies regarding this side effect since the 1990s [11, 24]. Pruritus is the consequence of the neuronal deposition of HES in the skin. This accounts for its characteristic delayed onset of pruritus of usually 1–6 weeks after HES exposure as well as dose-dependency in frequency and severity of the pruritus. However, 15% of the patients developed itching at 30 g, which is about one tenth of the usual mean cumulative dose known to induce itching [25].

Primary skin lesions are not observed. In the majority of the patients the itching is generalized and severe with a negative impact on quality of life. The severity of the itching as quantified by the visual analogue scale demonstrated a median score of 9 out of 10, showing extreme discomfort in the affected patients [25]. Itching may be triggered by heat, sweat, mental stress, and characteristically by mechanical stimuli. The itching lasts on average 9–15 weeks or longer. Most of the currently available forms of therapy for itch are not effective. Gradual attenuation and cessation of the itching over a period of several weeks to months is expected with the concomitant disappearance of HES deposits in cutaneous tissues. Some patients respond to topical capsaicin, UV therapy, and naltrexone [26, 27].

Biological Cancer Treatments (Targeted Anticancer Therapies) and Itch

In the past decade the advent of targeted anticancer drugs has significantly increased the survival rate of patients with various malignancies. Since these novel agents target molecular pathways specific and crucial for cancer growth and metastasis, they have reduced the risk of systemic toxicities such as myelosuppression, infection, nausea, vomiting, and diarrhea seen with conventional cytotoxic chemotherapies. They are, however, associated with a wide spectrum of significant dermatologic adverse events (dAEs), which include acneiform rash, dry skin, hand-foot syndrome, paronychia, and pruritus. Pruritus may occur independently or is often associated with dry skin and acneiform rash [28]. In a survey of 379 cancer survivors, 36% reported experiencing pruritus during treatment, with 44% of them reporting reduced quality of life [29]. Among these new drugs, epidermal growth factor receptor (EGFR) inhibitors such as cetuximab, erlotinib, and panitumumab are known to commonly induce itching. The incidence of all-grade pruritus and high-grade pruritus of EGFR inhibitors as a whole is reported to be 17.4–31% and 1.4–2.0%. Other targeted anticancer drugs where the incidence of itch is relatively high are monoclonal antibody to cytotoxic T-lymphocyte antigen 4, mammalian target of rapamycin inhibitors, Raf kinase inhibitors, Bcr-Abl inhibitors, EGFR-HER2 inhibitors, and monoclonal antibodies to CD20 [30].

The pathogenesis of itching induced by EGFR inhibitors remains unclear. Binding of these drugs to EGFRs in keratinocytes of the epidermal basal layers may result in abnormal proliferation, migration, differentiation, and increased apoptosis of these cells, leading to skin barrier dysfunction, dry skin, and an inflammatory response characterized by increased production and release of cytokines. EGFR inhibitors might also induce secretion of stem cell factors and increase dermal mast cells suggesting the roles of histamine and substance P in the onset of itching.

Table 2. Morphological classification of drug eruptions in connection with itch occurrence and intensity

Types of eruption	Typical causative drugs or agent groups	Itch occurrence	Itch intensity
Maculopapular rash	antimicrobials, antiepileptics, NSAIDs, iohexol, iomeprol	often	− to ++
Fixed drug eruptions	antimicrobials, NSAIDs, allylisopropylacetyl urea, barbiturates	always	+
Urticaria	NSAIDs, antimicrobials, iohexol	always	++
SJS/TEN	NSAIDs, antimicrobials, antiepileptics, phenobarbital, carbamazepine	sometimes	+ to ++
Acneiform eruption	EGFR Inhibitors, vemurafenib, ipilimumab, corticosteroids	sometimes	− to +
Erythema multiforme	imatinib, antiepileptics, NSAIDs, antimicrobials, anti-anxiety drugs	often	+ to ++
Erythroderma	carbamazepine, cyanamide, allopurinol, ampicillin	always	++
Photosensitivity	pyridinecarboxylic acid, NSAIDs, griseofulvin	often	+ to ++
Systemic contact dermatitis	mercury, chloramphenicol, procaine, chlorpheniramine	always	++
Lichenoid eruption	tiopronin, captopril, interferon-α	often	− to +
Purpura	sodium aurothiomalate, sulfamethoxazole, penicillin, aspirin	rarely	− to +
DRESS or DIHS	carbamazepine, mexiletine, phenobarbital, phenytoin, allopurinol, sulpha	sometimes	− to ++
Red man syndrome	vancomycin	dependent on infusion rate	++
AGEP	antimicrobials, NSAIDs, diltiazem, terbinafine	sometimes	− to +

SJS = Stevens-Johnson syndrome; TEN = toxic epidermal necrolysis; DRESS = drug rash with eosinophilia and systemic symptoms; DIHS = drug-induced hypersensitivity syndrome; AGEP = acute generalized exanthematous pustulosis; NSAIDs = nonsteroidal anti-inflammatory drugs. Itch intensity: − = none, + = mild, ++ = severe.

These dAEs or dermatologic toxicities, though usually not extremely severe and life-threatening, result in a negative impact on quality of life and may interfere with the cancer therapy by necessitating dose reduction and treatment interruption. Interestingly, increased severity of dAEs is positively correlated with increased response and/or survival. Therefore, the full knowledge of these dAEs and effective supportive care for them is important for better cancer therapy. It should be borne in mind that severe immunologic reactions to these drugs may also occur, which necessitates the cessation of drug administration.

Drug-Induced Skin Reactions (Drug Eruptions)

Mucocutaneous eruptions are among the most common ADRs. Itching is often associated with drug eruptions [6]. Though this is not categorized as drug-induced itch, it is sometimes difficult to distinguish these two categories. For example, acute generalized itching of which the onset is from minutes to a few hours after drug intake may be an early sign of anaphylaxis before the emergence of urticaria. Prompt systemic therapies with epinephrine, corticosteroids, and antihistamines together with symptomatic treatment in case of shock should be initiated as soon as other signs of anaphylaxis become prominent.

Cutaneous ADRs are morphologically classified into several types [31] (table 2). The occurrence of itching associated with drug eruptions depends on these types. However, the incidence and causative agents of drug eruptions may vary among countries and with the trend of the times. In general, urticaria, erythroderma, and systemic contact dermatitis (eczema type) induce severe itching in almost all cases. Other types such as lichenoid, erythema multiforme, photosensitivity, and fixed drug eruptions also cause itch in the majority of patients. In the most common maculopapular type, itching varies in severity and occurrence. Most of the patients itch, but usually it is not severe.

In the early stage of toxic epidermal necrolysis, itching is sometimes associated with pain, which suggests the existence of severe epidermal inflammation. They do not start with apparent itching, but sometimes the sudden onset of strong itching is observed in association with the formation of vesicles. These changes in itching and association of pain may predict progress to toxic epidermal necrolysis and suggest the need to consider intensive therapies. Drug rash with eosinophilia and systemic symptoms [32] and drug-induced hypersensitivity syndrome [33, 34] have recently been described as a group of severe cutaneous ADRs characterized by late onset, long-lasting rash with fever, eosinophilia, multiorgan involvement, and reactivation of herpesviruses HHV-6, HHV-7, EBV, and cytomegalovirus. They are caused by limited classes of drugs (table 2). The incidence of itching varies, but in some cases severe itch occurs.

Management of Drug-Induced Itch

Diagnosis
The lack of apparent skin lesions makes the diagnosis of drug-induced itch extremely difficult. It can be suspected empirically in cases where the drugs known to induce itching without skin lesions have been administered. But even when a certain drug is suspected to be the cause of the itching, there is no reliable way to prove it except for the positive results from discontinuation and rechallenge of the suspected drug. This may also be obscure for chronic drug-induced itch.

It is essential to do a complete history and physical examination of the patients who complain of itching. The detailed anamnesis of the intensity, onset, time course, quality, localization, and triggering factors of their itching should be obtained. Together with the anamnesis of preexisting diseases, allergies, and atopic diathesis, it is important to ask about current and recent drug intake including medications in the operation room or within emergency situations, over-the-counter drugs, and dietary and herbal supplements [35].

The physical examination of patients complaining about itch should include a thorough inspection of the entire skin together with the mucous membrane, scalp, hair, nails, and anogenital region. Care should be taken to avoid judging the primary skin lesions as the secondary changes induced by rubbing and scratching. And through the necessary laboratory tests and diagnostic imaging, all of the categories of systemic diseases that can cause itching should be carefully ruled out. Skin biopsy is considered when it is necessary to exclude other dermatological diseases. For example, mastocytosis and pemphigoid can be ruled out by applying the direct immunofluorescent antibody technique. Electron microscopy provides definitive evidence of HES storage in the skin, confirming the diagnosis of HES-induced itch.

The most reliable method to establish drug-induced itch is discontinuation and rechallenge with the suspected medicine. However, the adequate length of a break for diagnosis is difficult to determine. Furthermore, the fact that many patients take multiple medications makes this test complicated. Rechallenge or a drug provocation test is basically contraindicated when itching is associated with liver dysfunction.

Treatment
The principle of treatment of drug-induced itch is to identify and withdraw the responsible agent, which usually resolves itching shortly afterwards except for chronic itch, e.g. HES-induced itch and some cases of itching associated with drug-induced cholestasis. On the other hand, discontinuation is not the choice for itch caused by anticancer drugs. One should continue with anticancer therapy with the aid of symptomatic antipruritic treatment in order to avoid dose reduction and discontinuance of anticancer drugs, which leads

Table 3. Proposed antipruritic treatment for specific types of drug-induced itch

Type	First-line treatment	Second-line treatment	Third-line treatment
Opioid-induced	MOR antagonist κ-opioid receptor agonist	dopamine receptor antagonist	serotonin 5-HT$_3$ antagonist sedating antihistamines
Chloroquine-induced	antihistamines	MOR antagonist	prednisolone
HES-induced	MOR antagonist	phototherapy	topical capsaicin
Drug-induced cholestasis	ursodeoxycholic acid rifampicin	cholestyramine	MOR antagonist
EGFRi-induced	antihistamines topical corticosteroids and menthol	gabapentin, pregabalin systemic corticosteroids	aprepitant
Other types of drug-induced itch	high doses of antihistamines	MOR antagonist	gabapentin, paroxetine, amitryptiline

EGFRi = EFGR inhibitor. Modified from Reich et al. [9, table III].

to poor prognosis. A short-term systemic cortisone application should also be considered as a symptomatic treatment.

If itching is not sufficiently reduced after discontinuation of the suspected drug, symptomatic treatment should be applied. Instructions on the general itch-relieving measures are also important. These are application of moisturizers, cooling of the skin, and the elimination of worsening factors of itching such as dryness of the skin, excessive rubbing and scratching, bathing with hot water for long periods of time, mental stress, spicy food, and irregular lifestyle habit of sleep and meals.

First-line symptomatic treatment includes topical moisturizers, systemic H$_1$-antihistamines, and topical corticosteroids in case secondary eczematous lesions exist. Further antipruritic symptomatic measures that follow are topical capsaicin, topical calcineurin inhibitors, naltrexone, gabapentin, pregabalin, cyclosporine, and UV phototherapy. Specific treatments for different types of drug-induced itch are shown in table 3. Caution should be taken as most of these therapies are not approved. Informed consent must be obtained before prescribing.

References

1 Weisshaar E, Greaves MW: Pruritus; in Williams H, Bigby M, Diepgen T, Herxheimer A, Naldi L, Rzany B (eds): Evidence-Based Dermatology, ed 2. Oxford, Blackwell, 2008, pp 650–670.

2 Szepietowski J, Reich A: Drugs; in Misery L, Ständer S (eds): Pruritus. London, Springer, 2010, pp 195–204.

3 Patel TK, Thakkar SH, Sharma DC: Cutaneous adverse drug reactions in Indian population: a systematic review. Indian Dermatol Online J 2014;5(suppl 2):s76–s86.

4 Sarno AM, Bernhard JD: Drug-induced pruritus without a rash; in Bernhard JD (ed): Itch Mechanisms and Management of Pruritus. New York, McGraw-Hill, 1994, pp 329–335.

5 Bigby M, Jick S, Jick H, Arndt K: Drug-induced cutaneous reactions. A report from the Boston Collaborative Drug Surveillance Program on 15,438 consecutive inpatients, 1975 to 1982. JAMA 1986;256:3358–3363.

6 Raksha MP, Marfatia YS: Clinical study of cutaneous drug eruptions in 200 patients. Indian J Dermatol Venereol Leprol 2008;74:80.

7 Szarvas S, Harmon D, Murphy D: Neuraxial opioid-induced pruritus: a review. J Clin Anesth 2003;15:234–239.

8 Ajayi AA, Oluokun O, Sofowora O, Akinleye A, Ajayi AT: Epidemiology of antimalarial-induced pruritus in Africans. Eur J Clin Pharmacol 1989;37:539–540.

9 Reich A, Ständer S, Szepietowski JC: Drug-induced pruritus: a review. Acta Derm Venereol 2009;89:236–244.

10 Ständer S, Weisshaar E, Mettang T, Szepietowski JC, Carstens E, Ikoma A, Bergasa NV, Gieler U, Misery L, Wallengren J, Darsow U, Streit M, Metze D, Luger TA, Greaves MW, Schmelz M, Yosipovitch G, Bernhard JD: Clinical classification of itch: a position paper of the International Forum for the Study of Itch. Acta Derm Venereol 2007;87:291–294.

11 Bork K: Pruritus precipitated by hydroxyethyl starch: a review. Br J Dermatol 2005;152:3–12.

12 Levy C, Lindor KD: Drug-induced cholestasis. Clin Liver Dis 2007;7:311–330.

13 Kremer AE, van Dijk R, Leckie P, Schaap FG, Kuiper EM, Mettang T, Reiners KS, Raap U, van Buuren HR, van Erpecum KJ, Davies NA, Rust C, Engert A, Jalan R, Oude Elferink RP, Beuers U: Serum autotaxin is increased in pruritus of cholestasis, but not of other origin, and responds to therapeutic interventions. Hepatology 2012;56:1391–1400.

14 Kowdley KV, Keeffe EB, Fawaz KA: Prolonged cholestasis due to trimethoprim sulfamethoxazole. Gastroenterology 1992;102:2148–2150.

15 Ballantyne JC, Loach AB, Carr DB: Itching after epidural and spinal opiates. Pain 1988;33:149–160.

16 Ko MC: Neuraxial opioid-induced itch and its pharmacological antagonism. Handb Exp Pharmacol 2015;226:315–335.

17 Jannuzzi RG: Nalbuphine for treatment of opioid-induced pruritus: a systematic review of literature. Clin J Pain 2016;32:87–93.

18 Braga CB, Martins AC, Cayotopa AD, Klein WW, Schlosser AR, DaSilva AF, de Souza MN, Andrade BW, Filgueira-Junior JA, Pinto Wde J, da Silva-Nunes M: Side effects of chloroquine and symptom reduction in malaria endemic area (Mancio Lima, Brazil). Interdiscip Perspect Infect Dis 2015;2015:346853.

19 Bussaratid V, Walsh DS, Wilairatana P, Krudsood S, Silachamroon U, Looareesuwan S: Frequency of pruritus in *Plasmodium vivax* malaria patients treated with chloroquine in Thailand. Trop Doct 2000;30:211–214.

20 Spencer HC, Poulter NR, Lury JD, Poulter CJ: Chloroquine-associated pruritus in a European. Br Med J (Clin Res Ed) 1982;285:1703–1704.

21 Ajayi AA, Kolawole BA, Udoh SJ: Endogeneous opioids, μ-opiate receptors and chloroquine-induced pruritus: a double-blind comparison of naltrexone and promethazine in patients with malaria fever who have an established history of generalized choroquine-induced itching. Int J Dermatol 2004;43:972–977.

22 Adebayo RA, Sofowora GG, Onayemi O, Udoh SJ, Ajayi AA: Chloroquine-induced pruritus in malaria fever: contribution of malaria parasitaemia and the effects of prednisolone, niacin, and their combination, compared with antihistamine. Br J Pharmacol 1997;44:157–161.

23 Liu Q, Tang Z, Surdenikova L, Kim S, Patel KN, Kim A, Ru F, Guan Y, Weng HJ, Geng Y, Undem BJ, Kollarik M, Chen ZF, Anderson DJ, Dong X: Sensory neuron-specific GPCR Mrgprs are itch receptors mediating chloroquine-induced pruritus. Cell 2009;139:1353–1365.

24 Wiedermann CJ, Joannidis M: Accumulation of hydroxyethyl starch in human and animal tissues: a systematic review. Intensive Care Med 2014;40:160–170.

25 Ständer S, Richter L, Osada N, Metze D: Hydroxyethyl starch-induced pruritus: clinical characteristics and influence of dose, molecular weight and substitution. Acta Derm Venereol 2014;94:282–287.

26 Szeimies RM, Stolz W, Wlotzke U, Korting HC, Landthaler M: Successful treatment of hydroxyethyl starch-induced pruritus with topical capsaicin. Br J Dermatol 1994;131:380–382.

27 Metze D, Reimann S, Beissert S, Luger T: Efficacy and safety of naltrexone, an oral opiate receptor antagonist, in the treatment of pruritus in internal and dermatological diseases. J Am Acad Dermatol 1999;41:533–539.

28 Fischer A, Rosen AC, Ensslin CJ, Wu S, Lacouture ME: Pruritus to anticancer agents targeting the EGFR, BRAF, and CTLA-4. Dermatol Ther 2013;26:135–148.

29 Gandhi M, Oishi K, Zubal B, Lacouture ME: Unanticipated toxicities from anticancer therapies: survivors' perspectives. Support Care Cancer 2010;18:1461–1468.

30 Ensslin CJ, Rosen AC, Wu S, Lacouture ME: Pruritus in patients treated with targeted cancer therapies: systematic review and meta-analysis. J Am Acad Dermatol 2013;69:708–720.

31 Fukuda H, Fukuda H: Collected Report of Drug Eruptions in Japan, ed 16 (in Japanese). Fukuoka, Fukuda Dermatology Clinic, 2015, pp 37–468.

32 Bocquet H, Bagot M, Roujeau JC: Drug-induced pseudolymphoma and drug hypersensitivity syndrome (drug rash with eosinophilia and systemic symptoms: DRESS). Semin Cutan Med Surg 1996;15:250–257.

33 Tohyama M, Yahata Y, Yasukawa M, Inagi R, Urano Y, Yamanishi K, Hashimoto K: Severe hypersensitivity syndrome due to sulfasalazine associated with human herpes virus 6. Arch Dermatol 1998;134:1113–1117.

34 Suzuki Y, Inagi R, Aono T, Yamanishi K, Shiohara T: Human herpesvirus 6 infection as a risk factor for the development of severe drug-induced hypersensitivity syndrome. Arch Dermatol 1998;134:1108–1112.

35 Weisshaar E, Szepietowski JC, Darsow U, Misery L, Wallengren J, Mettang T, Gieler U, Lotti T, Lambert J, Maisel P, Streit M, Greaves MW, Carmichael A, Tschachler E, Ring J, Ständer S: European Guideline on Chronic Pruritus. Acta Derm Venereol 2012;92:563–581.

Toshiya Ebata, MD
Department of Dermatology, The Jikei University School of Medicine, Chitofuna Dermatology Clinic
5-17-13 Sakuragaoka
Setagaya, Tokyo 156-0054 (Japan)
E-Mail ebatoshi@nifty.com

Szepietowski JC, Weisshaar E (eds): Itch – Management in Clinical Practice.
Curr Probl Dermatol. Basel, Karger, 2016, vol 50, pp 164–172 (DOI: 10.1159/000446087)

Itch in Pregnancy Management

Julien Lambert

Department of Dermatology, University Hospital of Antwerp, University of Antwerp, Edegem, Belgium

Abstract

Pruritus is common in pregnancy. It deserves an elaborated work-up of the patient. It is frequently a symptom of a dermatosis that coincides by chance with pregnancy or a preexisting dermatosis that can flare during pregnancy. In some cases, it is due to the group of pregnancy-specific dermatoses. Work-up requires a prudent consideration of the diagnostic tests as well as the choice of treatment because of the potential effects on the fetus. This chapter will focus on the specific dermatoses of pregnancy and the local and systemic treatment of pruritus in general during pregnancy.

© 2016 S. Karger AG, Basel

Pruritus is an important symptom in pregnancy. It deserves a thorough work-up of the patient. Among the pruritic skin diseases during pregnancy, we have to distinguish the dermatoses that coincide by chance with pregnancy or preexisting dermatoses that can flare during pregnancy (table 1) on the one hand, and the four specific dermatoses of pregnancy on the other hand.

The work-up of a pruritus problem starts with a thorough medical history and clinical examination to rule out dermatological diseases as well as internal pathology besides the specific dermatoses of pregnancy. Indeed, 1 out of every 5 consultations for pruritus in pregnancy is not related to the specific dermatoses of pregnancy [1].

The work-up also requires a prudent consideration of the diagnostic tests as well as for the choice of treatment because of the potential effects on the fetus. For example, prick tests and patch tests are not indicated during pregnancy [2]. There are no guidelines for every test and in every case the risk-benefit for mother and fetus has to be considered. If a biopsy is needed, both lidocaine and adrenaline are considered safe in small amounts for local anesthesia [3]. There is some discussion about the addition of adrenaline, but the benefits of using small amounts seem to outweigh potential risks. This chapter focuses on the specific dermatoses of pregnancy and the local and systemic treatment of pruritus in general during pregnancy.

Table 1. Pruritic disease that can flare up during pregnancy

Psoriasis[1]
Atopic dermatitis[1]
Dyshidrosis and dyshidrotic eczema
Dermatomyositis
HIV/AIDS
Urticaria (also dermographism)
Mastocytosis[1]
Lichen ruber planus
Neurofibromatosis
Bacterial, mycological, and viral infections
Pityriasis rosea

[1] May also improve.

Specific Dermatoses of Pregnancy

Pruritus is a very prominent symptom of the specific dermatoses of pregnancy. The most recent classification includes pemphigoid gestationis (PG), polymorphic eruption of pregnancy (PEP), intrahepatic cholestasis of pregnancy (ICP), and atopic eruption of pregnancy – a new 'umbrella' concept comprising atopic dermatitis in pregnancy, prurigo of pregnancy, and pruritic folliculitis of pregnancy [4]. Taking into consideration the moment of onset, the medical history (primigravida, multiple gestation pregnancy), the clinical presentation, and the results of diagnostic tests will help to establish the correct diagnosis, which is essential for the therapeutic strategy and the prognosis for mother and fetus.

Polymorphic Eruption of Pregnancy

PEP, previously known as 'pruritic urticarial papules and plaques of pregnancy' (this term is still preferred in the American literature), occurs in the third trimester of pregnancy (most frequently in the 35th to 39th week) or immediately postpartum [5]. PEP is a common pregnancy-specific dermatosis with an incidence of

1 in 160 pregnancies [6, 7]. It is associated with primigravida, excessive maternal weight gain (not fetal weight), and multiple pregnancies. The etiopathogenesis is unknown, but a relationship with damage of the collagen fibers due to distension and overstretching of skin is suspected [8]. This damage with subsequent conversion of nonantigenic molecules to antigenic ones could trigger an inflammatory response [5]. The relevance of a statistically significant reduction in serum cortisol among 44 patients with PEP in a prospective study of 200 women with dermatoses of pregnancy remains unclear [9]. Finally, the authors of a study of 181 patients with PEP, which revealed a frequency of atopy among 55% of the included patients, speculate that the atopic background may influence the natural course of PEP [6]. This high frequency was especially pronounced in patients with a longer disease duration.

In nearly all patients the clinical examination shows intensely pruritic urticarial papules and plaques in the beginning, and later on a polymorphous aspect is seen in more than 50% of the patients with vesicular, targetoid, and eczematous lesions [6]. The lesions start on the lower abdomen and/or proximal thighs, especially within or adjacent to the striae distensae, and spread in most cases to the buttocks, legs, arms, chest, and back. The rash usually spares the umbilical region (fig. 1–3), and generally resolves within 6 weeks. The eruption may persist for a longer time in patients with early onset of PEP, multigravidae, and atopic women [6]. Recurrences are very rare and have only been reported in case of multiple pregnancies. The diagnosis is based on the clinical picture with the typical characteristics. The association of skin lesions with striae distensae and the sparing of the umbilicus is important in the differentiation from pemphigoid gestation in which lesions present independently from striae distensae and frequently involve the umbilical region. Histopathology is not specific and varies with the stage of the disease. Direct immunofluo-

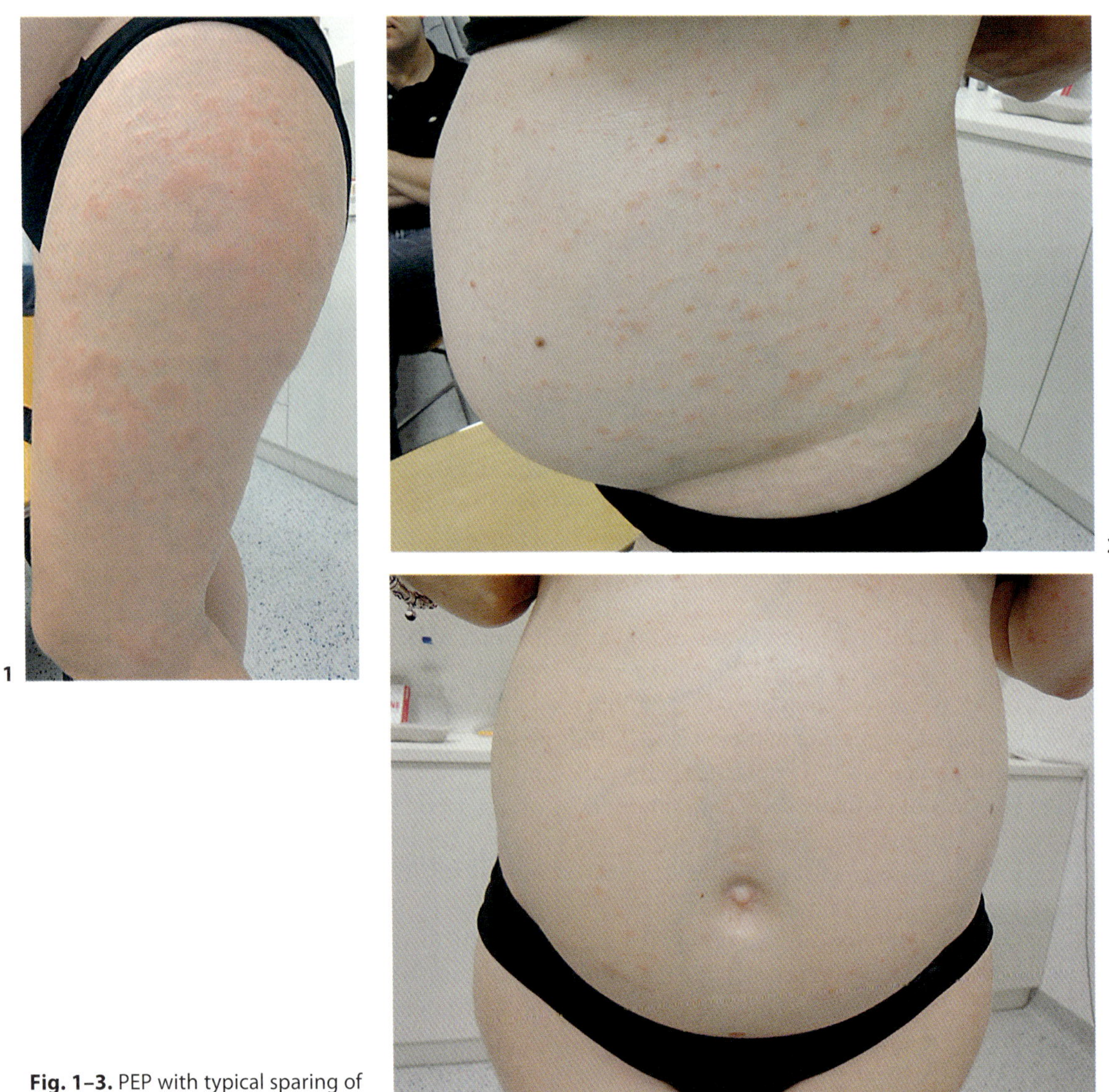

Fig. 1–3. PEP with typical sparing of the umbilical region.

rescence and indirect immunofluorescence are negative. Generally, PEP is neither regarded as being associated with cutaneous manifestations or risk to the fetus, nor with maternal morbidity. Treatment consists of topical corticosteroids with or without oral antihistamines. In severe cases, a short course of systemic corticosteroids may be necessary.

Pemphigoid Gestationis

PG, formally known as herpes gestationis, is a rare bullous autoimmune disease that normally occurs in the second half of the pregnancy or immediately postpartum. The incidence is approximately 1 in 60,000 pregnancies and PG has a worldwide distribution [10, 11]. The pathogene-

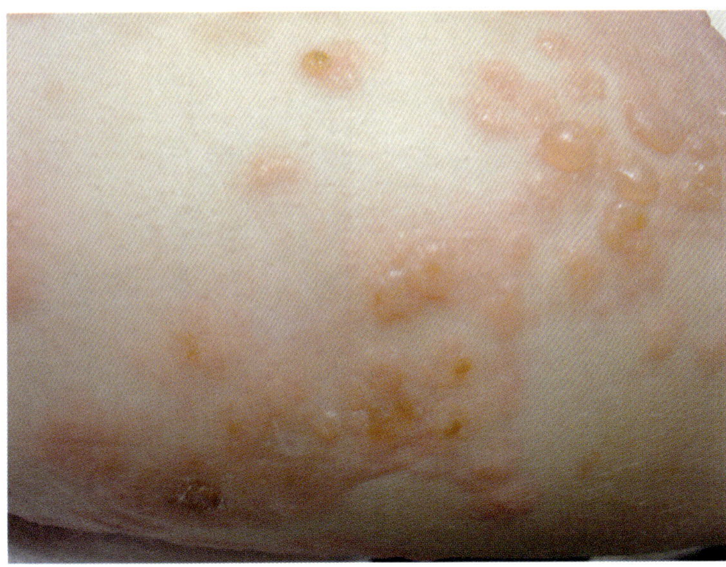

Fig. 4. Pemphigoid gestationis.

sis of this disease is based on the production of circulating antiplacental immunoglobulin G antibodies that bind to bullous pemphigoid antigen 2 (BP-180) and BP-230 in the hemidesmosomes of the dermoepidermal junction, which results in membrane damage and production of tense bullae. Recently, both IgA and IgE antibodies to either BP180 or BP230 have also been detected in PG [12].

Clinical examination shows initially pruritic urticarial papules and annular plaques, followed by vesicles, and finally large tense bullae on an erythematous background. The lesions start on the abdomen, especially the periumbilical region, and do not spare the umbilical region; there is also no association with the striae distensae. The lesions spread to the rest of the abdomen and may involve the total body, but spare the face and scalp (fig. 4–6). There is no mucosal involvement. The diagnosis is confirmed by histology and especially direct immunofluorescence, which shows a linear deposition of IgG and C3 along the dermoepidermal junction. C3 is reported in up to 100% of cases, while IgG is seen in 25–50% [13]. PG tends to resolve within weeks to months of delivery, but will often return in subsequent pregnancies. There is a higher risk of premature and small-for-gestational age babies [8]. Because of the passive transfer of IgG1 antibodies from the mother to the fetus, approximately 10% of newborns develop a mild clinical picture consisting of urticaria-like or vesicular skin lesions [7]. Treatment consists of oral corticosteroids with a daily dose of 0.5 mg/kg. Depending on the activity of the disease, the dose will be gradually tapered to a maintenance dose [11]. In case of mild disease, potent local corticosteroids and oral histamines are the first choice.

Intrahepatic Cholestasis of Pregnancy

ICP, also known as pruritus gravidarum, is a condition that has not always been included in the classifications of pregnancy dermatoses because it is a liver disorder, which is not associated with primary skin lesions.

Patients present secondary skin lesions caused by scratching. It is a hormonally triggered reversible cholestasis, occurring in late pregnancy (late

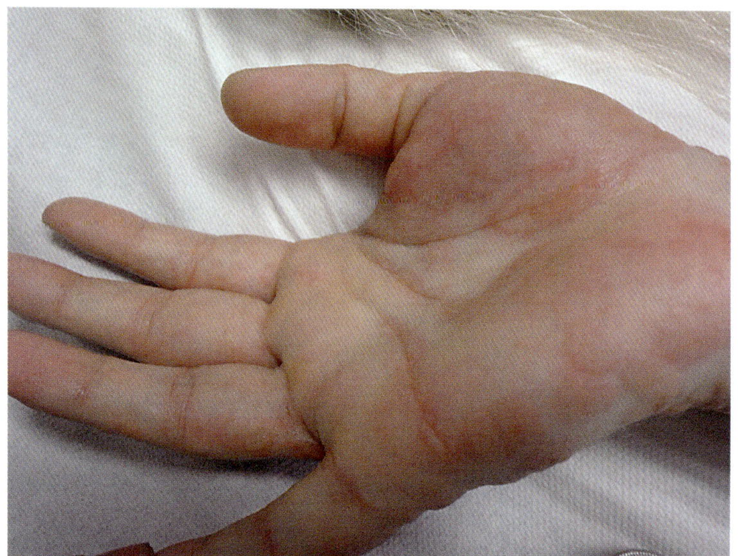

Fig. 5. Pemphigoid gestationis.

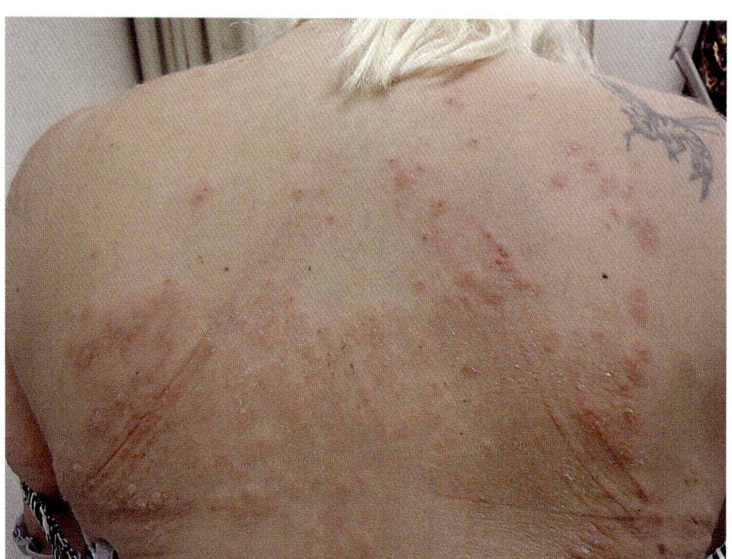

Fig. 6. Pemphigoid gestationis.

second or third trimester) in genetically predisposed women. The prevalence is around 1%, but is variable: it is higher in Scandinavia, South America, and South Africa [11]. The etiopathogenesis is multifactorial and involves genetic, hormonal, and environmental factors, such as seasonal variability and dietary factors [14]. ICP is characterized by an inability to excrete bile salts, causing elevated serum bile acid levels, responsible for pruritus in the mother, and negatively influencing the fetal prognosis. There is an increased risk of prematurity (20–60%), intrapartal fetal distress (20–30%), and stillbirth (1–2%) [7, 14]. In severe or prolonged ICP, cholestasis might cause vitamin K deficiency and coagulopathy in patients and their children [11].

Patients present a sudden-onset pruritus that starts in the palmoplantar regions, but very quickly becomes generalized to the entire body. Due to scratching and rubbing, patients present secondary linear excoriations and prurigo nodularis lesions on the extensor surfaces of the arms and legs. Signs of icterus are seen in approximately 10% of the cases 1–4 weeks after the onset of pruritus. Diagnosis is made after the exclusion of other clinical entities included in the differential diagnosis of cholestasis and hepatic disease and by the rise of serum bile acid levels >11 μmol/l [8, 14, 15]. Normal levels are 6 μmol/l, but during pregnancy 11 μmol/l is tolerated. Liver function tests are normal in 30% of the cases. The elevation of the serum bile acid levels has a prognostic value; in case of levels >40 μmol/l, the fetal risk is markedly higher [15, 16]. A very recent study proposes three sulfated progesterone metabolites as a prognostic indicator for ICP. The serum levels of these compounds were significantly higher at 9–19 weeks of gestation and prior to symptom onset [17]. Treatment consists of ursodeoxycholic acid (15 mg/kg/day or 500 mg/twice a day), which reduces serum bile acid levels. This treatment reduces maternal pruritus and also improves fetal prognosis. No maternal or fetal adverse effects have been reported. Phototherapy with UVB can be used in refractory cases [11]. The symptoms usually disappear 1–2 days after delivery, accompanied by normalization of serum bile acid concentrations and other liver enzyme levels. Recurrences occur in subsequent pregnancies (risk: 50–70%) and in cases of oral contraceptive treatment.

Atopic Eruption of Pregnancy

Ambros-Rudolph et al. [4] introduced the term 'atopic eruption of pregnancy' in 2005 to cover all patients formerly given a diagnosis of eczema of pregnancy, prurigo of pregnancy, and pruritic folliculitis of pregnancy. A prospective study on pruritic skin diseases in pregnancy had demonstrated a higher prevalence of atopic eczema [9]. This finding was not taken into consideration in former classifications. They observed a considerable overlap among patients with eczema of pregnancy, prurigo of pregnancy, and pruritic folliculitis, both clinically and histopathologically, so they grouped them within a new disease complex: atopic eruption of pregnancy. There is still controversy regarding this terminology [18, 19].

Atopic eruption of pregnancy is the most common pregnancy dermatosis and is noted in almost 50% of the patients [4]. Only 20% of the patients suffered from exacerbation of a preexisting atopic dermatitis, as 80% experienced atopic skin lesions for the first time during their pregnancy [4]. Concerning this discussion about the concept of atopic eruption of pregnancy, Koutroulis et al. [20] raised the question of whether pregnant patients with 'new atopic dermatitis' have 'pure atopy' or instead present a transient eczematiform eruption that may not recur postpartum or may recur only in pregnancy.

These eczematous lesions could be related to the typical dominance of the Th2 immunity observed during pregnancy. In order to prevent fetal rejection, normal pregnancy is characterized by lower Th1 cytokine production and enhanced Th2 cytokine production [21]. Atopic dermatitis is considered to be a Th2-dominant disease. The Th2 shift associated with pregnancy may explain the exacerbation of atopic dermatitis during pregnancy. In contrast to the other specific dermatoses of pregnancy, the onset occurs in 75% of the cases before the third trimester, usually early in the first or second trimester. The skin lesions can be divided in either eczematous-type skin changes or prurigo-type lesions [4]. The eczematous-type lesions are located in the classic localizations like the face, neck, presternal region, and flexure sides. The prurigo lesions occur on the extensor surfaces of the extremities. Elevated serum IgE levels are present in 30–70% of the cases [8]. However, according to Koutroulis et al. [20], serum IgE levels should not be used in the diagnosis of atopic dermatitis in pregnancy because the regulation of IgE in normal pregnancy has not been clarified.

Fetal prognosis is unaffected. Recurrences in later pregnancies are to be expected. Treatment depends on the severity of the condition and first consists of topical corticosteroids. In severe cases, systemic corticosteroids, antihistamines, and UVB phototherapy may be considered.

Treatment of Pruritus during Pregnancy

Treating pruritus in pregnancy remains frequently a challenge, requiring prudent consideration due to potential effects on the fetus. In addition to the specific topical and systemic treatments for the underlying etiology, general pruritus-relieving measures, which include avoidance of factors that foster dryness of the skin, use of mild soaps, moisturizing syndets, and shower or bathing oils, also have to be taken into consideration [22]. In case of damaged or inflamed skin, patients should dab their skin dry without rubbing after contact with water. Patients should be advised to moisturize their skin on a daily basis, especially after showering and bathing. Topicals containing antipruritic additives such as menthol, camphor, and polidocanol are also indicated.

Topical corticosteroids are the most frequently used drugs for treating skin conditions and are prescribed to more than 6% of pregnant women [23]. However, little is known about the effects of local corticosteroids on the fetus. A European evidence-based guideline suggests the following recommendations [24]: mild/moderate topical corticosteroids are preferred to more potent corticosteroids, and potent/very potent local corticosteroids as a second-line therapy should be limited as much as possible and appropriate obstetric care should be provided because there is an increased risk of fetal growth restriction. A recent study showed a significantly increased risk of low birth weight in cases where >300 g of potent or

very potent topical corticosteroids were applied over the course of the entire pregnancy [23]. There are no data available to determine if newer lipophilic topical corticosteroids (mometasone furoate, fluticasone propionate, and methylprednisolone aceponate) are associated with a lower risk of fetal growth restriction. On theoretical grounds they have a more favorable side-effect profile. Finally, a very recent Cochrane Review update adds more evidence showing no causal associations between maternal exposure to topical corticosteroids of all potencies and pregnancy outcomes including mode of delivery, congenital abnormalities, preterm delivery, fetal death, and low Apgar score [25]. This update also identified the probable association between low birth weight and maternal use of large cumulative dosage of potent to very potent topical corticosteroids. A possible protective effect of mild-to-moderate topical corticosteroids on fetal death was also found.

Systemic corticosteroids have a greater potential for fetotoxicity than local corticosteroids because of a greater bioavailability. They are associated with a reduction in fetal birth weight and an increase in preterm delivery. In case systemic corticosteroids are necessary, nonhalogenated corticosteroids should be administered [26]. In the placenta, cortisol, prednisone, and prednisolone are inactivated, but not betamethasone and dexamethasone. Prednisolone is the corticosteroid of choice in pregnancy. The usual initial dose is 0.5–2 mg/kg/day according to the nature and severity of the disease. A maintenance dose should not exceed 10–15 mg/day in the first trimester, so as to avoid a slightly increased risk of cleft lips/cleft palates.

There is also a lack of knowledge concerning the use of antihistamines during pregnancy. The older, sedating antihistamines such as dimetindene and clemastine are considered safe because they have already been prescribed for very long time [2]. Regarding the use of hydroxyzine during the first trimester, reports concerning a slightly higher risk of malformation [27] and risk of neonatal seizures in case of use in late pregnancy [28] call for cautiousness. The antihistamines of the second generation such as cetirizine, loratadine, fexofenadine, desloratadine, levocetirizine, and bilastine, which provoke low or no sedation, are categorized as medications of which we do not have extensive information about use in humans, but animal studies have not shown evidence of embryotoxicity or teratogenicity [2, 29]. Loratadine and cetirizine are among the best studied second-generation antihistamines. They can be prescribed after the first trimester in case of well-considered indications. Smedts et al. [30] recently presented the results of two case-control studies which showed a rise of congenital heart defects in early pregnancy exposure to antihistamines. Administration just before or after birth has to be avoided.

Narrowband as well as broadband UVB phototherapy are safe [3]. Folic acid levels may decrease with both narrowband and broadband therapy. Folate deficiency in the first trimester predisposes to the development of neural tube defects. A follow-up of the folic acid levels is indicated. Psoralen is a known mutagen and teratogen. PUVA treatment is therefore contraindicated during pregnancy.

Permethrin, benzoyl benzoate, and crotamiton are considered safe for scabies treatment [3]. Lindane is potentially neurotoxic and is contraindicated. For ivermectin, no teratogenicity has been shown in humans. Topical calcineurin inhibitors are poorly absorbed systemically [3]. There are no studies on safety in human pregnancies. If no alternatives exist, topical use on small surfaces is permissible. The use of coal tar is not indicated, but there are no indications of teratogenic effects in humans [3, 30]. The use of capsaicin is also contraindicated [31].

References

1 Roger D, Vaillant L, Fignon A, Pierre F, Dacq Y, Bréchot JF, Grangeponte MC, Lorette G: Specific pruritic diseases of pregnancy. A prospective study of 3192 pregnant women. Arch Dermatol 1994; 130:7234–7239.
2 Treudler R: Allergische Erkrankungen bei Schwangeren. Hautarzt 2010;61: 1027–1033.
3 Murase JE, Heller MM, Butler DC: Safety of dermatological medications in pregnancy and lactation: part I. Pregnancy. J Am Acad Dermatol 2014;70: 401.e1–14.
4 Ambros-Rudolph CM, Mullegger RR, Vaughan-Jones SA, Kerl H, Black MM: The specific dermatoses of pregnancy revisited and reclassified: results of a retrospective two center study on 505 pregnant patients. J Am Acad Dermatol 2006;54:395–404.
5 Matz H, Orion E, Wolf R: Pruritic urticarial papules and plaques of pregnancy: polymorphic eruption of pregnancy (PUPPP). Clin Dermatol 2006;24:105–108.
6 Rudolph CM, Al-Fares S, Vaughan-Jones SA, Mulleger RR, Kerl H, Black MM: Polymorphic eruption of pregnancy. Clinicopathology and potential trigger factors in 181 patients. Br J Dermatol 2006:154:54–60.
7 Roth MM: Pregnancy dermatoses: diagnosis, management and controversies. Am J Clin Dermatol 2011;12:25–41.
8 Ambros-Rudolph CM: Spezifische Schwangerschaftsdermatosen. Hautarzt 2010;61:1014–1020.
9 Vaughan-Jones SA, Hern S, Nelson-Piercy C, Seed PT, Black MM: A prospective study of 200 women with dermatoses of pregnancy correlating clinical findings with hormonal and immunopathological profiles. Br J Dermatol 1999;141:71–81.
10 Shornick JK, Bangert JL, Freeman RG, Gillian JN: Herpes gestationis: clinical and histologic features of twenty-eight cases. J Am Acad Dermatol 1983;8:214–224.
11 Saverall C, Sand FL, Thomsen SF: Dermatological diseases associated with pregnancy: pemphigoid gestationis, polymorphic eruption of pregnancy, intrahepatic cholestasis of pregnancy and atopic eruption of pregnancy. Dermatol Res Pract 2015;2015:979635.
12 Beard MP, Millington GWM: Recent developments in the specific dermatoses of pregnancy. Clin Exp Dermatol 2011; 37:1–5.
13 Intong LRA, Murrell DF: Pemphigoid gestationis: pathogenesis and clinical features. Dermatol Clin 2011;29:447–452.
14 Ozkan S, Ceylan Y, Ozkan OV, Yildirim S: Review of a challenging clinical issue: intrahepatic cholestasis of pregnancy. World J Gastroenterol 2015;21:7134–7141.
15 Lehrhoff S, Pomeranz MK: Specific dermatoses of pregnancy and their treatment. Dermatol Ther 2013;26:274–284.
16 Glantz A, Marschall HU, Mattsson LA: Intrahepatic cholestatis of pregnancy: relationships between bile acid levels and fetal complication rates. Hepatology 2004;40:467–474.

17 Abu-Hayyeh S, Ovadia C, Lieu T, et al: Prognostic and mechanistic potential of progesterone sulfates in intrahepatic cholestasis of pregnancy and pruritus gravidarum. Hepatology 2016;63:1287–1298.

18 Ingber A: Atopic eruption of pregnancy. J Eur Acad Dermatol Venereol 2010;24:984.

19 Cohen LM, Kroumpouzos G: Pruritic dermatoses of pregnancy: to lump or to split? J Am Acad Dermatol 2007;56:708–709.

20 Koutroulis I, Papoutsis J, Kroumpouzos G: Atopic dermatitis in pregnancy: current status and challenges. Obstet Gynecol Surv 2011;66:654–663.

21 Garcia-Gonzalez E, Ahued-Ahued R, Arroyo E, Montes-De Oca D, Granados J: Immunology of the cutaneous disorders of pregnancy. Int J Dermatol 1999;38:721–729.

22 Weisshaar E, Szepietowski JC, Darsow U, et al: European guideline on chronic pruritus. Acta Derm Venereol 2012;92:563–581.

23 Chi CC, Wang SH, Mayon-White R, Wojnarowska F: Pregnancy outcomes after material exposure to topical corticosteroids: a UK population-based cohort study. JAMA Dermatol 2013;149:1274–1280.

24 Chi CC, Kirtschig G, Aberer W, Gabbud JP, Lipozencic J, Karpati S, Haustein UF, Zubervier T, Wojnarowska F: Evidence-based (S3) guideline on topical corticosteroids in pregnancy. Br J Dermatol 2011;165:943–952.

25 Chi CC, Wang WH, Wojnarowska F, Kirtschig G, Davies E, Bennett C: Safety of topical corticosteroids in pregnancy. Cochrane Database Syst Rev 2015;10:CD007346.

26 Ambros-Rudolph CM: Dermatoses of pregnancy – clues to diagnosis, fetal risk and therapy. Ann Dermatol 2011;23:265–275.

27 Gilboa SM, Strickland MJ, Olshan AF, Werler MM, Correa A; National Birth Defects Prevention Study: Use of antihistamine medications during early pregnancy and isolated main malformations. Birth Defects Res A Clin Teratol 2009;85:137–150.

28 Serreau R, Komiha M, Blanc F, Guillot F, Jacqz-aigrain E: Neonatal seizures associated with maternal hydroxyzine hydrochloride in late pregnancy. Reprod Toxicol 2005;20:573–574.

29 Lucero ML, Arteche JK, Sommer EW, Casadesus A: Preclinical toxicity profile of oral bilastine. Drug Chem Toxicol 2012;35(suppl 1):25–33.

30 Smedts HPM, De Jonge L, Bandola SJG, Baardman ME, Bakker MK, Stricker BHC, Steegers-Theunissen RPM: Early pregnancy exposure to antihistamines and risk of congenital heart defects results of two case-control studies. Eur J Epidemiol 2014;29:653–661.

31 Weisshaar E, Witteler R, Diepgen TL, Luger TA, Ständer S: Pruritus in der Schwangerschaft. Eine häufige diagnostische und therapeutische Herausforderung. Hautartz 2005;56:48–57.

Dr. Julien Lambert
Department of Dermatology, University Hospital of Antwerp
Wilrijkstraat 10
BE–2650 Edegem (Belgium)
E-Mail Julien.Lambert@uza.be

Szepietowski JC, Weisshaar E (eds): Itch – Management in Clinical Practice.
Curr Probl Dermatol. Basel, Karger, 2016, vol 50, pp 173–191 (DOI: 10.1159/000446090)

Itch Management in Childhood

Regina Fölster-Holst

Klinik für Dermatologie, Venerologie und Allergologie, Universitätsklinikum Schleswig-Holstein, Kiel, Germany

Abstract

Itch in children is a very common symptom and is mainly related to a skin disease rather than an underlying systemic disorder. The most common dermatoses include atopic dermatitis, contact dermatitis, insect bites, scabies, and pediculosis capitis. There are specific diagnostic patterns which require the evaluation of a careful history and dermatological examination. For dermatological treatment, we have to consider that children, especially infants, show differences in physiology and pathophysiology, and also in pharmacokinetics and pharmacodynamics compared with adults.　　© 2016 S. Karger AG, Basel

usually included case reports. Pruritus in childhood is mainly associated with dermatoses. Systemic diseases and drug reactions are rare compared with adults. Itchy dermatoses in childhood include eczematous diseases (especially atopic dermatitis), exanthemas, infestations/infections, urticaria/mastocytosis, autoimmune diseases, as well as genodermatoses. For dermatologic treatment (topical and systemic), we have to consider special features in childhood regarding physiology and pathophysiology, and also pharmacokinetics and pharmacodynamics, which differ from those of adults.

Itch (pruritus) is a common symptom in children and therefore it is surprising that there are no data on the prevalence of itch in childhood regarding the general population. After searching for 'itch and children' and 'pruritus and children' in PubMed (up to March 9, 2016) there were 2,629 and 2,136 publications, respectively, but in the majority they were related to specific diseases and

Special Features of Skin Physiology, Pathophysiology, and Skin Care of Early Childhood That Should Be Considered in Treatment

We have to consider special features regarding skin physiology and pathophysiology in childhood, mainly in young infants. The high ratio of

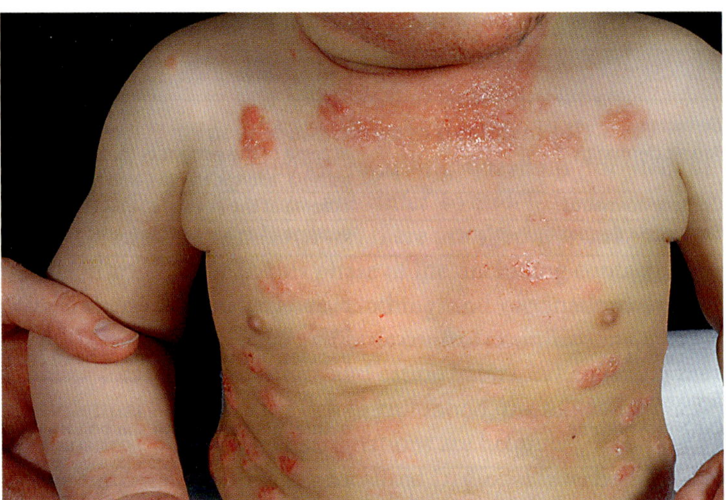

Fig. 1. Nummular form of atopic dermatitis, extreme exudative.

itching. This is associated with disruption of sleep and concentration as well as social stigmatization [11]. During the first days of life, pruritus is sometimes difficult to recognize. Compared with older children and adults, these young infants show different predilection sites and morphology. First, the head and the face are affected followed by the extensor of the extremities [4]. These lesions are very exudative with prominent erythema, papules, pustules, crusts, and oozing.

The typical lichenifications in the folds of the extremities, which are probably related to permanent scratching are seen in later childhood. A very special form in childhood is nummular dermatitis, which may be very exudative (fig. 1) and is seen not only at the extremities but also on the trunk compared to adults (lower limbs are the predilection sites). Many children show a very early onset and atopic dermatitis may manifest as an erythroderma with fine scaling. In these cases, various differential diagnoses should be considered (table 1). It is recommended to cut some hair (scalp hair or eye lashes or eye brows) from these neonates for the microscopic analysis of the hair shaft to exclude Netherton syndrome with the pathognomonic feature of trichorrhexis invagi-

nata (bamboo hair). The diagnosis can be verified by molecular analysis which show the mutation of *SPINK 5* gene coding for LEKTI, a serine protease inhibitor [12]. Netherton syndrome shares many symptoms of atopic dermatitis and other atopic diseases including excessive pruritus [4, 13]. This is also the case for the generalized peeling skin syndrome (fig. 2) related to mutations in the *CDSN* gene. This leads to complete loss of corneodesmosin, resulting in severe epidermal barrier defect. Clinically, erythroderma, generalized desquamation, and unendurable itch are the typical features [14].

Another eczematous disease is the infantile seborrheic dermatitis, which is like atopic dermatitis common in early infancy. The itch is only mild or absent and compared with atopic dermatitis the disease shows the predilection site of the diaper area. This is typically spared in atopic dermatitis due to hyperhydration and occlusive conditions of the diaper. There are a lot of other differential diagnoses [15] including further inflammatory skin diseases such as psoriasis and immunodeficiency disorders like Omenn syndrome and Wiskott-Aldrich syndrome, malignancies such as Langerhans cell histiocytosis and infestations like scabies. All

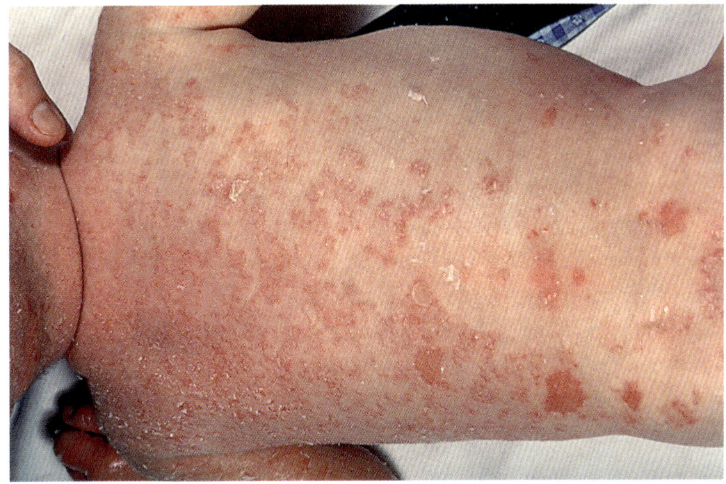

Fig. 2. Generalized peeling skin syndrome.

these differential diagnoses require different therapeutic measurements.

The most important therapeutic measurement in patients with atopic dermatitis is the regularly use of emollients to repair the defective epidermal barrier [16]. This may prevent re-exacerbation of the disease and provide a steroid-sparing effect [17, 18]. It also helps to reduce the itch sensation [19].

In addition to the use of moisturizers, topical anti-inflammatory drugs (topical corticosteroids and calcineurin inhibitors) are components of the standard therapy of patients with atopic dermatitis. They are used both for reactive and proactive therapy to control skin inflammation. This has also been well documented for children [20].

Although topical corticosteroids are still the therapy of choice [21], calcineurin inhibitors are indicated for the management of atopic dermatitis in children. They are recommended for the use in sensitive areas like face, folds, and genitoanal areas, and they provide antipruritic properties [22]. In addition, they are indicated in cases with intolerance against corticosteroids and thus can spare corticosteroid use. Recently, it was once again highlighted that calcineurin inhibitors are safe, also for treatment in children. Even though they are not licensed in many countries, including Germany, before the second year of life, there are many studies that have shown its effectiveness and safety in the infantile stage [23, 24].

If patients do not respond to topical therapy despite considering the trigger factors, systemic therapy is indicated. Cyclosporine (licensed from 16 years on) is the only on-label-used drug in Germany; mycophenolate mofetil, methotrexate, and azathioprine are off-label-used drugs. All of them have antipruritic properties.

Recently, a Canadian group [25] pointed out the excellent antipruritic effect of the combination of clonidine (adrenergic agonist) and trimeprazine (phenothiazine) in a 6-year-old boy with severe atopic dermatitis and refractory pruritus. There are other interesting antipruritic drugs also in development. Draelos et al. [11] showed the positive effect of the topical phosphodiesterase-4 inhibitor crisaborole in children and adolescents with mild-to-moderate atopic dermatitis based on data from four studies. A 4-point rating was used to assess the pruritus severity. The therapy resulted in statistically significant reductions in pruritus severity measured at days 8 and 29. Furthermore, there are many new drugs, especially biologics, in the phase of clinical trials [26]. In addition to the severity score, the pruritus severity will also be assessed. Adult studies will be followed by child studies; for example, studies with the interleukin (IL)-4/IL-13-receptor-α dupilumab are already underway in children [27].

There are many known factors that trigger atopic dermatitis, which is associated with pruritus. One of these factors is contact allergens. De Waard-van der Spek and Oranje [28] showed that 55% children with positive reactions to one or more contact allergen suffered from atopic dermatitis. They recommend that there is an indication for patch testing in children with atopic dermatitis, especially in recalcitrant cases. Other authors also raise the diagnostic significance of patch tests in refractory forms of atopic dermatitis [29].

Contact Dermatitis
Allergic contact dermatitis in children is more frequent than was previously thought, even in very young children [30]. The evaluation of contact sensitization in 321 children younger than 3 years of age with suspected allergic contact dermatitis were patch tested from 2002 to 2008. The most common positive reactions were to metals, cocamidopropyl betaine, neomycin, and methylchloroisothiazolinone/methylisothiazolinone. There was no difference in the prevalence of contact sensitization between children with and without atopic dermatitis.

Mainly in childhood we have to consider the following sources for possible allergic or irritative toxic contact dermatitis: temporary henna tattoos and hair dye (common trigger: paraphenylenediamine, paratoluenediamine), game consoles (most common trigger: rubber components), shin pads and bandages (common trigger: rubber components, welding, friction), mobile phones and tablets (most common trigger: nickel), and cosmetics (common triggers: fragrances, preservatives such as methylisothiazolinone, natural cosmetics) [31].

Exanthemas

Mainly in early infancy there are extremely itchy exanthemas of unknown causes. These include infantile eosinophilic pustular folliculitis and infantile acropustulosis (table 2).

Infantile Eosinophilic Pustular Folliculitis
Infantile eosinophilic pustular folliculitis is a typical but rare rash occurring in infancy [32]. The predilection site is the scalp with the development of extremely itchy vesiculopustular lesions. A characteristic finding is a chronic relapsing course, which may persist for up to 3 years. In this age we have to consider differential diagnoses, which also go along with itchy vesiculopustular rashes. Of these, infantile scabies is common and involves the scalp at this early age compared to older children and adults. Other differential diagnoses are very rare and include infantile acropustulosis (see below), incontinentia pigmenti (arranged along the Blaschko lines, usually not itchy), and Langerhans cell histiocytosis, which requires a biopsy for histological/immunohistochemical analysis [33]. Whether the infantile eosinophilic pustular folliculitis is a variant of the classic eosinophilic pustular folliculitis of Ofuji [34] in adults remains controversial. Special forms of eosinophilic pustular folliculitis are due to AIDS, drugs, silicone injections, and leukemia [35]. They are seen more in adults than in children [35].

The unendurable itch is extremely stressful. The therapy of choice is the combination of topical corticosteroids and antihistamines [36]. Alternative topical calcineurin inhibitors may be used [37, 38].

Infantile Acropustulosis
Infantile acropustulosis occurs mainly in older infants [39] and more in black than in white patients [40]. Like infantile eosinophilic pustular folliculitis, it is rare and shows a recurrent course of an intensely pruritic vesiculopustular rash. However, it is not follicular oriented and is typi-

Table 2. Itchy exanthematous diseases (selection)

Diseases	Clinical pattern	Age of onset
Exanthemas in early childhood		
Infantile eosinophilic pustular folliculitis	chronic relapsing course of vesiculopustular lesions on the scalp	infancy
Infantile acropustulosis	chronic relapsing course of vesiculopustular lesions on hands and feet	infancy
Exanthema due to direct viral effect		
Varicella	polymorphous exanthema, secondary impetiginization, involvement of scalp and oral mucous membranes	mainly in infancy
Paraviral exanthemas		
Papular purpuric gloves and socks syndrome	edema and erythema with petechiae on hands and feet, enanthem	adolescents and young adults
Pityriasis rosea	primary medallion, exanthema along the Langer lines, collarette scaling of all lesions	adolescents
Gianotti-Crosti syndrome	monomorphic papules or papulovesicles on the cheeks, extremities, and buttocks	infants and preschoolers

cally located on the hands and feet (fig. 3). For some authors the rash is due to a persistent hypersensitivity of the immune system in infants who were successfully treated for scabies infection [40–43]. However, there is no consensus regarding this hypothesis. The sterile subcorneal pustules contain neutrophilic and eosinophilic granulocytes. Differential diagnoses include scabies, infections such as impetigo, candidiasis, and neonatal rash of transient neonatal pustular melanosis [44]. In addition, the local form of DIRA (deficiency of the IL-1-receptor antagonist) should be considered when there are sterile pustules on the hands and feet [45].

The children with infantile acropustulosis are very restless due to the extreme itch and require adequate therapy. Topical corticosteroids provide an anti-inflammatory effect and are also antipruritic. If there is no response, it can be combined with antihistamines. Some rare cases require systemic treatment. The therapy of choice is dapsone, which reduces itch, but there are rare side effects such as hemolytic anemia and methemoglobinemia.

Exanthemas in general are very common in childhood and mainly related to virus infections. Pathogenetically, we have to differentiate between exanthemas, which are related to direct viral effect (e.g. varicella) and those related to the response of the immune system to a viral infection (e.g. Gianotti-Crosti syndrome). The latter is known as paraviral exanthemas [46].

Varicella (Exanthema due to the Direct Effect of Varicella Zoster Virus with the Skin and Mucous Membranes)

Varicella (chickenpox) is the initial manifestation of the varicella zoster virus (HHV-3) and occurs many in childhood; however, there has been a shift to adolescents and young adults. The pruritic polymorphous exanthema (eruption of new effloresces, from the maculae to papules, papulovesicles, vesicles, pustules, and crusts) spreads from the hairline to the caudal and lower extremities and typically involves the scalp and oral mucosa. The involvement of the scalp and the oral mucous membranes is a characteristic finding. The disease is accompanied by elevated temperature and mild fatigue.

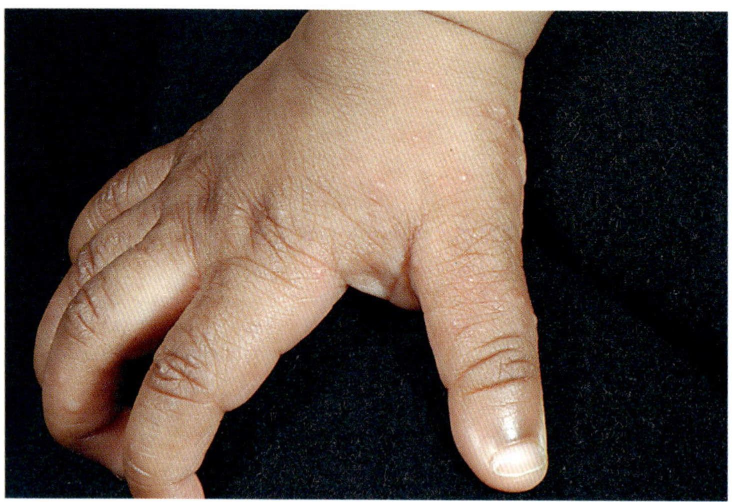

Fig. 3. Infantile acropustulosis with multiple vesiculopustules.

Scratching promotes secondary infections with *Streptococcus pyogenes* and *Staphylococcus aureus*. Complications include local and systemic infections and neurologic involvement.

Therapeutically it is very important to prevent the complication of secondary infections. In particular, this means relieving the itch by symptomatic therapy using drying agents such as tanning agents or lotio alba/calamine lotion in combination with antihistamines. In severe cases, especially in immunocompromised children, antiviral drugs like acyclovir, alternative famciclovir, and valacyclovir can be used [47].

Papular-Purpuric Gloves and Socks Syndrome (Paraviral Exanthema)

Papular-purpuric gloves and socks syndrome is mainly related to parvovirus B, less often to other viruses such as cytomegalovirus, coxsackie B6 virus, and measles viruses [48]. The exanthema occurs mainly in adolescents and young adults and is characterized by edema and erythema of the hands and feet, which may present very purpuric and petechial. The lesions are accompanied by intense itch and burn. In addition, many patients show an enanthem with petechiae and erosions. Fever and arthralgia are often associated with it. The disease is self-limiting and requires only symptomatic therapy.

Pityriasis Rosea (Paraviral Exanthema)

Pityriasis rosea is a common exanthema and affects mainly adolescents. The disease is mainly associated with human herpes viruses 6 and 7 [49]. The clinic shows a typical pattern: primary medallion (herald patch), which is followed by an exanthema that is seen along the lines of skin creases (Langer lines). Primary and secondary lesions present as ovular red-brownish plaques with typical collarette scaling (fig. 4). The exanthema is predominantly located on the trunk and the proximal extremities. Patients show an extremely irritable skin, which is especially apparent after bathing, and it can lead to eczema and severe pruritus [50]. Therefore, skin irritation such as vigorous washing and using too much soap should be avoided. If patients follow the recommendation, many of them will not need a specific therapy. In severe cases there are different therapy options: combination of mild topical glucocorticoids and low-dose UVB radiation (for patients aged 12 years and older) [50], erythromycin [51], and acyclovir [52].

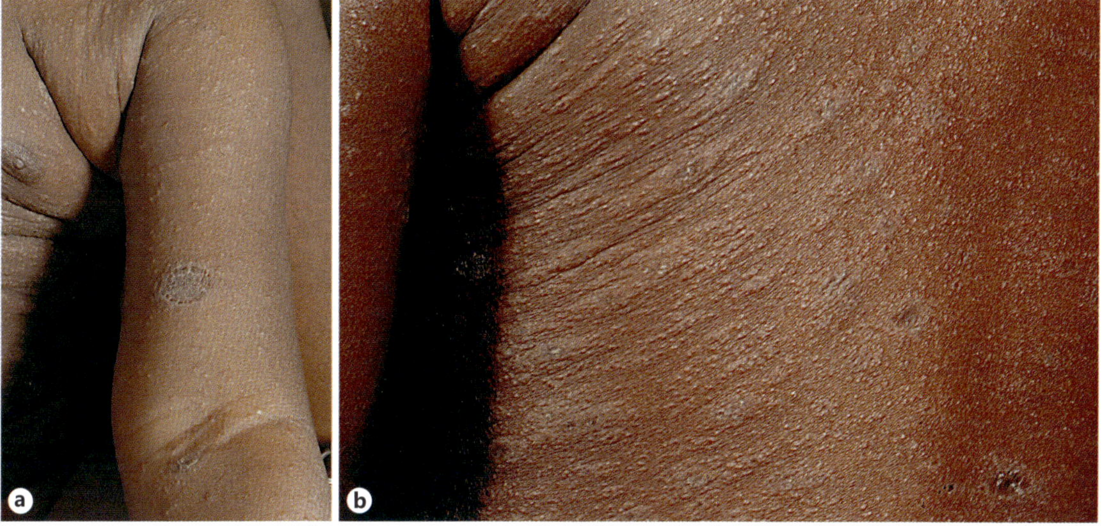

Fig. 4. Pityriasis rosea: primary medallion (**a**) and exanthema along Langer lines (**b**).

Gianotti-Crosti Syndrome (Paraviral Exanthema)

Gianotti-Crosti syndrome is a distinct exanthema of infants, which is mainly associated with Epstein-Barr virus. At the predilection sites of cheeks, extremities and buttocks (fig. 5) the children present a monomorphic exanthema, which consist of small papules or papulovesicles. The exanthema may be accompanied by pruritus. In general, emollients should be used. In cases of severe pruritus sedative systemic histamine antagonist might be considered [53]. In refractory cases ribavirin may be an option [54].

Infestations

Scabies

Scabies is a very common infestation in every age group. After a sensitization phase of 2–3 weeks, in primary infestation skin lesions will be seen at the predilection sites of the flexural surface of the wrist, axillary folds, and interdigital webs of the hands. They consist of papules and nodules and are related to a cellular immune response to *Sarcoptes scabiei* mites, eggs, and feces. The immune response is also the cause of pruritus that is most severe at night [55]. Cutaneous burrows which are dug by the female mites in the stratum corneum are pathognomonic. Patients in early infancy show involvement of the face and head compared to older children and adults. Furthermore, infants have more of a tendency to develop polymorphic eczematous lesions with vesicles, papules, pustules, and scaling [56]. In addition, young infants typically present pustules in the plantar region. The clinical diagnosis of scabies can be verified by microscopic and/or dermoscopic examination of mites, eggs, and/or burrows. While the most important differential diagnoses is atopic dermatitis (also polymorphic eczematous lesions), others include infantile acropustulosis, infantile eosinophilic follicular pustulosis, and Langerhans cell histiocytosis. 5% permethrin is the standard therapy. After a successful therapy some patients present with very itchy reddish-brown papules/nodules, which are free of scabies mites. These are postscabious

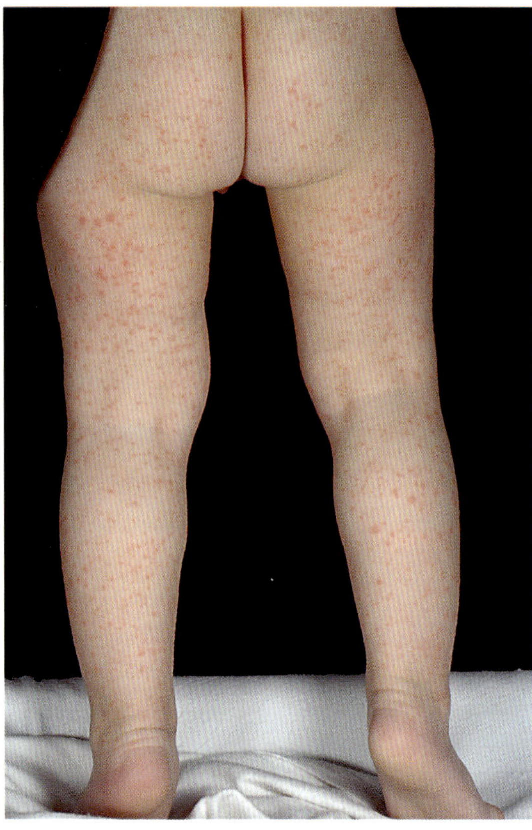

Fig. 5. Gianotti-Crosti syndrome, monomorphic aspect of papulovesicles.

granulomas, which respond to mild topical corticosteroids; in some cases emollients are sufficient.

Pediculosis Capitis

Pediculosis capitis, due to an infestation with *Pediculus humanus capitis,* is the most common form of lice and affects mainly school children. The transmission occurs from head to head; transmission from other subjects as combs, brushes or towels is rare. Pruritus is the most common clinical symptom, which is due to a cellular immune reaction to proteins of the saliva of the louse. Patients respond with scratching, which increases the risk of bacterial infec-

tion with *Staphylococcus aureus* or *Streptococcus pyogenes.* This may result in impetiginization and cervical and suboccipital lymphadenopathy [57]. The therapy of choice is topical pyrethroids like permethrin or silicone oil. Recently, there were studies published which showed resistance of head lice to pyrethroids in Europe [58]. However, the molecular resistance (mutation of gene in the α-subunit of the voltage-gated sodium channel, the so-called knockdown resistance (kdr)-like gene) did not correlate with failure using permethrin or pyrethrin in the treatment of pediculosis capitis in German children [58]. However, the possibility of resistance should be kept in mind.

Cercarial Dermatitis

Cercarial dermatitis ('swimmer's itch') is a cutaneous hypersensitivity reaction to nonhuman *Schistosoma* parasites, which penetrate the skin. This happens while swimming or wading in lakes or ponds and is facilitated by the release of proteolytic enzymes [59]. The most relevant parasites are the *Trichobilharzia* species [60]. The actual hosts are water birds, which release along with their feces the eggs of the parasites into the water. The larvae (miracidiae) hatch from the eggs and penetrate aquatic snails (intermediate hosts). After development to cercariae they leave the snail and search for their actual hosts again. However, they infest erroneously humans, which are final hosts. Cercariae die in our stratum corneum because they are not able to reach the blood vessels.

On exposed skin areas patients develop very itchy papules and papulovesicles, which occur some hours after the contact with the cercariae (fig. 6). Antihistamines and topical corticosteroids are helpful to relieve itch.

There are many other itchy dermatoses to be considered: insect bites, human schistosomiasis (especially in Africa, Asia, and South America), contact dermatitis (especially from poison ivy), and sea bather's eruption.

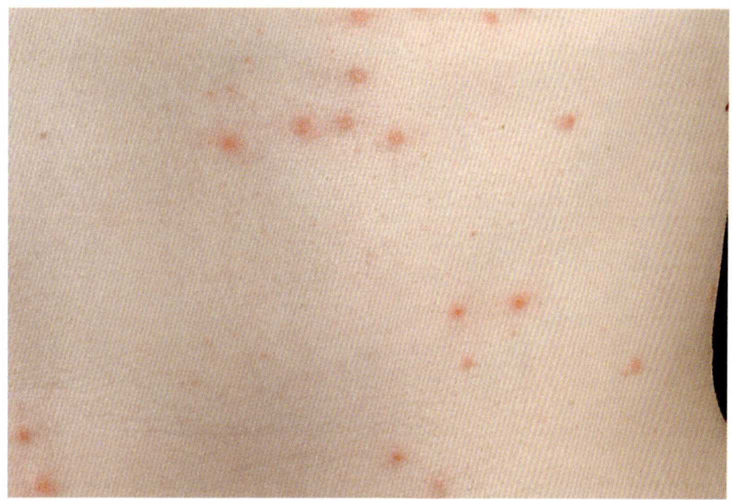

Fig. 6. Cercarial dermatitis: dermatitis with multiple eroded papulovesicles.

The Itchy Diaper Area in Childhood

Many dermatoses in the diaper area are accompanied by itch. These include inflammatory dermatoses (e.g. psoriasis), infections/parasitoses (e.g. bullous impetigo, candidiasis), metabolic disorders (e.g. acrodermatitis enteropathica), autoimmune diseases (e.g. lichen sclerosus), and neoplasia (e.g. Langerhans cell histiocytosis). These are listed in table 3. The following section focuses on lichen sclerosus.

Genital Lichen Sclerosus
Genital lichen sclerosus is an uncommon autoimmune disease which occurs mainly in adult women. Premenarchal girls are affected to a lesser extent, and lichen sclerosus is also known in boys associated with acquired phimosis [61]. The hallmark of the dermatosis is the unbearable itching resulting in a huge impact on quality of life [62]. The dermatosis shows a typical 'figure 8 pattern' involving the area around the vulva and the anus [63]. Morphologically porcelain white papules and plaques are prominent. The skin of lichen sclerosus is extremely fragile, with bleeding and fissures caused by rubbing or scratching [62]. The

hemorrhagic skin lesions may mimic sexual abuse. Further differential diagnoses include infections and eczema (contact eczema, atopic dermatitis) [63] (table 1).

The disease is poorly recognized and misdiagnosed by clinicians [64]. On average a year passes before the correct diagnosis is made, with the children usually receiving antimycotic drugs during this time [63].There is evidence that lichen sclerosus does not resolve after puberty [64]. A retrospective chart review and follow-up telephone interview [65] were done for 36 premenarchal girls (mean age at diagnosis 7 years) diagnosed with lichen sclerosus from 1989 to 2010. The mean duration of follow-up was 5.3 years. Thirty-three girls developed an improvement of their symptoms within an average of 14 weeks (range: 2 weeks to 2 years) by using topical corticosteroids. While 83% showed a remission after initial treatment, 16 patients experienced relapses requiring further therapy. It is recommended to follow the children at least until puberty [66]. Lichen sclerosus et atrophicus should be treated with potent corticosteroids or calcineurin inhibitors [63]. The benefits include relief of pruritus, pain, and inflammation [67]. Sequelae such as

Table 3. Itchy diaper area and their causes (selection)

Diseases	Clinical pattern	Age of onset
Inflammatory diseases		
Psoriasis	erythema and scaling on the scalp and large body folds	any age
Atopic dermatitis	eczema on scalp, face, extremities, atopy; diaper area often free of lesions; in later childhood eczema possible in the genitoanal area	mainly during the first year of life
Autoimmune diseases		
Lichen sclerosis (genital)	'figure 8 pattern' in girls with porcelain white papules and plaques	premenarchal girls, less frequent in preschool boys; associated with phimosis
Linear IgA dermatosis	bullae-forming annular or rosette-like lesions on legs, feet, trunk	preschoolers
Epidermolysis bullosa	dependent on the form: erosions, bullae, scars triggered by trauma	dependent on the form: at birth or in early childhood
Infections and infestations		
Candidiasis	intertrigo and satellite papulopustules	infants, premenarchal and adolescent females (vulvovaginitis)
Perianal streptococcal (or staphylococcal) dermatitis	erythema perianal with wet surface, perianal and rectal itching, painful defecation	prepubertal children
Scabies	burrows, disseminated eczema including face and head, pustules plantar	anytime
Metabolic disorder		
Acrodermatitis enteropathica	triad of eczematous lesions (periorificial, fingers and toes), alopecia, and diarrhea	2 weeks after weaning
Neoplasia		
Langerhans cell histiocytosis	brownish papules, papulovesicles, impetigo-like lesions of the axillae and groin, seborrheic lesions on the scalp	at birth or during the first 2 years

vulvar stenosis or squamous cell carcinoma are very rare in childhood [63].

Bullous and Urticarial Dermatoses

Epidermolysis bullosa
Epidermolysis bullosa, a heterogenous group of bullous dermatoses triggered by trauma, is associated with severe pruritus. There are the acquired and the hereditary form, with the latter divided into the scarring (dystrophic) and nonscarring forms (intraepidermal and junctional separation). These can be defined on the basis of clinical features, the mode of inheritance, histopathology, and molecular biology measurements. The therapy is symptomatic with the aim to prevent infections.

Some publications focus on pruritus in patients with epidermolysis bullosa. The most important messages, based on clinical studies, are [68]:

1 Pruritus is a common and burdensome symptom in patients with epidermolysis bullosa

2 The average daily frequency of pruritus increase with self-reported epidermolysis bullosa severity
3 Pruritus is most frequent at bedtime and interferes with sleep
4 Factors that aggravate pruritus include healing wounds, dry skin, infected wounds, stress, heat, dryness, and humidity

The management of patients with epidermolysis bullosa requires interdisciplinary cooperation (ophthalmologists, gastroenterologists, otolaryngologists, plastic surgeons, dentists, and physical therapists) to address extracutaneous involvement.

Prevention measurements include avoidance of trauma and infections of the skin and mucous membranes as well as using appropriate clothing and wound dressings that provide sufficient hydration and allow for a painless changes of bandages. In addition, educational programs should be included in the therapeutic management to give patients instructions on how to develop better self-control in tolerating pruritus [68].

Recently it was shown that the use of saltwater baths can lead to significant improvement in quality of life [69]. After starting saltwater baths, patients reported a significant reduction in pain, pain medication use, skin odor, and skin discharge by using a standardized questionnaire. Another study [70] focused on the evaluation of different treatment modalities using a questionnaire. The questions relate to bathing products, moisturizers, topical products, oral medications, dressings, and alternative therapies. In order of the frequency, greasy ointments, lotions, creams, and oral hydroxyzine (39.0%) were the most frequently used treatments for pruritus. The most effective were topical corticosteroids, oral hydroxyzine, topical diphenhydramine, and vaporizing rub (menthol, camphor, eucalyptus). It was noticed that systemic opioids, adherent bandages, and bleach baths slightly increased pruritus.

Mastocytosis
Mastocytosis (accumulation of mast cells) in pediatric patients present mainly as mastocytoma and urticarial pigmentosa (fig. 7). The other forms (bullous, diffuse) including the involvement of extracutaneous organ systems like gastrointestinal tract, skeletal, and bone marrow are rare compared to adults [71]. The diagnosis is made by morphology and positive Darier sign. In particular infants tend to develop strong reactions by the mechanical irritation of the Darier sign, which can lead not only to the formation of urticae and bullae, but also to flush. Besides the mechanical trigger, there are extreme temperature (heat, cold), exercise, foods, drugs, and venoms that may lead to mast cell degranulation. Compared with adults, children show a very good prognosis and remission is very common. Therapy is symptomatic, including the avoidance of trigger factors and administration of type 1 antihistamines.

There is a useful scoring system (SCORMA) that correlates with serum tryptase level and includes surface area involvement and intensity of the lesions as well as subjective symptoms as pruritus [72, 73].

Urticaria
Urticaria is defined as the sudden appearance of very itchy wheals, which mainly last for a few hours up to 24 h. Based on duration and etiology, urticaria is classified into the following types: spontaneous acute urticaria, spontaneous chronic urticaria, physical urticaria, and other urticaria types [74, 75]. These types require different management.

The disease is very common in childhood and presents most often as an acute urticaria (less than 6 weeks' duration), which is frequently related to viral infections. In a study of 54 children with urticaria, Sackesen et al. [76] found that 68.5% suffered from the acute form. In around half of these patients infection was the cause (48.6%), while physical factors were the leading cause in the group of chronic urticaria (52.94%).

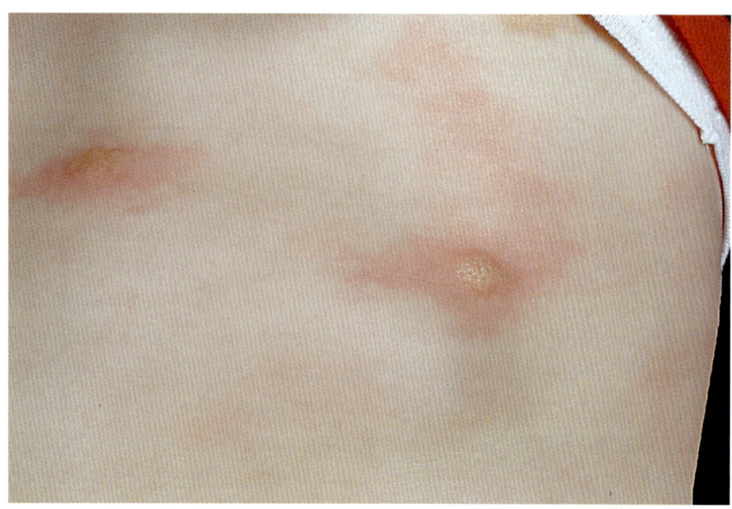

Fig. 7. Mastocytoma: positive Darier sign.

The authors recommend the diagnostic measurements of certain infectious agents in addition to a detailed history. The identification rate of a cause in children with chronic urticarial is documented with 20–50% [77]. However, in 30–47% of these children the urticaria is related to an autoreactive form (verified by the positive autologous serum skin test) which is caused by IgG antibodies against the high-affinity IgE receptor (FcεRIα) [78].

Second-generation antihistamines are the mainstay of pharmacological treatment [75, 77]. Omalizumab is recommended in refractory cases, especially in children with autoreactive chronic urticaria [79].

Tumors as the Cause of Localized Itch

Localized pruritus may be due to tumors of the nervous system. Soltani-Arabshahi et al. [80] recommend neurologic examination and neuroimaging in children with persistent localized pruritus in the absence of any other causes of pruritus. The results of their literature research showed that astrocytoma and glioma are the most common intramedullary neoplasms associated with pruritus in the pediatric population. In addition, they noted 6 articles reported children suffering from persistent localized pruritus in the head and neck or upper extremities due to brainstem or spinal cord tumors [80]. Five of these children showed café-au-lait macules associated with neurofibromatosis. The next section focuses on neurofibromatosis 1, which is associated with itchy dermal neurofibromas most likely due to the presence of mast cells. These tumors do not appear before puberty.

Neurofibromatosis 1 (von Recklinghausen Disease)

Neurofibromatosis 1 is an autosomal dominant disease due to a mutation in the *NF1* tumor suppressor gene (17q11.2) encoding a Ras-GTPase-activating protein neurofibromin, which is expressed throughout the nervous system [81]. The inactivation of the tumor suppressor gene is associated with a high risk for certain types of tumors arising from embryonic neural crest. The diagnosis of NF1 is made when there are at least 2 of 7 clinical criteria: ≥6 café-au-lait macules >0.5 cm, axillary and inguinal freckling, ≥2 neurofibromas or 1 plexiform neurofibroma, ≥2 Lisch nodules, optic glioma, a characteristic

Table 4. Topical antipruritic therapy in childhood (based on Lucas et al. [1] and Eichenfield [85])

Active substance/approval by age	Dosage	Indication (selection)	Side effects/particularities
Urea pura 5 – 10%/not for infants	2–3 times a day	Eczematous diseases Ichthyoses Psoriasis vulgaris	In infancy and acute lesions 'stinging effect'
Calcineurin inhibitors/ licensed from 2 years on			
Pimecrolimus	2 times a day	Mild to moderate atopic dermatitis	Transient burning at the site of application/requires sun protection
Tacrolimus	2 times a day	Moderate to severe atopic dermatitis	
		Off-label use of both in Lichen sclerosus	
Corticosteroids			
Methylprednisolonaceponate/ licensed from 3 years on	Once (if needed twice) a day	Exacerbation of atopic dermatitis, other inflammatory dermatoses	If used properly no side effects/no applying intertriginous
Mometasonfuroate/licensed from 2 years on	Once (if needed twice) a day	Exacerbation of atopic dermatitis, other inflammatory dermatoses	If used properly no side effects/no applying intertriginous
Prednicarbate/in infancy only after careful consideration	Once (if needed twice) a day	Exacerbation of atopic dermatitis, other inflammatory dermatoses	If used properly no side effects/no applying intertriginous
Antiparasitic drugs			
Benzylbenzoate 10%/not for preterms	Once a day for 3 days, wash off on day 4	Scabies	Irritation of skin and mucous membranes/sensitization possible, Gasping syndrome in preterms
Crotamiton/no age limit	Once a day for 3–5 days	Scabies	Effectiveness lower than other scabicides
Permethrin 5%/no age limit	Scabies: once a day for 8 h pediculosis capitis: once after washing hairs for 30–45 min	Scabies Pediculosis capitis	Visit of institutions (kindergarten, school) 1 day after lege artis guided therapy
Dimeticone	Different products have different times for leave on, see instructions for use	Pediculosis capitis	Visit of institutions (kindergarten, school) 1 day after lege artis guided therapy

bone lesion (pseudarthrosis or sphenoid dysplasia), or a first-degree family relative with NF1 [82].

Approximately every 5th patient suffers from pruritus [83]. Brenaut et al. [81] evaluated the characteristics of pruritus in 40 patients (adults) with NF1 by using a questionnaire. The most important findings were that one third of the patients suffer from pruritus daily, the sensation tends to appear more frequently in the evening, only 5 patients were treated for their pruritus (emollients, antihistamine), the intensity of pruritus was assessed by a visual analogic scale (0–10): worst (6.7/10), mild (1/10), with a mean intensity of pruritus of 3.8/10. 23.5% and 17.6% of the patients also suffered from pain and heat sensation, respectively. For half of the patients, pruritus was localized on neurofibromas.

In a large cohort of adult and pediatric patients the presence of facial plexiform neurofibromas and pruritus in children was significantly associated with mortality in univariate analysis [83]. The authors recommend a close follow-up for patients presenting with subcutaneous neurofibromas.

Systemic Diseases and Drugs

Pruritus related to systemic diseases or adverse events to drugs are uncommon in childhood compared with adults. However, they occur and

Table 5. Systemic antipruritic therapy in childhood (based on Lucas et al. [1], Cuvillo [86], and Fitzsimons [87])

Active substance/approval by age	Dosage	Indication (selection)	(Possible) side effects/particularities
H₁-Antihistamines			
Acrivastine/12–18 years	12–18 years: 8 mg 3×/day	Urticaria	The most common side effects of the listed H_1-antihistamines (all of the second generation): fatigue, dizziness, dry mouth, headache/no cardiovascular side effects
Ceterizine/1–18 years	1–2 years: 250 µg/kg 2×/day 2–6 years: 2.5 mg/kg 2×/day 6–12 years: 5 mg/kg 2×/day 12–18 years: 10 mg/kg 1×/day	Urticaria, atopic dermatitis, infantile acropustulosis	
Desloratidine/1–18 years	1–6 years: 1.25 mg 1×/day 6–12 years: 2.5 mg 1×/day 12–18 years: 5 mg 1×/day	Urticaria	
Fexofenadine/6–18 years	6–12 years: 30 mg 2×/day 6–18 years: 120 mg 1×/day	Urticaria	
Levozetericine Liquid: 2–18 years Tablets: 6–18 years	2–6 years: 1.25 mg 2×/day 6–18 years: 5 mg 1×/day	Urticaria	
Loratidine/2–18 years	2–12 years <30 kg: 5 mg 1×/day >30 mg: 10 mg 1×/day 12–18 years: 10 mg 1×/day	Urticaria	
Cyclosporine (microemulsion)/from 16 years	3–5 mg/kg/day	Atopic dermatitis, refractory urticaria	Most common in children: gastrointestinal symptoms and headache; in addition: hypertension, nephrotoxicity, gingiva hyperplasia, hypertrichosis, myalgia, hyperlipidemia/interaction with other drugs
Dapsone (sulfones)/not approved for children, recommendation: do not use in early infancy	0.5 mg/kg/day	Infantile acropustulosis that does not respond to the standard therapy of topical corticosteroids and H_1-antihistamines, autoimmune diseases	Headache, hemolytic anemia, methemoglobinemia, nausea, hypersensitivity reactions/baseline blood counts and glucose-6-phosphate dehydrogenase
Ivermectin (antiparasitic drug)	Single dose of 150–200 µg/kg, repeat after 8–10 days	In refractory cases of parasitoses (amongst others, pediculosis capitis, scabies)	Fever, pruritus, skin rash; interaction with other drugs

involve the same organ systems like adults. The difference is that these diseases are typical childhood disorders which mainly include genodermatoses [84]. Weisshaar et al. [84] provide an overview of the systemic diseases in childhood associated with pruritus.

The following questions are helpful making the correct diagnosis:

- Is there a history of any systemic disease?

- Are genetic diseases and/or diseases in the family known which are associated with liver diseases such as biliary atresia or hypoplasia, the Alagille syndrome (absence of interlobular bile ducts), choledochal cysts, and familial hyperbilirubinemia syndrome, such as Byler disease (intrahepatic cholestasis) and hemolytic icterus [84]?

- Does the child suffer from polycystic kidney disease?
- Is the serum iron level in the normal range?
- Does the child show lymphadenopathy (e.g. Hodgkin's disease)?
- Is the blood count in normal range (i.e. leukemia or polycythemia vera)?
- Are there signs of AIDS such as recurrent viral (mainly molluscum contagiosum), bacterial, and mycotic infections, or seborrheic dermatitis?
- Has the child taken drugs, especially antibiotics, anticonvulsive drugs, nonsteroid antiphlogistics, or morphine?

Table 4 and table 5 provide an overview of the topical and systemic medications most commonly used in childhood.

References

1 Lukas A, Wolf G, Fölster-Holst R: Special features of topical and systemic dermatologic therapy in children (in German). J Dtsch Dermatol Ges 2006;4: 658–678.

2 Stamatas GN, Nikolovski J, Mack MC, Kollias N: Infant skin physiology and development during the first years of life: a review of recent findings based on in vivo studies. Int J Cosmet Sci 2011;33: 17–24.

3 Nikolovski J, Stamatas GN, Kollias N, Wiegand BC: Barrier function and water-holding and transport properties of infant stratum corneum are different from adult and continue to develop through the first year of life. J Invest Dermatol 2008;128:1728–1736.

4 Fölster-Holst R: Management of atopic dermatitis: are there differences between children and adults? J Eur Acad Dermatol Venereol 2014;28(suppl 3):5–8.

5 Fölster-Holst R, Dähnhardt-Pfeiffer S, Dähnhardt D, Proksch E: The role of skin barrier function in atopic dermatitis: an update. Expert Rev Dermatol 2012;7:247–257.

6 Fernandes JD, Machado MC, Oliveira ZN: Children and newborn skin care and prevention. An Bras Dermatol 2011; 86:102–110.

7 Ronayne C, Bray G, Robertson G: The use of aqueous cream to relieve pruritus in patients with liver disease. Br J Nurs 1993;2:527–528.

8 Lodén M: Role of topical emollients and moisturizers in the treatment of dry skin barrier disorders. Am J Clin Dermatol 2003;4:771–788.

9 Fölster-Holst R: Management of atopic dermatitis: are there differences between children and adults? J Eur Acad Dermatol Venereol 2014;28(suppl 3):5–8.

10 Morris V, Murphy L, Rosenberg M, Rosenberg L, Holzer C, Meyer W: Itch Assessment Scale for the Pediatric Burn Survivor. Itch assessment scale for the pediatric burn survivor. J Burn Care Res 2012;33:419–424.

11 Draelos ZD, Stein Gold LF, Murrell DF, Hughes MH, Zane LT: Post hoc analyses of the effect of crisaborole topical ointment, 2% on atopic dermatitis: associated pruritus from phase 1 and 2 clinical studies. J Drugs Dermatol 2016;15:172–176.

12 Raghunath M, Tontsidou L, Oji V, et al: SPINK5 and Netherton syndrome: novel mutations, demonstration of missing LEKTI, and differential expression of transglutaminases. J Invest Dermatol 2004;123:474–483.

13 Fölster-Holst R, Swensson O, Stockfleth E, Mönig H, Mrowietz U, Christophers E: Comèl-Netherton syndrome complicated by papillomatous skin lesions containing human papillomaviruses 51 and 52 and plane warts containing human papillomavirus 16. Br J Dermatol 1999; 140:1139–1143.

14 Oji V, Eckl KM, Aufenvenne K, et al: Loss of corneodesmosin leads to severe skin barrier defect, pruritus, and atopy: unraveling the peeling skin disease. Am J Hum Genet 2010;87:274–281.

15 Jenneck C, Foelster-Holst R, Hagemann T, Novak N: Associated diseases and differential diagnostic considerations in childhood atopic eczema (in German). Hautarzt 2007;58:163–174; quiz 175–176.

16 Fölster-Holst R, Dähnhardt-Pfeiffer S, Dähnhardt D, Proksch E: The role of skin barrier function in atopic dermatitis: an update. Expert Rev Dermatol 2012;7:247–257.

17 Daehnhardt-Pfeiffer S, Surber C, Wilhelm KP, Daehnhardt D, Springmann G, Boettcher M, Foelster-Holst R: Noninvasive stratum corneum sampling and electron microscopical examination of skin barrier integrity: pilot study with a topical glycerin formulation for atopic dermatitis. Skin Pharmacol Physiol 2012;25:155–161.

18 Gahli FE: Improved clinical outcomes with moisturization in dermatologic disease. Cutis 2005;76:13–18.

19 Oszukowska M, Michalak I, Gutfreund K, Bienias W, Matych M, Szewczyk A, Kaszuba A: Role of primary and secondary prevention in atopic dermatitis. Postepy Dermatol Alergol 2015;32:409–420.

20 Werfel T, Heratizadeh A, Aberer W, Ahrens F, Augustin M, Biedermann T, Diepgen T, Fölster-Holst R, Gieler U, Kahle J, Kapp A, Nast A, Nemat K, Ott H, Przybilla B, Roecken M, Schlaeger M, Schmid-Grendelmeier P, Schmitt J, Schwennesen T, Staab D, Worm M: S2k guideline on diagnosis and treatment of atopic dermatitis – short version. J Dtsch Dermatol Ges 2016;14:92–105.

21 Fröschl B, Arts D, Leopold C: Corticosteroid therapy in the treatment of pediatric patients with atopic dermatitis. GMS Health Technol Assess 2007;20; 3:Doc09.

22 Ständer S, Luger TA: Antipruritic effects of pimecrolimus and tacrolimus (in German). Hautarzt 2003;54:413–417.

23 Cury Martins J, Martins C, Aoki V, Gois AF, Ishii HA, da Silva EM: Topical tacrolimus for atopic dermatitis. Cochrane Database Syst Rev 2015;7:CD009864.

24 Sigurgeirsson B, Boznanski A, Todd G, Vertruyen A, Schuttelaar ML, Zhu X, Schauer U, Qaqundah P, Poulin Y, Kristjansson S, von Berg A, Nieto A, Boguniewicz M, Paller AS, Dakovic R, Ring J, Luger T: Safety and efficacy of pimecrolimus in atopic dermatitis: a 5-year randomized trial. Pediatrics 2015;135:597–606.

25 Genois A, Haig M, Des Roches A, Sirard A, Le May S, McCuaig CC: Case report of atopic dermatitis with refractory pruritus markedly improved with the novel use of clonidine and trimeprazine. Pediatr Dermatol 2014;31:76–79.

26 Montes-Torres A, Llamas-Velasco M, Pérez-Plaza A, Solano-López G, Sánchez-Pérez J, Barbarot S: Biological treatments in atopic dermatitis. J Clin Med 2015;4:593–613.

27 Notaro ER, Sidbury R: Systemic agents for severe atopic dermatitis in children. Paediatr Drugs 2015;17:449–457.

28 De Waard-van der Spek FB, Oranje AP: Allergic contact dermatitis: a prospective study and review of the literature patch tests in children with suspected allergic contact dermatitis. Dermatology 2009;218:119–125.

29 Akan A, Toyran M, Vezir E, Azkur D, Kaya A, Erkoçoğlu M, Civelek E, Misirlioğlu ED, Kocabaş CN: The patterns and clinical relevance of contact allergen sensitization in a pediatric population with atopic dermatitis. Turk J Med Sci 2015;45:1207–1213.

30 Belloni Fortina A, Romano I, Peserico A, Eichenfield LF: Contact sensitization in very young children. J Am Acad Dermatol 2011;65:772–779.

31 Fölster-Holst R: Eczematous disorders in adolescence (in German). Hautarzt 2016;67:287–292.

32 Hernández-Martín Á, Nuño-González A, Colmenero I, Torrelo A: Eosinophilic pustular folliculitis of infancy: a series of 15 cases and review of the literature. J Am Acad Dermatol 2013;68:150–155.

33 Fölster-Holst R, Höger P: Pustular diseases of the newborn (in German). J Dtsch Dermatol Ges 2004;2:569–579.

34 Ofuji S, Ogino A, Horio T, Oseko T, Uehara M: Eosinophilic pustular folliculitis. Acta Derm Venereol 1970;50:195–203.

35 Rotoli M, Carlesimo F, Cavalieri S: Eosinophilic pustular folliculitis and Ofuji disease. A case report (in Italian). Recenti Prog Med 1995;86:386–390.

36 Darmstadt GL, Tunnessen WW Jr, Swerer RJ: Eosinophilic pustular folliculitis. Pediatrics 1992;89:1095–1098.

37 Zitelli K, Fernandes N, Adams BB: Eosinophilic folliculitis occurring after stem cell transplant for acute lymphoblastic leukemia: a case report and review. Int J Dermatol 2015;54:785–789.

38 Patel NP, Laguda B, Roberts NM, Francis ND, Agnew K: Treatment of eosinophilic pustulosis of infancy with topical tacrolimus. Br J Dermatol 2012;167:1189–1191.

39 Antaya RJ: Infantile acropustulosis; in Irvine AD, Hoeger PH, Yan AC (eds): Harpers Textbook of Pediatric Dermatology, ed 3. Hoboken, Wiley-Blackwell, 2011, pp 1–4.

40 Laude TA: Skin disorders in black children. Curr Opin Pediatr 1996;8:381–385.

41 Jarratt M, Ramsdell W: Infantile acropustulosis. Arch Dermatol 1979;115:834–836.

42 Prendiville JS: Infantile acropustulosis – how often is it a sequela of scabies? Pediatr Dermatol 1995;12:275–276.

43 Good LM, Good TJ, High WA: Infantile acropustulosis in internationally adopted children. J Am Acad Dermatol 2011;65:763–771.

44 Mazereeuw-Hautier J: Infantile acropustulosis (in French). Presse Med 2004;33:1352–1354.

45 Aksentijevich I, Masters SL, Ferguson PJ, Dancey P, Frenkel J, van Royen-Kerkhoff A, et al: An autoinflammatory disease with deficiency of the interleukin-1-receptor antagonist. N Engl J Med 2009;360:2426–2437.

46 Lipsker D, Saurat JH: A new concept: paraviral eruptions. Dermatology 2005;211:309–311.

47 Paller AS, Mancini AJ: Exanthematous diseases of childhood; in Paller AS, Mancini AJ (eds): Hurwitz Clinical Pediatric Dermatology: A Textbook of Skin Disorders of Childhood and Adolescence. Amsterdam, Elsevier, 2016, p 384.

48 Smith PT, Landry ML, Carey H, Krasnoff J, Cooney E: Papular-purpuric gloves and socks syndrome associated with acute parvovirus B19 infection: case report and review. Clin Infect Dis 1998;27:164–168.

49 Drago F, Broccolo F, Ciccarese G, Rebora A, Parodi A: Persistent pityriasis rosea: an unusual form of pityriasis rosea with persistent active HHV-6 and HHV-7 infection. Dermatology 2015;230:2326.

50 Fölster-Holst R, Kreth HW: Viral exanthems in childhood. Part 3: parainfectious exanthems and those associated with virus-drug interactions. J Dtsch Dermatol Ges 2009;7:506–510.

51 Sharma PK, Yadav TP, Gautam RK, Taneja N, Satyanarayana L: Erythromycin in pityriasis rosea: a double-blind, placebo-controlled clinical trial. J Am Acad Dermatol 2000;42:241–244.

52 Rassai S, Feily A, Sina N, Abtahian S: Low dose of acyclovir may be an effective treatment against pityriasis rosea: a random investigator-blind clinical trial on 64 patients. J Eur Acad Dermatol Venereol 2011;25:24–26.

53 Chuh AAT: Pediatric viral exanthems; in Thiers B (ed): Yearbook of Dermatology and Dermatologic Surgery. Mosby, Elsevier, 2005, pp 16–43.

54 Zawar V, Chuh A: Efficacy of ribavirin in a case of long lasting and disabling Gianotti-Crosti syndrome. J Dermatol Case Rep 2009;2:63–66.

55 Leone PA: Scabies and pediculosis pubis: an update of treatment regimens and general review. Scabies and pediculosis pubis: an update of treatment regimens and general review. Clin Infect Dis 2007;44(suppl 3):S153–S159.

56 Panzer R, Fölster-Holst R: Eczematous skin lesions of a suckling (in German). J Dtsch Dermatol Ges 2009;7:913–914.

57 Paller AS, Mancini AJ: Viral diseases of the skin; in Paller AS, Mancini AJ (eds): Hurwitz Clinical Pediatric Dermatology: A Textbook of Skin Disorders of Childhood and Adolescence. Amsterdam, Elsevier, 2016, pp 436–439.

58 Bialek R, Zelck UE, Fölster-Holst R: Permethrin treatment of head lice with knockdown resistance-like gene. N Engl J Med 2011;364:386–387.

59 Fölster-Holst R, Disko R, Röwert J, Böckeler W, Kreiselmaier I, Christophers E: Cercarial dermatitis contracted via contact with an aquarium: case report and review. Br J Dermatol 2001;145:638–640.

60 Paller AS, Mancini AJ: Infestations, bites, and stings; in Paller AS, Mancini AJ (eds): Hurwitz Clinical Pediatric Dermatology: A Textbook of Skin Disorders of Childhood and Adolescence. Amsterdam, Elsevier, 2016, pp 445–446.

61 Becker K: Lichen sclerosus in boys. Dtsch Arztebl Int 2011;108:53–58.

62 Jensen LS, Bygum A: Childhood lichen sclerosus is a rare but important diagnosis. Dan Med J 2012;59:A4424.

63 Fölster-Holst, R, Held I: Lichen sclerosus et atrophicus. Monatsschr Kinderheilkd 2011;159:468–474.

64 Dendrinos ML, Quint EH: Lichen sclerosus in children and adolescents. Curr Opin Obstet Gynecol 2013;25:370–374.

65 Focseneanu MA, Gupta M, Squires KC, Bayliss SJ, Berk D, Merritt DF: The course of lichen sclerosus diagnosed prior to puberty. J Pediatr Adolesc Gynecol 2013;26:153–155.

66 Ellis E, Fischer G: Prepubertal-onset vulvar lichen sclerosus: the importance of maintenance therapy in long-term outcomes. Pediatr Dermatol 2015;32:461–467.

67 Boms S, Gambichler T, Freitag M, Altmeyer P, Kreuter A: Pimecrolimus 1% cream for anogenital lichen sclerosus in childhood. BMC Dermatol 2004;4:14.

68 Danial C, Adeduntan R, Gorell ES, Lucky AW, Paller AS, Bruckner A, Pope E, Morel KD, Levy ML, Li S, Gilmore ES, Lane AT: Prevalence and characterization of pruritus in epidermolysis bullosa. Pediatr Dermatol 2015;32:53–59.

69 Petersen BW, Arbuckle HA, Berman S: Effectiveness of saltwater baths in the treatment of epidermolysis bullosa. Pediatr Dermatol 2015;32:60–63.

70 Danial C, Adeduntan R, Gorell ES, Lucky AW, Paller AS, Bruckner AL, Pope E, Morel KD, Levy ML, Li S, Gilmore ES, Lane AT: Evaluation of treatments for pruritus in epidermolysis bullosa. Pediatr Dermatol 2015;32:628–634.

71 Paller AS, Mancini AJ: Viral diseases of the skin; in Paller AS, Mancini AJ (eds): Hurwitz Clinical Pediatric Dermatology: A Textbook of Skin Disorders of Childhood and Adolescence. Amsterdam, Elsevier, 2016, pp 215–218.

72 Heide R, van Doorn K, Mulder PG, van Toorenenbergen AW, Beishuizen A, de Groot H, Tank B, Oranje AP: Serum tryptase and SCORMA (SCORing MAstocytosis) Index as disease severity parameters in childhood and adult cutaneous mastocytosis. Clin Exp Dermatol 2009;34:462–468.

73 Carter MC, Clayton ST, Komarow HD, Brittain EH, Scott LM, Cantave D, Gaskins DM, Maric I, Metcalfe DD: Assessment of clinical findings, tryptase levels, and bone marrow histopathology in the management of pediatric mastocytosis. J Allergy Clin Immunol 2015;136:1673–1679.

74 Zuberbier T, Asero R, Bindslev-Jensen C, Walter Canonica G, Church MK, Gimenez-Arnau A, et al: EAACI/GA(2) LEN/EDF/WAO guideline: definition, classification and diagnosis of urticaria. Allergy 2009;64:1417–1426.

75 Pite H, Wedi B, Borrego LM, Kapp A, Raap U: Management of childhood urticaria: current knowledge and practical recommendations. Acta Derm Venereol 2013;93:500–508.

76 Sackesen C, Sekerel BE, Orhan F, Kocabas CN, Tuncer A, Adalioglu G: The etiology of different forms of urticaria in childhood. Pediatr Dermatol 2004;21:102–108.

77 Choi SH, Baek HS: Approaches to the diagnosis and management of chronic urticaria in children. Korean J Pediatr 2015;58:159–164.

78 Paller AS, Mancini AJ: Hypersensitivity syndromes; in Paller AS, Mancini AJ (eds): Hurwitz Clinical Pediatric Dermatology: A Textbook of Skin Disorders of Childhood and Adolescence. Amsterdam, Elsevier, 2016, p 468.

79 Poddighe D, De Amici M, Marseglia GL: Spontaneous (autoimmune?) chronic urticaria in children: current evidences, diagnostic pitfalls and therapeutical managemen. Recent Pat Inflamm Allergy Drug Discov 2016, Epub ahead of print.

80 Soltani-Arabshahi R, Vanderhooft S, Hansen CD: Intractable localized pruritus as the sole manifestation of intramedullary tumor in a child: case report and review of the literature. JAMA Dermatol 2013;149:446–449.

81 Brenaut E, Nizery-Guermeur C, Audebert-Bellange S, Ferkal S, Wolkenstein P, Misery L, Abasq-Thomas C: Clinical characteristics of pruritus in neurofibromatosis 1. Acta Derm Venereol 2016;96:398–399.

82 National Institutes of Health Consensus Development Conference. Neurofibromatosis: conference statement. Arch Neurol 1988;45:575–578.

83 Khosrotehrani K, Bastuji-Garin S, Riccardi VM, Birch P, Friedman JM, Wolkenstein P: Subcutaneous neurofibromas are associated with mortality in neurofibromatosis 1: a cohort study of 703 patients. Am J Med Genet A 2005;132A:49–53.

84 Weisshaar E, Diepgen TL, Luger TA, Seeliger S, Witteler R, Ständer S: Pruritus in pregnancy and childhood – do we really consider all relevant differential diagnoses? Eur J Dermatol 2005;15:320–323.

85 Eichenfield LF, Tom WL, Berger TG, Krol A, Paller AS, Schwarzenberger K, Bergman JN, Chamlin SL, Cohen DE, Cooper KD, Cordoro KM, Davis DM, Feldman SR, Hanifin JM, Margolis DJ, Silverman RA, Simpson EL, Williams HC, Elmets CA, Block J, Harrod CG, Smith Begolka W, Sidbury R: Guidelines of care for the management of atopic dermatitis: section 2. Management and treatment of atopic dermatitis with topical therapies. J Am Acad Dermatol 2014;71:116–132.

86 Del Cuvillo A, Sastre J, Montoro J, Jáuregui I, Ferrer M, Dávila I, Bartra J, Mullol J, Valero A: Use of antihistamines in pediatrics. J Investig Allergol Clin Immunol 2007;17(suppl 2):28–40.

87 Fitzsimons R, van der Poel LA, Thornhill W, du Toit G, Shah N, Brough HA: Antihistamine use in children. Arch Dis Child Educ Pract Ed 2015;100:122–131.

Prof. Dr. med. Regina Fölster-Holst
Klinik für Dermatologie, Venerologie und Allergologie, Universitätsklinikum Schleswig-Holstein, Campus Kiel
Arnold-Heller-Strasse 3, Haus 19
DE–24105 Kiel (Kiel)
E-Mail rfoelsterholst@dermatology.uni-kiel.de

Szepietowski JC, Weisshaar E (eds): Itch – Management in Clinical Practice.
Curr Probl Dermatol. Basel, Karger, 2016, vol 50, pp 192–201 (DOI: 10.1159/000446094)

Itch Management in the Elderly

Tabi Anika Leslie

Department of Dermatology, Royal Free Hospital, London, UK

Abstract

Itch is a common symptom in the elderly population over 65 years old, and is often a chronic condition lasting more than 6 weeks. As in all age groups, but especially in the elderly, there can be a significant effect on the general health status and quality of life, with impaired daily activities and lack of sleep, which can also lead in some cases to depression or anxiety. The cause of chronic itch in the elderly is often multifactorial due to physiological changes in the aging skin, including impaired skin barrier function, and also due to decline in immunological (immunosenescence), neurological, and psychological changes associated with age. Common causes of chronic pruritus in the aging skin include xerosis (dry skin), dermatological disorders (eczema, psoriasis, lichen planus), and systemic (renal, hepatic, endocrine), neurodegenerative, and psychological diseases. Comorbidities in the elderly population lead to polypharmacy, increasing the potential risk of drug side effects, which can result in causing or exacerbating itch in the elderly patient. It is essential to obtain a detailed history, including drugs, as well as a thorough clinical examination with appropriate subsequent investigations. Management of the elderly patient with chronic pruritus should include treatment with topical therapies such as emollients as well as other agents for symptomatic relief. Systemic therapies should be directed at any underlying cutaneous or systemic diseases. Often the cause of itch in the elderly cannot be found and some systemic treatments can be used for symptomatic control of the itch, including antihistamines, gabapentin, and selective antidepressants. A holistic approach needs to be taken on an individual basis to relieve chronic pruritus, as the management of itch in the elderly can be a challenge.

The clinical management of itch in the elderly can be complicated due to multiple considerations, which must be taken into account as a result of the aging process. This chapter reviews and summarises the management of itch in the elderly, defined as patients over 65 years of age. More detailed aspects of itch pathophysiology and management in other specific conditions have been discussed elsewhere in this book. In the older population, therapies should be aimed at both cutaneous and central mechanisms, and, as in all age groups, there is no standard or universal recommendation [1]. The management of itch must be

History
Establish history of pruritus or rash, identify associated systemic disorders, past medical history including psychiatric disorders, drug history, allergies, family history; itch may occur without a rash

Examination
There may be evidence of skin disease, or signs of systemic disorders should be looked for; examine all areas – finger webs (scabies), scalp (lice/fungal infection), and mucosae; look for evidence of urticaria (wheals), symptomatic dermographism, cholinergic urticaria (small inducible papules), and cold urticaria (ice cube test), which should be tested for when suggested by the history

Baseline investigations
Full blood count, erythrocyte sedimentation rate, iron, serum ferritin, renal function, liver function, thyroid function, blood glucose, chest X-ray

Other investigations where appropriate
Calcium, serum electrophoresis and urine test, stool for ova, cysts and parasites, HIV testing, hepatitis B, hepatitis C, cancer screening, serum C-reactive protein, autoantibodies, antinuclear factor

Diagnostic investigation
Skin biopsy, histopathology and consider direct immunofluorescence

Questionnaire assessment
Visual analogue scales, quality-of-life measurements

tailored to the individual and the aetiology of itch if known, whether it is dermatological, systemic, neurological, or psychological. Chronic pruritus, defined as itch lasting more than 6 weeks, is a common symptom in the elderly [2]. The prevalence of chronic pruritus has been estimated to be 12% in patients over 65 years of age and almost 20% in patients over 85 years of age [3]. Xerosis is an uncomfortable and often distressing condition that is common in the elderly with symptoms including itching, dryness, and scaling of the skin, along with cracks or fissures [4]. More than 50% of people aged 65 years and over are affected by xerotic eruptions since the rate of repair and function of the epidermal water barrier declines with age [5].

Itch is often a debilitating symptom with a significant impact on quality of life, impairing daily activities and sleep especially in the elderly. The pathophysiology of chronic itch in the elderly may be multifactorial due to physiological changes in the skin, which occur with age, including impaired barrier function, immunological decline (immunosenescence), and neurodegenerative changes [6]. Chronic itch, especially in the elderly, is frequently a symptom of xerosis (dry skin), which can be caused by atrophy of the skin barrier and diminished hydration. Other common causes in the older population also include dermatoses, such as eczema, psoriasis, lichen planus, urticaria, and bullous pemphigoid. Underlying systemic diseases include renal, hepatic, and endocrine disorders as well as neurological and psychological disorders [7–9]. Elderly patients often have comorbidities, which may require polypharmacy [10]. The metabolism and pharmacokinetics of these drugs may also be altered in the elderly, leading to increased side effects causing or exacerbating the itch. Specific to the elderly population, itch can be caused by thiazides (hydrochlorothiazide) and calcium channel blockers [11]. In the elderly, itch frequently presents without a rash or identifiable cause, thus requiring topical and systemic therapies for symptomatic relief.

Itch Management

General Management of Itch in the Elderly
With general principles of itch management discussed in the chapter by Misery [this vol., pp. 35–39], there are particular considerations for the elderly population. It is important to obtain a detailed history including medications and a thorough clinical examination, directing the clinician to investigate with the most appropriate tests (table 1). Cutaneous and systemic causes of itch should be identified (table 2) and treated accordingly, keeping in mind that neuropathic and psychogenic disorders are also more frequent in the elderly [9]. If one potential cause for pruritus is found early on, a full evaluation should nevertheless be completed since the cause of itch in the elderly is regularly multifactorial. Topical (table 3) and systemic therapies (table 4) should be directed at symptomatic relief. Cutaneous diseases associated with chronic pruritus are often more prevalent in the aging population, such as dry skin and dermatitis, especially in patients with dementia and other neurological diseases. Scabies is frequently acquired by elderly people in long-term care homes, and is suggested by itching and skin lesions in the finger webs, wrists, genitals, and soles of the feet [12]. Systemic diseases in the elderly frequently include chronic renal, liver, and endocrine diseases, including thyroid disorders. Iron and vitamin deficiencies are also common in the elderly. Medications often prescribed for elderly patients are also likely to contribute to pruritus, including non-steroidal anti-inflammatory drugs, as well as codeine products (opioid analgesics) and antihypertensives. Polypharmacy in the elderly presents particular challenges, as the pathophysiology of drug-induced pruritus may be multifactorial and clinical presentation varies widely [13]. It can occur on the first dose or after years of being on a particular regimen. If the pruritus is drug induced, symptoms may persist even after cessation of the suspected medication [14]. All elderly patients with pruritus should

have their drug regime reviewed. Elderly patients are also more likely to present with chronic pruritus as a manifestation of underlying malignancy, including myelodysplastic disorders, which may require further investigations. Older patients with chronic pruritus that has commenced within the past 6 months should be examined and tested for cancers associated with itch. There may be several triggers of chronic pruritus in cancer patients, including xerosis and psychogenic causes, as well as the effect of the underlying disease. Therefore, they may need combined topical and systemic therapies agents such as selective se-

Table 2. Classification and common causes of pruritus [39]

Dermatological
Most inflammatory dermatoses
    Atopic dermatitis, lichen simplex, lichen planus, urticaria, drug hypersensitivity, scabies, xerosis, mycosis fungoides

Systemic
Hepatic
    Primary biliary cirrhosis, biliary obstruction, cholestasis during pregnancy, hepatitis B and C
Renal
    Chronic renal failure, dialysis
Endocrine
    Hypothyroidism
Malignancies
    Lymphoma, myeloma, central nervous system, tumours
Haematological
    Polycythaemia rubra vera, para-proteinaemia, iron deficiency

Neurological
Multiple sclerosis, brachioradial pruritus, notalgia paresthetica, post-herpetic neuralgia

Psychogenic/psychosomatic
Parasitophobia

Mixed
Co-existence of different diseases

Other
Pruritus of undetermined origin

Table 3. Common topical treatments for pruritus [1]

Agent	Indications	Major adverse effects
Coolants: menthol, camphor, phenol	Most pruritic conditions	Skin irritation
Capsaicin 0.025–0.1%	Neuropathic itch Prurigo nodularis Aquagenic pruritus Uraemic pruritus	Initial burning sensation
Anaesthetics	Neuropathic itch	Numbness
Calcineurin inhibitors	Eczema (various types) and anogenital pruritus	Transient burning sensation
N-palmitoylethanolamine	Atopic dermatitis, dry skin	Skin irritation
Doxepin	Atopic dermatitis Localized pruritus	Drowsiness in 25% of patients Allergic contact dermatitis
Aspirin and salicylates	Lichen simplex chronicus	Transient burning sensation

rotonin reuptake inhibitors which may also be effective [15] in symptomatic control of the itch.

In the general management of pruritus, the distinct limitations of old age mean that, once decided upon, therapy must be carefully planned and facilitated. Polypharmacy and the possibility of drug interactions are extremely important factors to take into account when proposing treatments, but considerations must also be given to the challenges of mobility that face older people. For example, bath oils and moisturisers may increase the risk of falls, or may be difficult to apply to certain areas. The application of emollient may present difficulties in older patients, especially those with arthritis. They may require the assistance of a carer or partner, or instead use devices, such as body creamers or sticks, available to help moisturize body parts that are hard to reach. Packaging should also be easy to open and contents easy to extract. Also problematic is possibly impaired cognitive function in the elderly which can affect compliance with advice. In these cases, caregivers should be aware of the treatment plan. Frequently, the use of soap may be ingrained an older person's cleansing regime, and might prove difficult to relinquish. It is important to acknowledge the concern of an elderly patient who claims not to feel clean if they have not used soap, and emphasize that emollient will also cleanse the skin without drying it. If there is anxiety about bacteria remaining on the skin, then an antimicrobial emollient with chlorhexidine may be prescribed as a soap or shower gel substitute. Patient education has an important place and has been shown in the general population to significantly reduce the frequency and intensity of itching and scratching [16]. Older people and their carers should be taught about the itch-scratch cycle, and how it may be interrupted by simple measures, such as keeping fingernails short and wearing loose clothing.

Since xerosis is the most common cause of pruritus in the elderly, it is important to educate patients upon how to manage this condition effectively. The focus must be twofold: healing the damage already within the stratum corneum and preventing further skin barrier deterioration [11]. Patients should bathe in tepid water, use cleanser that is non-irritating, and avoid high pH soaps or those containing alcohol. Instead, acidic pH

Table 4. Current systemic therapies for pruritus [1]

Medication class	Medication and dosages	Main indication	Major side effect
Anti-histamines	1st generation: usually only given at night due to their sedative effect Hydroxyzine Adults: 30–100 mg/day in 3 divided doses Diphenhydramine Adults: 25–50 mg b.d. Chlorpheniramine maleate Adults: 4 mg 6–8 h	Nocturnal itch	Sedation
	2nd generation: Loratadine Adults and children ≥12 years: 10 mg q.d. Cetirizine Adults and children ≥6 years: 10 mg q.d. or 5 mg b.d. Renal or hepatic insufficiency: reduce dosages by half Fexofenadine Adults and children ≥12 years: 60 mg b.d. or 180 mg q.d. Renal impairment: consider lower dose of 60 mg q.d.	Urticaria Mastocytosis Insect bite reactions	Infrequent: Drowsiness Dry mouth
Anti-convulsants	Gabapentin 300–3,600 mg/day in 3 divided doses Reduced dose in renal impairment In dialysis patients, 100–300 mg after each dialysis	Neuropathic itch Uraemic pruritus Prurigo nodularis Post-burn pruritus	Drowsiness Leg swelling Blurred vision Constipation Ataxia
	Pregabalin 150–450 mg/day in 2–3 divided doses Dose reduction in renal impairment		
μ-Opioid receptor antagonists	Naltrexone 25–50 mg o.m.	Pruritus associated with cholestasis, atopic dermatitis, chronic urticaria	Nausea and vomiting Insomnia Reversal of opioid analgesia Hepatotoxicity rarely
κ-Opioid receptor agonists	Butorphanol 1–4 mg intranasally o.n.		Drowsiness Nausia Vomiting
	Nalfurafine 2.5–5 μg o.m.	Uraemic pruritus	Insomnia
Anti-depressants	Mirtazapine 7.5–15 mg o.n. initially, up to 45 mg o.n.	Malignancy-associated pruritus Nocturnal pruritus in atopic dermatitis	Drowsiness Weight gain
	SSRIs Paroxetine 10–40 mg q.d. Sertraline 75–100 mg q.d. Fluvoxamine 25 mg for 3 days, then 50–150 mg q.d.	Consider in pruritus associated with depression and/or anxiety Pruritus associated with haematological malignancies and solid tumours (paroxetine) Cholestatic pruritus (sertraline)	Drowsiness Insomnia Sexual dysfunction
	Tricyclic antidepressants Doxepin 10–100 mg o.n. Amitriptyline 25–75 mg o.n.	Chronic idiopathic urticaria (doxepin) Neuropathic itch (amitriptyline)	Anticholinergic effects: Drowsiness Dry eyes and mouth Blurred vision Urinary retention Cardiovascular effects: Orthostatic hypotension Conduction disturbances

Medication class	Medication and dosages	Main indication	Major side effect
Thalidomide	100–200 mg q.d.	Prurigo nodularis Uraemic pruritus Actinic prurigo	Teratogenicity Peripheral neuropathy Drowsiness
Neurokinin 1 receptor antagonist	Apretitant 80 mg q.d.	Itch associated with: Haematological malignancies Solid tumours Biological cancer drugs Prurigo nodularis	Nausea Dizziness
Phototherapy	UVB, broadband and narrowband UVA Combined UVA and UVB PUVA, oral and topical	Atopic dermatitis Psoriasis Uraemic pruritus Cholestatic pruritus	Tanning Increased itch Skin malignancies

SSRIs = Selective serotonin reuptake inhibitors; b.d. = twice daily; q.d. = 4 times a day; o.m. = on morning; o.n.= on night.

products are recommended. Skin should be gently patted dry and moisturiser applied generously immediately afterwards, so that its efficacy in improving barrier function is maximised. Fluctuations in temperature and humidity should be avoided; therefore, air conditioning and dehumidifying units may be helpful. Where xerosis is severe or secondary to underlying medical conditions (HIV, thyroid disease, diabetes), systemic treatments may be necessary [4]. In cases where elderly patients' medications are contributing to dry skin, it may be unviable to discontinue them, unless the xerosis is extremely severe [8]. Where pruritus due to xerosis or other inflammatory dermatoses is refractory, the itch may be reduced with 'soak and smear' hydration techniques [17]. Patients bathe for 10–20 min, apply moisturiser, and then occlude the skin with kitchen cling film (plastic wrap). Particularly frail patients prone to falling may prefer to use wet wraps, where a moist garment is worn and covered with a dry garment following bathing and moisturisation [2].

There is no single therapeutic agent that is consistently successful in treating itch, especially in the elderly patient, where each patient must be considered individually [7]. Management of the itch must be tailored to the individual aetiology whether dermatologic or systemic. Topical and systemic management of itch, discussed in detail in the chapters by Metz and Staubach [this vol., pp. 40–45] and Pongcharoen and Fleischer [this vol., pp. 46–53], will now be reviewed with specific relevance to the elderly population.

Topical Treatments in the Elderly

An emollient may be useful where the pruritus occurs in otherwise healthy elderly people. Topical treatments including emollients (table 3) are the first-line therapy for xerosis, as they help prevent transepidermal water loss and improve skin barrier function [1]. Moisturisers and cleansers with a low pH should be used, and alkaline soaps avoided, so that the secretion of pruritic serine proteases on the skin surface is reduced [18]. For treatment of xerosis, moisturisers should be applied 1–3 times per day and immediately after bathing, while the skin is still wet [19]. Colloidal oatmeal topically applied may be effective at reducing itch responses since oats contain avenanthramides that inhibit the release of inflammatory cytokines [20]. Bathing with oatmeal may also be a useful therapy in elderly patients [11]. Pruritus in the elderly may also be relieved with cooling agents such as menthol with aqueous cream, especially in palliative care. This can be useful for short-term alleviation of itch, and its effects can last for up to 70 min. Calamine also has an antipruritic effect, which is attributed to the cooling and anaesthetic effect of the ingredient phenol. Topical calcineurin inhibitors pimecrolimus and tacrolimus are recommended in elderly patients to reduce itch in inflammatory skin conditions. If the symptoms are relieved, then topical calcineurin inhibitors may be used indefinitely [8].

Other preparations that are often helpful in reducing pruritus in the general population are less suitable for use in the elderly and must be used carefully. Lactic acid 12%, neutralised with ammonium hydroxide and pramoxine hydrochloride 1%, has been shown to effectively moisturise and reduce pruritus in dry itchy skin [21], but such high concentrations of lactic acid may irritate inflamed elderly skin with the effect of worsening pruritus, and so its practicality in this population is ambiguous. Topical capsaicin, derived from chilli peppers, exerts an antipruritic effect on chronic localized itch [22]. Elderly sufferers of neuropathic itch may find it beneficial, although the initial burning sensation at the site of application can last for 2 weeks and may lessen compliance. While topical corticosteroids may control itch of inflammatory conditions, prolonged daily treatment should be limited due to local adverse effects [23]. Elderly patients are particularly susceptible to thinning of the skin, and should be monitored closely if using topical steroids long term [11]. Doxepin 5% cream, a topical antihistamine, is not recommended in the elderly due to an increased risk of sensitisation with localised stinging, burning, and drowsiness caused by absorption through the skin [1, 23].

Systemic Treatments in the Elderly

Second-generation non-sedating antihistamines such as fexofenadine, cetirizine, and loratadine may be effective in managing the itch of urticaria [24]. First-generation sedating antihistamines such as hydroxyzine may be useful for nocturnal itch that disturbs sleep, although increased drowsiness may be problematic in the elderly [25]. Oral doxepin, a tricyclic antidepressant with H_1 and H_2 antagonist activity, is an effective antipruritic that is usually well tolerated; however, doxepin has anticholinergic side effects, including confusion, dry mouth, and constipation, which are more pronounced in the elderly with an increased risk of hypotension and hyponatremia, and therefore must be used with caution [2, 26]. The use of antihistamines is not recommended in pruritic conditions that are not mast cell mediated [9, 24], but may be used for their sedating properties to help break the itch-scratch cycle. It is preferable to avoid long-term use of systemic steroids in the elderly, particularly because of medical comorbidities and impaired immune surveillance. Potential side effects include headaches, gastrointestinal problems, and neuropathy, and there is further risk of infection, malignancy, and re-activation of herpes zoster when treating older patients [8].

Gabapentin and pregabalin are antiepileptic drugs that have been beneficial in neuropathic disorders causing itch or pain [27]. Although these agents are reasonably well-tolerated, there are dose-dependent side effects that may be hazardous in the elderly, such as dizziness, blurred vision, and sedation [8, 27]. Therefore, a low initial gabapentin dose on 100–300 mg depending on frailty of the patient that gradually commences, up to 1,800 mg in divided doses, is judicious [28]. Similarly, pregabalin cessation should be tapered down to avoid withdrawal symptoms [11].

Mirtizapine is a selective norepinephrine reuptake inhibitor that has been effective in reducing the nocturnal itch of leukaemia, lymphoma, cholestasis, chronic kidney disease, and atopic dermatitis [29]. Compliance in the elderly is facilitated by using a fixed once-daily low dose of 15 mg. Paroxetine and fluvoxamine are selective serotonin reuptake inhibitors that have been used to improve itch associated with atopic dermatitis, systemic lymphoma, and solid carcinoma [30], although some side effects of paroxetine, such as insomnia and sexual dysfunction, may worsen these conditions in the elderly [31]. Sertraline may be suitable for older people as an effective treatment of cholestatic itch, especially as it is well tolerated. Amitriptyline and doxepin (also acting as H_1 and H_2 antagonists) are tricyclic antidepressants that have been beneficial in treating neuropathic and psychogenic itch [1]. However, amitriptyline in particular has anticholinergic side effects that indicate dosages in the elderly population should start low and taper up [9, 11, 28].

The perception of itch may be reduced with μ-opioid receptor antagonists and κ-opioid receptor agonists [32, 33]. There are potential adverse effects, such as nausea, dizziness, and drowsiness, and μ-opioid antagonists in particular are associated with hepatotoxicity, diarrhoea, and analgesia reversal [11]. Therefore, treatment in the elderly should proceed with caution at lower initial doses. Butorphanol is a κ-opioid agonist/partial μ-antagonist and antimigraine agent administered intranasally (initial dose of 1 mg/day) that has been effective in case reports against intractable nocturnal itch of different types [1, 34]. It may be a helpful treatment option for the elderly population with fewer hazardous side effects than μ-opioid antagonists, as well as ease of use. Thalidomide is an immunomodulator and neuromodulator that has demonstrated considerable efficacy as an antipruritic agent, and may be considered as an alternative treatment for elderly patients who do not otherwise find relief, or used in combination with other treatments such as phototherapy [35].

Physical Treatments in the Elderly

Physical treatments, fully discussed in the chapter by Chan and Murrell [this vol., pp. 54–63], include narrowband TL01 UVB light phototherapy. This is known to be effective in treating chronic pruritus of different types, with the advantage for the elderly population of avoiding adverse drug reactions [9, 36]. Because polypharmacy is a likely factor in the elderly, phototherapy is an especially attractive option, avoiding further systemic medication. Phototherapy in the elderly population can be safe and effective, but caution must be exercised in its administration, particularly where there is multiple drug intake, since photosensitivity and phototoxicity may be increased with longer-lasting, more intense erythema [9, 11, 37]. If photosensitizing medications are being taken, then it is important to check the minimal erythema dose before therapy commences [38]. While this mode of therapy overcomes some physical and cognitive concerns that can cause non-compliance in other treatments, patients should be deemed able to attend regular therapy and stand in a booth for a number of minutes, as well as be able to follow instructions. UV therapy can be offered using a sunbed if standing presents an obstacle to treatment.

Other holistic approaches such as acupuncture may have positive effects on some forms of chronic itch in the elderly. Acupuncture has been beneficial for itch associated with chronic kidney disease. Although there is not strong evidence for this mode of therapy, it may be reasonably offered as a treatment with no adverse effects to elderly patients not responding to first-line treatments [39].

Conclusion

The management of itch in the elderly remains a challenge. A holistic approach is required for each individual patient, based on a detailed history, including comorbidities and polypharmacy, which are common in the older population. A thorough clinical examination and assessment of the patient will help direct the clinician to perform the necessary investigations required. For the treatment of itch in the elderly, the changes associated with the aging skin should be taken into account including changes in barrier skin function, the immune system (immunosenescence), and neurological and psychological decline. Underlying cutaneous and systemic diseases should be treated and the elderly patient should be provided with symptomatic relief of the itch using topical and systemic therapies. There is no single therapeutic intervention in the management of itch in the elderly, but an individual care plan is essential.

References

1 Leslie TA, Greaves MW, Yosipovitch G: Current topical and systemic therapies for itch. Handb Exp Pharmacol 2015; 226:337–356.

2 Berger TG, Shive M, Harper GM: Pruritus in the older patient: a clinical review. JAMA 2013;310:2443–2450.

3 Yalcin B, Tamer E, Toy GG, Oztas P, Hayran M, Alli N: The prevalence of skin diseases in the elderly: analysis of 4099 geriatric patients. Int J Dermatol 2006;45:672–676.

4 Norman RA: Xerosis and pruritus in the elderly: recognition and management. Dermatol Ther 2003;16:254–259.

5 Paul C, Maumus-Robert S, Mazereeuw-Hautier J, Guyen CN, Saudez X, Schmitt AM: Prevalence and risk factors for xerosis in the elderly: a cross-sectional epidemiological study in primary care. Dermatology 2011;223:260–265.

6 Berger TG, Steinhoff M: Pruritus in elderly patients – eruptions of senescence. Semin Cutan Med Surg 2011;30:113–117.

7 Leslie TA: Itch. Medicine 2013;41:367–371.

8 Garibyan L, Chiou AS, Elmariah SB: Advanced aging skin and itch: addressing an unmet need. Dermatol Ther 2013;26:92–103.

9 Patel T, Yosipovitch G: The management of chronic pruritus in the elderly. Skin Therapy Lett 2010;15:5–9.

10 Farage MA, Miller KW, Berardesca E, Maibach HI: Clinical implications of aging skin: cutaneous disorders in the elderly. Am J Clin Dermatol 2009;10:73–86.

11 Valdes-Rodriguez R, Stull C, Yosipovitch G: Chronic pruritus in the elderly: pathophysiology, diagnosis and management. Drugs Aging 2015;32:201–215.

12 Suwandhi P, Dharmarajan TS: Scabies in the nursing home. Curr Infect Dis Rep 2015;17:453.

13 Reich A, Stander S, Szepietowski JC: Drug-induced pruritus: a review. Acta Derm Venereol 2009;89:236–244.

14 Joly P, Benoit-Corven C, Baricault S, et al: Chronic eczematous eruptions of the elderly are associated with chronic exposure to calcium channel blockers: results from a case-control study. J Invest Dermatol 2007;127:2766–2771.

15 Weisshaar E: Intractable chronic pruritus in a 67-year-old man. Acta Derm Venereol 2008;88:488–490.

16 van Os-Medendorp H, Ros WJ, Eland-de Kok PC, et al: Effectiveness of the nursing programme 'Coping with Itch': a randomized controlled study in adults with chronic pruritic skin disease. Br J Dermatol 2007;156:1235–1244.

17 Gutman AB, Kligman AM, Sciacca J, James WD: Soak and smear: a standard technique revisited. Arch Dermatol 2005;141:1556–1559.

18 Steinhoff M, Neisius U, Ikoma A, et al: Proteinase-activated receptor-2 mediates itch: a novel pathway for pruritus in human skin. J Neurosci 2003;23:6176–6180.

19 Elmariah SB, Lerner EA: Topical therapies for pruritus. Semin Cutan Med Surg 2011;30:118–126.

20 Sur R, Nigam A, Grote D, Liebel F, Southall MD: Avenanthramides, polyphenols from oats, exhibit anti-inflammatory and anti-itch activity. Arch Dermatol Res 2008;300:569–574.

21 Grove G, Zerweck C: An evaluation of the moisturizing and anti-itch effects of a lactic acid and pramoxine hydrochloride cream. Cutis 2004;73:135–139.

22 Boyd K, Shea SM, Patterson JW: The role of capsaicin in dermatology. Prog Drug Res 2014;68:293–306.

23 Weisshaar E, Szepietowski JC, Darsow U, et al: European guideline on chronic pruritus. Acta Derm Venereol 2012;92:563–581.

24 O'Donoghue M, Tharp MD: Antihistamines and their role as antipruritics. Dermatol Ther 2005;18:333–340.

25 Patel T, Ishiuji Y, Yosipovitch G: Nocturnal itch: why do we itch at night? Acta Derm Venereologica 2007;87:295–298.

26 Greaves MW: Itch in systemic disease: therapeutic options. Dermatol Ther 2005;18:323–327.

27 Ehrchen J, Stander S: Pregabalin in the treatment of chronic pruritus. J Am Acad Dermatol 2008;58(2 suppl):S36–S37.

28 Yosipovitch G, Bernhard JD: Clinical practice. Chronic pruritus. N Engl J Med 2013;368:1625–1634.

29 Hundley JL, Yosipovitch G: Mirtazapine for reducing nocturnal itch in patients with chronic pruritus: a pilot study. J Am Acad Dermatol 2004;50:889–891.

30 Ständer S, Bockenholt B, Schurmeyer-Horst F, et al: Treatment of chronic pruritus with the selective serotonin re-uptake inhibitors paroxetine and fluvoxamine: results of an open-labelled, two-arm proof-of-concept study. Acta Derm Venereol 2009;89:45–51.

31 Gareri P, Castagna A, Francomano D, Cerminara G, De Fazio P: Erectile dysfunction in the elderly: an old widespread issue with novel treatment perspectives. Int J Endocrinol 2014;2014:878670.

32 Phan NQ, Bernhard JD, Luger TA, Stander S: Antipruritic treatment with systemic mu-opioid receptor antagonists: a review. J Am Acad Dermatol 2010;63:680–688.

33 Phan NQ, Lotts T, Antal A, Bernhard JD, Stander S: Systemic kappa opioid receptor agonists in the treatment of chronic pruritus: a literature review. Acta Derm Venereol 2012;92:555–560.

34 Dawn AG, Yosipovitch G: Butorphanol for treatment of intractable pruritus. J Am Acad Dermatol 2006;54:527–531.

35 Sharma D, Kwatra SG: Thalidomide for the treatment of chronic refractory pruritus. J Am Acad Dermatol 2016;74:363–369.

36 Steinhoff M, Cevikbas F, Ikoma A, Berger TG: Pruritus: management algorithms and experimental therapies. Semin Cutan Med Surg 2011;30:127–137.

37 Gloor M, Scherotzke A: Age dependence of ultraviolet light-induced erythema following narrow-band UVB exposure. Photodermatol Photoimmunol Photomed 2002;18:121–126.

38 Powell JB, Gach JE: Phototherapy in the elderly. Clin Exp Dermatol 2015;40:605–610.

39 Combs SA, Teixeira JP, Germain MJ: Pruritus in kidney disease. Semin Nephrol 2015;35:383–391.

Dr. Tabi Anika Leslie, BSc(Hons), MBBS, FRCP(London)
Department of Dermatology, Royal Free Hospital
Pond Street
London NW3 2QG (UK)
E-Mail tabi.leslie@doctors.org.uk

Author Index

Subject Index

HES, *see* Hydroxyethyl starch
Histamine, itch role 11, 20
HIV, *see* Human immunodeficiency virus
Hives, *see* Urticaria
Human immunodeficiency virus (HIV)
    diagnostic testing of itch 28
    epidemiology of itch 8
Hydroxyethyl starch (HES), drug-induced itch
    159

Incidence, *see* Epidemiology, itch
Infantile acropustulosis 178, 179
Infantile eosinophilic pustular folliculitis 178
Interleukin-21 receptor, itch role 22
Interleukin-31 receptor A antibody
    atopic dermatitis itch management 91
    clinical trials 72, 73
Itch intensity assessment
    monodimensional severity scales 30, 31
    overview 29, 30
    questionnaires 31, 32
    scratching activity measurement 32
    sensory threshold measurement 32

Laboratory examination, itch 25
Lactic acid, elderly itch management 198
Leukotriene receptor, antagonists for urticaria
    itch management 83
γ-Linolenic ointment, uremic itch management
    135–137
Liver transplantation, cholestatic itch
    management 146

Management principles, itch
    associated measures 37, 38
    etiological treatment 36
    overview 35, 36
    psychological support 38
    symptomatic treatment 36, 37
    topical therapy, *see* Topical therapy
Mas-related receptors, itch role 21
Massage, itch management 60
Mastocytosis, children 185
Medical history, itch 24, 25

Menthol
    elderly itch management 197
    topical therapy 37, 43
Methotrexate, prurigo nodularis itch
    management 99
Mirtazapine
    elderly itch management 198
    paraneoplastic itch management 151, 152
    prurigo nodularis itch management 98
    psoriatic itch management 107, 108
    psychogenic itch management 127, 128
    systemic therapy 48, 50

Nalfurafine
    systemic therapy 47, 49, 74
    uremic itch management 137
Nalmefene, systemic therapy 47, 48
Naloxone
    prurigo nodularis itch management 98
    systemic therapy 48, 49
Naltrexone
    prurigo nodularis itch management 98
    systemic therapy 47, 48
    uremic itch management 137
Nerve growth factor (NGF)
    psoriasis pathogenesis 106, 107
    therapeutic targeting 74
Neural pathways, *see* Central mechanisms, itch;
    Peripheral mechanisms, itch
Neurofibromatosis, children 186, 187
Neurokinin 1 receptor
    antagonist therapy 43, 51, 73, 64
    itch role 21
Neurologic itch
    clinical characteristics 117
    definition 117
    diagnostics 117–119
    treatment
        overview 119
        physical therapies 121
        systemic therapy 120, 121
        topical therapy 119, 120
Neurotrophin (NTP), atopic dermatitis itch
    management 88